Experimental cardiac hypertrophy and heart failure

International Erwin Riesch Symposium, Tübingen, April 3–7, 1979

EXPERIMENTAL CARDIAC HYPERTROPHY AND HEART FAILURE

Edited by
Prof. Dr. RUTHARD JACOB
Tübingen

With 103 figures and 35 tables

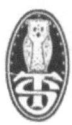

Springer-Verlag Berlin Heidelberg GmbH 1980

ISBN 978-3-7985-0577-3   ISBN 978-3-662-41468-2 (eBook)
DOI 10.1007/978-3-662-41468-2

1980 by Springer-Verlag Berlin Heidelberg
Originally published by Dr. Dietrich Steinkopff Verlag, Darmstadt in 1980.

Special Edition from Basic Research in Cardiology, Vol. 75, No. 1 (1980)

CIP-Kurztitelaufnahme der Deutschen Bibliothek

Experimental cardiac hypertrophy and heart failure / Internat. Erwin Riesch Symposium, Tübingen, April 3–7, 1979. Ed. by Ruthard Jacob. – Special ed. – Darmstadt: Steinkopff. 1980.

NE: Jacob, Ruthard [Hrsg.]; International Erwin Riesch Symposium (1979, Tübingen)

Contents · Inhalt

VI

Basic Research in Cardiology

Archiv für Kreislaufforschung

Official Journal of the German Association of Cardiovascular Research

Edited by R. Jacob, Tübingen, and W. Schaper, Bad Nauheim

| Volume 75 | January/February 1980 | Number 1 |

This issue contains papers of the
Erwin Riesch Symposium

Experimental cardiac hypertrophy and heart failure

in Tübingen, April 5–7, 1979,
sponsored by the Erwin-Riesch-Stiftung
zur Förderung der wissenschaftlichen Forschung

Organized by Prof. Dr. *R. Jacob*, Tübingen

The significance of hypertrophy research in biomedical sciences justifies the publication of this volume which contains the contributions of an international symposium focusing on experimental findings and pathophysiological aspects of cardiac hypertrophy. Structural and functional alterations which are directly or indirectly related to the process of hypertrophy are treated within the framework of fundamental questions of muscle mechanics, biochemistry and energetics. In addition, consideration is given to the effects of insufficiency of the overloaded heart on the entire circulation, particularly the electrolyte and water balance. Although this collection of papers cannot claim to cover the contents of all subfields of hypertrophy research, the contributions suffice to provide an introduction to the essential problems of an area of research which equally attracts the interest of pathologists, clinical cardiologists and sports specialists, as well as physiologists, biochemists and biophysicists. Hopefully, differences in results or scientific concepts of the individual contributions, e.g., with regard to the significance of different models of hypertrophy in clarification of specific questions, the criteria of pathological hypertrophy, the calcium dependence of unloaded shortening velocity, the elastic properties of myocardium in various models of hypertrophy, or the relation between substructure and enzymatic activity of myosin, etc., will stimulate further investigations leading to final clarification of these questions.

Basic Res. Cardiol. **75**, 2–12 (1980)
© 1980 Dr. Dietrich Steinkopff Verlag, Darmstadt
ISSN 0300–8428

Paper, presented at the Erwin Riesch Symposium, Tübingen, April 3–7, 1979

Max-Planck-Institut für medizinische Forschung,
Abteilung Physiologie, Heidelberg

Quantitative aspects of the calcium concept of excitation contraction coupling – a critical evaluation

Quantitative Aspekte des Calciumkonzeptes der Kopplung zwischen Erregung und Kontraktion – eine kritische Bewertung

W. Hasselbach

With 5 figures and 2 tables

Summary

The role of sarcoplasmic reticulum membranes in the calcium concept of muscle activation is critically evaluated applying data and findings obtained by in-vitro studies with isolated sarcoplasmic reticulum membrane vesicles.

At the Third European Congress on Cardiology in Rome 1960 we have reported that the activity of the physiological relaxing factor discovered by *Marsh* (1) resides in a vesicular membrane fraction. We showed that the relaxing activity of the vesicular material is closely related to its ability to store calcium ions. Calcium storage was found to be an active calcium transport process which requires ATP as energy donor and magnesium ions as cofactor (2). It was speculated that the system might interact with the contractile proteins via a calcium-sensitive soluble relaxing factor because calcium addition to the medium which transiently increases the total calcium concentration to 10^{-5}M, abolishes the relaxing effect. Yet, the idea of a soluble relaxing factor turned out to be wrong. *Ebashi* (3) proved that the relaxing factor was the stable native tropomyosin associated with actin. In 1964 the identity of the calcium storing vesicles with membrane fragments of the sarcoplasmic reticulum was proven (4). Subsequently, schemes were developed and widely accepted in which the interaction of calcium ions with various muscle constituents plays a crucial role (fig. 1). The main elements of these schemes are calcium channels, calcium gates and calcium pumps in different membrane systems, on the one hand, and calcium-sensitive target proteins, on the other hand. It could be shown that muscle activity depends on a calcium concentration transient in the myoplasma (5). The activating calcium ions are thought to be released from extra- und intracellular stores depending on the muscle. The calcium-sensitive target proteins are the C-components of troponin in striated muscles, and myosin itself in smooth muscles (6). Elimination of calcium is thought to be brought about by the combined effect of calcium

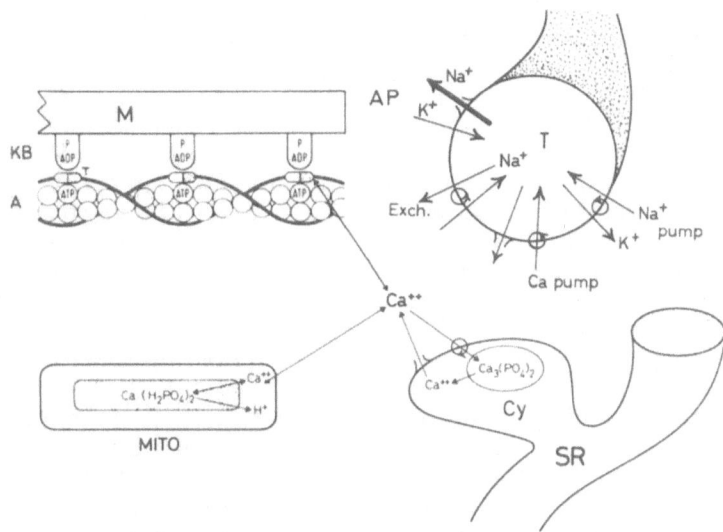

Fig. 1. Structures involved in the regulation of muscle activity by calcium release and removal.
T = Transverse tubule, SR = Sarcoplasmic reticulum with cisterna, MITO = Mitochondrium, M = Myosin filament with KB crossbridges, A = Actin filament with T Troponin
From *F. H. Degenring, Der Herzmuskel*, 1976, Springer-Verlag, Berlin-Heidelberg-New York, with some modifications.

transport systems in different membranes. Among the membrane structures which were considered to participate in calcium removal, the sarcoplasmic reticulum membranes exhibit the highest calcium transport activity. Therefore the sarcoplasmic reticulum membranes have become essential elements in the concept of excitation contraction coupling. In the following, the role of the sarcoplasmic reticulum in this concept will be evaluated critically on the basis of experiments performed with the isolated membranes.

Functional and structural characterizations of the sarcoplasmic reticulum membranes

The isolated sarcoplasmic membranes have been characterized by three activities on account of which they can clearly be distinguished from all other membranes in the muscles.
1. They catalyze the cleavage of ATP which is activated by low and inhibited by high concentrations of ionized calcium in the presence of magnesium ions.
2. They accumulate large quantities of calcium ions.
3. They are permeable for calcium-precipitating ions which makes it possible to visualize the accumulated calcium in the electron microscope as electron dense material (4, 7, 8).

All procedures used to isolate the sarcoplasmic reticulum membranes lead to the fragmentation of the complex membrane network which consists of a number of different structural entities: terminal cisterna, intermediate cisterna, fenestrated collar, and free reticulum. The fragmented membranes heal over and form closely sealed vesicles of very similar morphological appearance. On account of their size and shape it is not possible to determine from which part of the reticulum these vesicles originate. Attempts were made to designate the calcium-storing vesicles to certain structural elements in the sarcoplasmic reticulum by observing the formation of calcium precipitates in the membranes left in their natural arrangement in the muscle fiber. Calcium precipitates were mainly found in the cisternal elements indicating that the cisternal membranes themselves or limited areas thereof are able to transport calcium. Since, however, the longitudinal elements or the free sarcoplasmic reticulum are not preserved, the involvement of this important structure remains undecided in these experiments. Yet, according to *Winegrad's* experiments (9) with living muscle, calcium is stored at first in longitudinal elements and shifted inside towards the cisternae of the reticulum. Although the isolated membrane vesicles presumably originate from very different parts of the sarcoplasmic reticulum, their chemical composition proves to be very simple and similar, 70 % of the membrane mass consists of the calcium-transporting protein (10, 11). This finding can be taken as strong evidence that nearly the total surface of the sarcoplasmic reticulum can participate in calcium translocation. The surface of the sarcoplasmic reticulum has been evaluated only for the frog skeletal muscle. The estimated total surface of $10.000 \text{ cm} \cdot \text{ml}^{-1}$ (12) corresponds to the surface of 3–5 mg protein of isolated vesicles. This is approximately the yield of isolated vesicles from one gram of frog or rabbit skeletal muscle. The yield obtained depends very much on the animal and the type of muscle. For cardiac muscles (dog and rabbit) yields of approximately one milligram per gram of muscle have been reported (13). In conclusion: The sarcoplasmic reticulum membranes can be isolated from a great variety of muscles. All parts of the reticulum presumably take part in calcium transport.

The calcium-concentrating power of the isolated sarcoplasmic reticulum vesicles

The relaxation of the contracted muscle fibers in ATP-containing media brought about by the suspension of sarcoplasmic reticulum vesicles is the most convincing demonstration for the functional interrelationship between the two systems. Relaxation ist complete when the level of ionized calcium of the ATP-containing media has been reduced by the vesicles to below 10^{-7} M. This concentrations corresponds to the level of ionized calcium in the resting muscle (14). If calcium-precipitating anions are present, even lower calcium concentrations can be established in the external medium (2 nM).

Experimental evidence has been given in abundance showing that the described calcium depletion is the result of an ATP-driven calcium transport process and not brought about by the binding of calcium to the membranes energized by ATP (15). The transport of calcium from the external medium into the comparatively small volume of vesicles leads to a steep rise of the calcium concentration in the internal space if there are no calcium precipitating anions or other calcium binding material present. The storing capacity of the vesicles is reached when they have taken up approximately 100–150 nmol calcium · mg protein^{-1}. At an intravesicular volume of 10 µl · mg protein^{-1} (16) this quantity of stored calcium corresponds to a concentration of total calcium of 10 mM. This value is in good agreement with the recent estimates of the calcium concentration in the sarcoplasmic reticulum in the intact muscle (17). A great fraction of this calcium remains unliganded. Possible calcium-binding constituents in the interior of the vesicles are present only in relatively small quantities or have a relatively low affinity for calcium ions (18, 19). Consequently, a very high calcium concentration ratio is created by the calcium pump between intra- and extravesicular space. This calcium ratio observed in vitro corresponds quite well to the calcium ratio between intracellular and extracellular or intracellular and intrareticular space. This high concentration ratio is maintained at low energy expenditure by the sarcoplasmic reticulum membrane, because the passive calcium permeability of the membranes is very low. The lipid bilayer of the membranes which constitute approximately 30–50% of the vesicular surface is practically impermeable for calcium ions. The slow leakage which can be observed presumably occurs mainly through membrane defects and through the pump protein itself. The permeation through the calcium pump represents the reversal of the ATP-driven calcium influx and leads in the presence of ADP and phosphate to the synthesis of ATP. Therefore the osmotic energy stored in the calcium gradient is not lost when calcium ions move through the pump (cf. 15) (fig. 2).

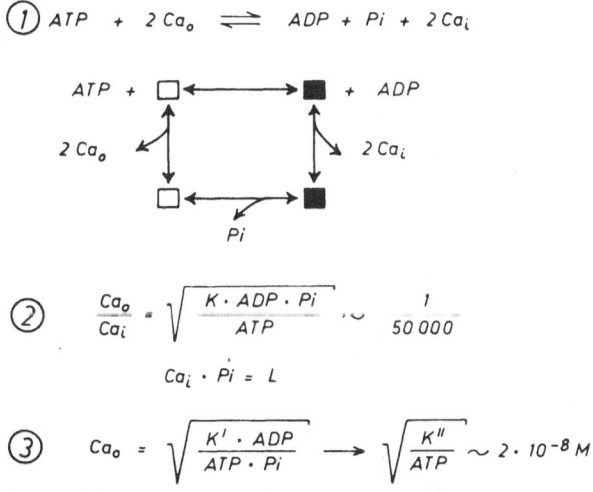

$$\text{(1)}\quad ATP + 2\,Ca_o \rightleftharpoons ADP + Pi + 2\,Ca_i$$

$$ATP + \square \longleftrightarrow \blacksquare + ADP$$

$$2\,Ca_o \qquad 2\,Ca_i$$

$$\square \longleftrightarrow \blacksquare$$

$$Pi$$

$$\text{(2)}\quad \frac{Ca_o}{Ca_i} = \sqrt{\frac{K \cdot ADP \cdot Pi}{ATP}} \sim \frac{1}{50\,000}$$

$$Ca_i \cdot Pi = L$$

$$\text{(3)}\quad Ca_o = \sqrt{\frac{K' \cdot ADP}{ATP \cdot Pi}} \longrightarrow \sqrt{\frac{K''}{ATP}} \sim 2 \cdot 10^{-8}\,M$$

Fig. 2. Working cycle of the sarcoplasmic reticulum calcium pump. When calcium uptake approaches equilibrium of the reaction, the concentration ratio calcium outside – calcium inside is given by equation 2. When calcium is precipitated inside the vesicles as calcium phosphate, equation 3 approximates the external calcium concentration.

Conclusion: The sarcoplasmic membranes can create and maintain the physiologically required high calcium ratio between myoplasma and the vesicular space at low energy cost.

Calcium elimination in the resting muscle

Due to the limited storing capacity of the sarcoplasmic menbranes, they cannot cope with the permanent influx of calcium ions during rest and activity in the living muscle. Mechanisms are required by which the stored calcium can be eliminated. There are only two possibilities by which this can be accomplished. A secretion of calcium through the transverse tubules or a slow elimination driven by the sodium-calcium exchange mechanism in the plasma membrane, whereby the calcium ions have to diffuse at a subthreshold concentration through the myoplasma. If calcium quantities are offered to isolated sarcoplasmic reticulum vesicles which exceed their storing capacity, the activity of the pump is suppressed by the high internal calcium concentration and a slow calcium turnover persists.

Conclusion: No mechanism has been established by which calcium ions can be eliminated from the sarcoplasmic reticulum in order to prevent overloading.

Calcium release for muscle activation

The calcium-filled sarcoplasmic reticulum membranes, especially their cisternal elements, are thought to function as stores from which calcium is released during activation. Such intracellular stores are a necessity for fast contracting muscles composed of thick fibers. In contrast, the contractile

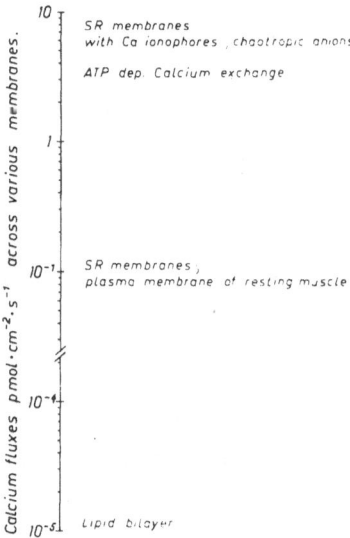

Fig. 3. Calcium fluxes across various membranes.

apparatus of thin fibers or cells in slowly contracting muscles can be supplied with activator calcium from the extracellular space. Cardiac muscles with their thin and relatively fast contracting fibers must be considered to be intermediates in which both mechanisms of calcium supply might be effective. The calcium supply from the extracellular space is thought to take place in analogy to the sodium influx during excitation through ion channels. Pharmacological agents by which the calcium influx together with its electrical equivalent, the calcium current, can be blocked specifically are in support of this mechanism (20).

As to the release of calcium from its intracellular stores there is only general agreement that the electrical signal which induces the release is conducted inward to the stores via the transverse tubules. Yet no experimentally supported concept has been worked out for the mechanism by which calcium is released from these stores by the electrical event in the complex of cisternal und tubular membranes. Experiments with isolated sarcoplasmic vesicles have contributed relatively little to this important problem. The passive efflux of calcium from calcium-loaded vesicles, as mentioned above, is a slow process (fig. 3).

It proceeds as slowly as the influx of calcium across the plasma membranes. Under the assumption that the contractile protein needs for activation 0.14–0.28 μmol calcium $\cdot$ ml^{-1} (21) in 5–50 ms, the calcium flux across the sarcoplasmic membranes must rise by more than a factor of 1000. If such an enhancement could be achieved in vitro, the calcium stored by the isolated sarcoplasmic reticulum vesicles (100 nmol $\cdot$ mg^{-1})

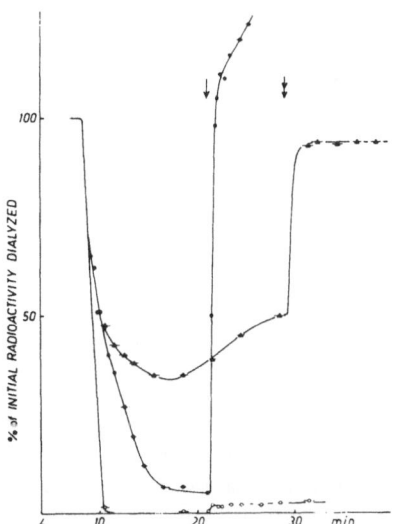

Fig. 4. Calcium release induced by the calcium ionophore X537A. ●——●. The assay medium contained 5 mM ATP and 100 nmol calcium. Calcium uptake occurred during 10 min. At 21 min 60 μg ionophore were added. ▲——▲ The assay medium contained 0.5 mM ATP. Calcium uptake is incomplete and followed by a spontaneous release of calcium. The addition of 60 μg ionophore at 29 min accelerates calcium release. ○——○ The assay medium contained 5 mM oxalate. The ionophore is ineffective.

should be set free in approximately 50 ms. Many attempts have been made to induce such a sudden release of calcium ions by changing the ionic environment of the vesicles (cf. 22). Changes supposed to charge the interior of the vesicles either positively or negatively induced a release of only insignificant calcium quantities. Likewise the attempt to induce a calcium release from calcium-loaded vesicles by suddenly increasing the external calcium level (calcium-induced calcium release) did not result in a rapid net release of calcium ions. On addition of unlabelled calcium to vesicles loaded with ^{45}calcium in a magnesium-ATP-containing medium a calcium exchange takes place. Yet the amount of calcium which leaves the vesicles never exceeds the added amount. In contrast, the addition of the calcium ionophore X 537 A causes a quite rapid net release of calcium (23) (fig. 4). However, even this greatly enhanced calcium efflux remains far below the value required for the muscle activation. As an alternative for an influx of calcium ions from calcium stores it has been suggested that the calcium ions might be supplied by a release of bound calcium. On account of recent results obtained by different groups (24, 25), this mechanism seems not very likely. Experiments were performed to measure the dissociation of the bound calcium from the reticular membranes, and half-times of approximately 20 ms at 30 °C were found, which indicates a relatively slow dissociation rate. Apart from the fact that we do not know any mechanism by which the high affinity of the sarcoplasmic reticulum membranes can be reduced markedly, the amounts which become avail-

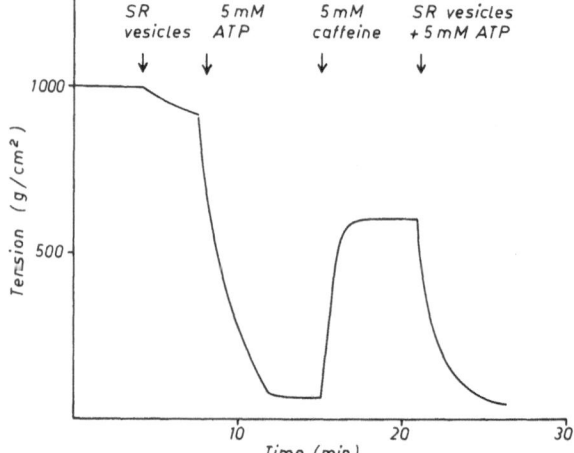

Fig. 5. Caffeine-induced contracture of glycerinated muscle fibers relaxed by sarco-plasmic reticulum vesicles.
The glycerinated muscle fiber develops tension in a solution containing 5 mM ATP and 5 mM magnesium. At zero time, the bath fluid was replaced by an ATP-free solution. The fiber maintains its tension. The addition of sarcoplasmic reticulum vesicles (Marsh-Bendall factor) does not markedly affect the developed tension. On addition of 5 mM ATP the fiber relaxes. The addition of 5 mM caffeine induces a rapid tension development. In a caffeine-free relaxing solution the fiber relaxes again. From *H. H. Weber*, Adenosine triphosphate and motility of living systems, 1953. *The Harvey Lectures*, Ser. XIL, Academic Press, New York, 1955.

able appear to be not sufficient. Furthermore, we must assume that in the resting muscle the external binding sites of the membranes are not occupied by calcium ions.

It has long been known that freshly glycerinated muscle fibers relaxed in ATP-containing solutions contract when caffeine is added to the bath fluid (fig. 5). Since caffeine is not effective after the reticular membranes persisting in the fiber have been destroyed, we have to assume that caffeine causes contraction by a release of calcium from reticular structures. Since, however, caffeine is not very effective as a calcium-releasing agent when applied to isolated sarcoplasmic membranes, the target structures of caffeine are presumably not removed from the muscle structures during isolation or have been destroyed. In conclusion, the results indicate that the calcium-transporting membranes of the sarcoplasmic reticulum membranes are not involved in the mechanism of calcium release.

Calcium removal during relaxation

According to the calcium concept of muscle activations, the performance of a given muscle should depend on the amount of ionized calcium which is released and the duration of its presence in the myoplasma. Both parameters can be affected by the activity of the sarcoplasmic calcium pump. At a given amount of activator calcium an activation of the calcium pump should shorten the active state of the muscle, and, therefore, reduce its mechanical output. The opposite effect can be expected, however, if an enhanced activity of the pump would lead to an increase of the amount of calcium in the stores. Similar opposite effects can be envisaged if the pump activity is inhibited. Evidently, it is very difficult to relate changes in muscle activity with changes in the activcity of the sarcoplasmic calcium pump. Nevertheless, an abundance of data has been collected in recent years dealing with the rate of calcium uptake of isolated reticular

Table 1. ATP-driven calcium uptake of canine cardiac sarcoplasmic reticulum vesicles.

ATP driven calcium uptake
of canine cardiac SR vesicles.
(n mol · mg^{-1} · min^{-1})

	control		stimulated activity	
Tada et al. (26)	100*	25°C	C AMP dep. prot. kinase	250
Schwartz et al. (27)	120*	30°C	C AMP dep. prot. kinase or phosphorylase b kinase	190
Suko (13)	450*	25°C	——	
Besch (28)	100	37°C	100 mM KCl	400
Scarpa (29)	200*	26°C	——	

x = 50 – 100 mM KCl present

Table 2. Calcium removal by transport and binding.

1 Calcium amounts to be removed during relaxation (n mol/ml)	15 – 150
2 Amounts of SR (mg/ml)	3 – 6
3 Rate of calcium uptake (nmol/mg·min)	1000
Required rate of calcium removal (nmol/ml·s)	1500
Rate obtained from 2 and 3 (nmol/ml·s)	100
Available calcium binding sites in SR membranes (nmol/ml)	50 – 100
Sites can be occupied at pCa 6 in ms ($k_1 = 5 \cdot 10^8 \cdot l\,mol^{-1} \cdot s^{-1}$)	1 – 2
Calcium release from troponin C half time in ms (Potter)	2

membranes, and many speculations concerning the interrelationship between pump and muscle activity were made. In table 1 results of such
measurements performed with isolated cardiac reticulum are compiled.
The data include the activating effects of various modulator systems and
possible activators. The results of these experiments provoke the question
as to the significance of the measured activities for the living muscle. For
an evaluation of this question we have to introduce information concerning the amount of calcium required for the activation of the contractile
system and the amount of the reticulum in the respective muscle.
Although the data compiled in table 2 are the most favourable approxima-
tions, it turns out that the calcium quantities which seem to be necessary
for muscle activation can hardly be removed during relaxation by the
sarcoplasmic membranes. An obvious way out of this apparent dilemma is
1) the assumption that the calcium transport system of the sarcoplasmic
reticulum might degenerate rapidly after isolation. Yet this degeneration
should mainly affect the rate of calcium uptake of the sarcoplasmic
reticulum membranes but not their concentrating power which corresponds to the physiological reqirement. Such a selective activity loss
seems to be not very probable. 2) The contractile protein in its natural
arrangement might need less calcium than the isolated proteins of the
regulator system. There are indications that the contractile protein possesses some kind of a calcium-saving mechanism. In favour of such a
mechanism is the observation that the tension of isolated fibers rises much
more steeply than calcium binding when the calcium level is elevated (30).
Other observations in support of such a mechanism were made by
Dancker (31) and *Weber* (32) who showed that actin-myosin interaction
can amplify itself after activity has been initiated by the interaction of

calcium with troponin C. 3) Calcium might be removed from the myoplasma much faster than it can be observed under steady-state conditions. A rapid binding to empty calcium binding places on the surface of the reticulum may occur prior to calcium translocation. Rapid calcium binding can quickly remove an amount of calcium which corresponds to the amount which the contractile protein might need for maximal activation. Yet such a mechanism requires that calcium movement occurs well ordered in time and space. Furthermore, during repetitive contractions the binding capacity of the sarcoplasmic reticulum would soon be exhausted and the slow ATP-dependent translocation would determine the rate of calcium removal. Since this process has to replenish the calcium stores in the reticulum from which calcium is released, calcium release, and as a consequence, the mechanical activity of the muscle must accommodate to the activity of the calcium pump.

Zusammenfassung

Die Rolle des sarkoplasmatischen Retikulums im Calciumkonzept der Muskelaktivierung wird anhand von Daten und Beobachtungen, die in In–vitro–Studien an der isolierten sarkoplasmatischen Membran erhoben wurden, kritisch bewertet.

References

1. *Marsh, B. B.:* A factor modifying muscle fibre synaeresis. Nature **167**, 1065–1066 (1951).
2. *Hasselbach, W., M. Makinose:* Die Calciumpumpe der „Erschlaffungsgrana" des Muskels und ihre Abhängigkeit von der ATP-Spaltung. Biochem. Z. **333**, 518–528 (1961).
3. *Ebashi, S., M. Endo:* Ca ion and muscle contraction. Progr. Biophys. Mol. Biol. **18**, 123–183 (1968).
4. *Hasselbach, W.:* Relaxation and the sarcotubular calcium pump. Fed. Proc. **23**, 909–912 (1964).
5. *Rüdel, R., S. R. Taylor:* Aequorin luminescence during contraction of amphibian skeletal muscle. J. Physiol. (London) **233**, 5P–6P (1973).
6. *Bremel, R. D.:* Myosin linked calcium regulation in vertebrate smooth muscle. Nature **252**, 405–407 (1974).
7. *Constantin, L. L., C. Franzini-Armstrong, R. J. Podolsky:* Localization of calcium-accumulating structures in striated muscle fibers. Science **147**, 158–160 (1965).
8. *Beil, F. U., D. von Chak, W. Hasselbach, H. H. Weber:* Competition between oxalate and phosphate during active calcium accumulation by sarcoplasmic vesicles. Z. Naturforsch. **32c**, 281–287 (1977).
9. *Wincgrad, S.:* The intracellular site of calcium activation of contraction in frog skeletal muscle. J. Gen. Physiol. **55**, 77–88 (1970).
10. *Hasselbach, W.:* in Mol. Bioenergetics and Macromolecular Biochemistry, Meyerhof Symposion 1970, pp.149–171: The sarcoplasmic calcium pump. (Berlin, Heidelberg, New York 1972).
11. *Meissner, G., S. Fleischer:* Characterization of sarcoplasmic reticulum from skeletal muscle. Biochim. Biophys. Acta **241**, 356–378 (1971).
12. *Peachey, L.D.:* The sarcoplasmic reticulum and transverse tubules of the frogs's sartorius. J. Cell. Biol. **25**, 209–231 (1965).
13. *Suko, J., W. Hasselbach:* Characterization of cardiac sarcoplasmic reticulum ATP-ADP phosphate exchange and phosphorylation of the calcium transport adenosine triphosphatase. Eur. J. Biochem. **64**, 123–130 (1976).

14. *Portzehl, H., R. C. Caldwell, J. C. Rüegg:* The dependence of contraction and relaxation of muscle fibres from the crab maia squinado on the internal concentration of free calcium ions. Biochim. Biophys. Acta **79**, 581–591 (1964).
15. *Hasselbach, W.:* The reversibility of the sarcoplasmic calcium pump. Biochim. Biophys. Acta **515**, 23–53 (1978)
16. *Duggan, P. I., A. Martonosi:* Sarcoplasmic reticulum. IX. The permeability of sarcoplasmic reticulum membranes. J. Gen. Physiol. **56**, 147–167 (1970).
17. *Wendt-Gallitelli, M. F., H. Wolburg, W. Schlote, M. Schwegler, C. Holubarsch, and R. Jacob:* Prospects of X-ray microanalysis in the study of pathophysiology of myocardial contraction. Basic Res. Cardiol. **75**, 66–72 (1980).
18. *Ikemoto, N., G. M. Bhatnagar, B. Nagy, J. Gergely:* Interaction of divalent cations with the 55,000 dalton protein component of the sarcoplasmic reticulum. Studies of fluorescence and circular dichronism. J. Biol. Chem. **247**, 7835–7837 (1972).
19. *König, V., W. Hasselbach:* Unpublished results.
20. *Fleckenstein, A.:* in: Calcium and the Heart. Ed. *P. Harris, L. H. Opie:* Specific inhibitors and promoters of calcium action in the excitation-contraction coupling of heart muscle and their role in the prevention on production of myocardial lesions (New York 1971).
21. *Potter, J. D., J. Gergely:* Troponin, tropomyosin, and actin interactions in the Ca^{2+} regulation of muscle contraction. Biochem. **13**, 2679–2703 (1974).
22. *Beeler, T., A. Martonosi,:* The relationship between membrane potential and Ca^{2+} fluxes in isolated sarcoplasmic reticulum vesicles. FEBS Lett. **98**, 173–176 (1979).
23. *Mermier, P., W. Hasselbach:* Comparison between strontium and calcium uptake by the fragmented sarcoplasmic reticulum. Eur. J. Biochem. **69**, 79–86 (1976).
24. *Rauch, B., D. von Chak, W. Hasselbach:* An estimate of the kinetics of calcium binding and dissociation of the sarcoplasmic reticulum transport ATPase. FEBS Lett. **93**, 65–68 (1978).
25. *Sumida, M., T. Wang, F. Mandel, J. P. Froehlich, A. Schwartz:* Transient kinetics of Ca^{2+} transport of sacoplasmic reticulum. J. Biol. Chem. **253**, 8772–8777 (1978).
26. *Tada, M., M. A. Kirchberger, A. M. Katz:* Phosphorylation of a 22,000-dalton component of the cardiac sarcoplasmic reticulum by adenosine 3':5'-monophosphate-dependent protein kinase. J. Biol. Chem. **250**, 2640–2647 (1975).
27. *Schwartz, A., M. L. Entman, K. Kaniike, L. K. Lane, W. B. van Winkle, E. P. Bornet:* The rate of calcium uptake into sarcoplasmic reticulum of cardiac muscle and skeletal muscle. Effects of cyclic AMP-dependent protein kinase and phosphorylase b kinase. Biochim. Biophys. Acta **426**, 57–72 (1976).
28. *Jones, L. R., H. R. Besch, jr., A. M. Watanabe:* Monovalent cation stimulation of Ca^{2+} uptake by cardiac membrane vesicles. J. Biol. Chem. **252**, 3315–3323 (1977).
29. *Scarpa, A., J. R. Williamson:* In: Calcium Binding Proteins. Eds. *W. Drabikowski* et al. pp. 547–584: Calcium binding and calcium transport by subcellular fractions of heart (Amsterdam 1974).
30. *Julian, F. J.:* The effect of calcium on the force-velocity relation of briefly glycerinated frog muscle fibres. J. Physiol. **218**, 117–145 (1971).
31. *Dancker, P.:* The modification of actomyosin ATPase activity by tropomyosin-troponin and its dependence on ionic strength, ATP-concentration, and actin-myosin ratio. Z. Naturforsch. **29c**, 496–505 (1974).
32. *Bremel, R. D., A. Weber:* Cooperation within actin filament in vertebrate skeletal muscle. Nature New Biology **238**, 97–101 (1972).

Author's address:

Prof. Dr. *W. Hasselbach,* Max-Planck-Institut für medizin. Forschung, Abt. Physiologie, Jahnstraße 29, D-6900 Heidelberg 1, Germany

Basic Res. Cardiol. **75**, 13–17 (1980)
© 1980 Dr. Dietrich Steinkopff Verlag, Darmstadt
ISSN 0300–8428

Paper, presented at the Erwin Riesch Symposium, Tübingen, April 3–7, 1979

Department of Medicine, University of Connecticut Health Center, Farmington
(U.S.A.)

Calcium-induced calcium release in sarcoplasmic reticulum vesicles purified from rabbit fast skeletal muscle*)

Ca^{2+}-induzierte Ca^{2+}-Freisetzung aus gereinigten Vesikeln vom sarkoplasmatischen Retikulum schneller Kaninchen-Skelettmuskeln

*R. Kupsaw, Ch. F. Louis**), and A. M. Katz*

With 2 figures

Summary

Addition of small amounts of CaCl$_2$ can induce calcium release from calcium-filled sarcoplasmic reticulum vesicles. The time of onset and rate of calcium release in the vesicular preparations, which occurs when ionized Ca^{2+} in the medium is increased from < 1 µM to 3–5 µM, are considerably slower than in skinned muscle fiber preparations.

The appearance of spontaneous calcium release[1] after calcium uptake[1] by sarcoplasmic reticulum vesicles in media containing a calcium-precipitating anion (1–3) depends in part on the amount of calcium initially presented to the vesicles (initial Ca/SR protein ratio) (fig. 1). Spontaneous calcium release is minimal or absent in reactions carried out at low initial Ca/SR protein ratios, where there is insufficient calcium for the vesicles to achieve their maximal capacity to take up calcium (calcium capacity) and calcium sequestration within the vesicles lowers Ca$_0$[1] to below 0.1 µM (2–4) (fig. 1A). At high initial Ca/SR protein ratios that exceed the calcium capacity, Ca$_0$ remains sufficiently high so as not to limit calcium pump activity throughout the calcium uptake reaction. Under these conditions initial calcium uptake can be followed by spontaneous calcium release (1, 2) and renewed calcium uptake (3) (fig. 1B). Unidirectional calcium efflux rates measured after initial calcium uptake are more

---

*) Supported by Research Grants HL-21812 and HL-22135 from the U.S. Public Health Service and also supported by a general Research Supply Account available to Medical Students doing research.
**) Muscular Dystrophy Association of America Fellow.

[1] *Calcium uptake* refers to a net increase in the calcium content of the vesicles; *calcium release* to a net decrease in calcium content; *Ca$_0$:* external Ca^{2+} concentration.

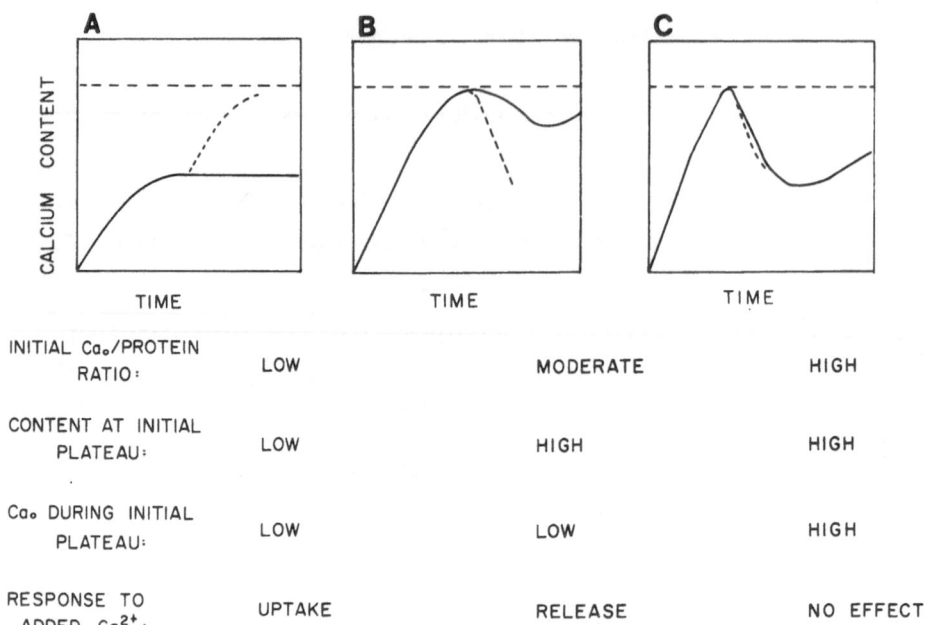

INITIAL Ca$_o$/PROTEIN RATIO:	LOW	MODERATE	HIGH
CONTENT AT INITIAL PLATEAU:	LOW	HIGH	HIGH
Ca$_o$ DURING INITIAL PLATEAU:	LOW	LOW	HIGH
RESPONSE TO ADDED Ca^{2+}:	UPTAKE	RELEASE	NO EFFECT

Fig. 1. Schematic diagram showing the patterns of spontaneous calcium uptake and release when sarcoplasmic reticulum vesicles are incubated at low (A), moderate (B) or high (C) initial Ca/SR protein ratios. At low ratios (A), calcium content cannot reach the calcium capacity of the vesicles (horizontal dashed line) and calcium uptake stops when the vesicles have lowered Ca$_0$. At high ratios (C) Ca$_0$ remains high when calcium content reaches the calcium capacity, and spontaneous calcium release occurs shortly after this capacity is reached. At moderate ratios (B) calcium content can approach the calcium capacity at low levels of Ca$_0$. Also shown are responses to added Ca^{2+} (see text and fig. 2).

rapid at higher Ca$_0$ (1, 2, 5–8), suggesting that the spontaneous calcium release seen with high initial Ca/SR protein ratios (fig. 1B–C) may be related to high Ca$_0$.

The present study demonstrates that calcium release from calcium-filled sarcoplasmic reticulum vesicles can be promoted when small amounts of CaCl$_2$ are added to reaction mixtures after calcium uptake had ceased at low levels of Ca$_0$ and calcium content had approached the calcium capacity of the vesicles (fig. 1B). Reaction conditions were selected to approach those depicted schematically in figure 1B by choosing an initial Ca/SR protein ratio that approximated the calcium capacity of the vesicles determined from a series of "pilot" reactions carried out at high initial Ca/SR protein ratios. Under these conditions, the initial maximum of calcium content approached the calcium capacity of the vesicle preparation when calcium sequestration by the vesicles had lowered Ca$_0$ to below 1 µM (fig. 2). Addition of a small amount of CaCl$_2$ during this initial maximum of calcium content, which increased Ca$_0$ less than 4 µM, promoted a calcium release that was more rapid and of greater magnitude than occurred later in the control reactions (fig. 2). In these experiments,

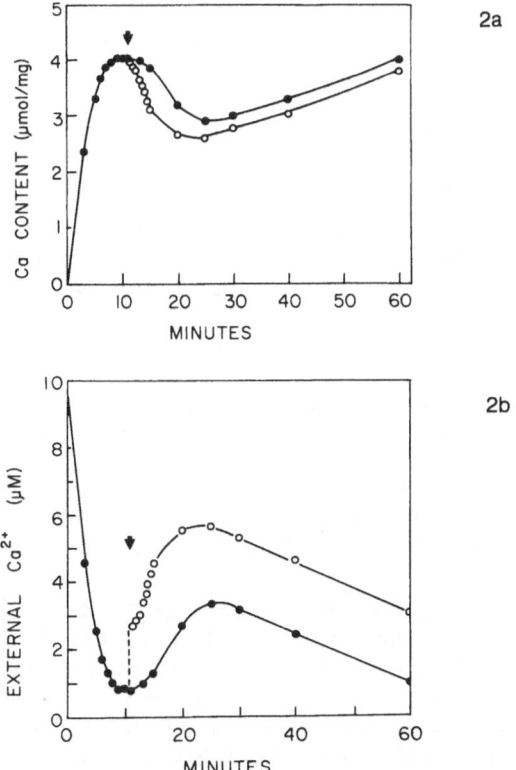

Fig. 2. Effects of increased Ca_0 on calcium release from rabbit vesicles. The control calcium uptake reaction (●——●) was carried out at 25 °C in 50 mM Tris phosphate (which stabilized internal Ca^{2+} at approximately 150 μM (1), 120 mM KCl, 40 mM histidine buffer (pH 6.8), 5 mM MgATP, 54 μM $^{45}CaCl_2$ and an ATP-regenerating system consisting of 5 mM phosphoenolpyruvate and 0.15 mg/ml pyruvate kinase. Reactions were started by addition of 12 μg/ml vesicles (1, 9). At appropriate times, samples were filtered through type HA (0.45 μm pore size) Millipore filters mounted in Swinny adapters, and the radioactivity of 50 μl aliquots of the filtrate was measured. At t = 11 minutes, Ca_0 was increased by the transfer of 7.5 ml of the reaction mixture to a tube containing 0.12 ml $^{45}CaCl_2$ (↓) of the same specific activity as that used in the original reaction mixture such that Ca_0 was increased by 1.8 μM (○——○). The use of $^{45}CaCl_2$ of a single specific activity simplified the calculations of vesicular calcium content from determinations of radioactivity. The radioactivity of 50 μl of the unfiltered reaction mixture was measured before and after transfer, and appropriate corrections were made to correct for the < 2% dilution of the initial reaction mixture by the added CaCl_2. Ca_0 was calculated from the total CaCl_2 concentrations taking into account binding of both Ca^{2+} and Mg^{2+} to ATP as described previously (10). Data plotted as calcium content (A) and Ca_0 (B).

Ca_0 remained well below that previously shown to inhibit the calcium pump (11).

The ability of increasing Ca_0 to promote calcium release was very sensitive to both the calcium content of the vesicles and Ca_0 at the time of the initial maximum of calcium content. In experiments conducted at initial Ca/SR protein ratios that greatly exceeded the calcium capacity of the vesicle preparation, Ca_0 remained high (> 6 µM) throughout the reaction, and rapid spontaneous calcium release occured immediately after the initial maximum of calcium content was reached (3). Under these conditions, $CaCl_2$ addition had little effect on this rapid calcium release (fig. 1C). Reduction of the initial Ca/SR protein ratio to below the calcium capacity of the vesicles was associated with renewed calcium uptake after $CaCl_2$ was added (1, 7, fig. 1A).

The calcium release shown in figure 2 could not be attributed to a mechanical artefact as transfer of aliquots of the reaction mixture to small volumes of water (2, 4) did not promote calcium release. Deterioration of the vesicles appears unlikely to explain the calcium release observed in these studies as a calcium reuptake phase was regulary observed (4, fig. 2), and preincubation of the vesicles at 25 °C for 1 hour in a complete reaction mixture lacking only calcium was not associated with significantly decreased calcium uptake activity when calcium was subsequently added. The possibility that ATP depletion or ADP accumulation slowed calcium influx and contributed to the calcium release was minimized by the use of a high ATP concentration, an ATP-regenerating system, and low concentrations of vesicles.

The present findings, which demonstrate that increasing Ca_0 in the micromolar range can accelerate calcium release from calcium-filled sarcoplasmic reticulum vesicles, are in accord with previous reports that unidirectional calcium efflux during the initial maximum of calcium content is increased at high levels of Ca_0 (1, 2, 5–8). *Inesi* and *Malan* (12) have reported that a much larger increase in Ca_0 (0.5 mM) can cause a net calcium release from calcium-filled sarcoplasmic reticulum vesicles.

Calcium-induced calcium release from the sarcoplasmic reticulum of skinned skeletal (13–16) and cardiac (17, 18) muscle fibers has been observed previously. In accord with observations in these skinned fiber preparations (15) the ability of small increases in Ca_0 to promote calcium release from sarcoplasmic reticulum vesicles requires preloading to a high calcium content and a low Ca_0 at the time of calcium addition. In the absence of sufficient calcium preload, skinned fibers (15) and sarcoplasmic reticulum vesicles (1, 7, fig. 1A) exhibit uptake of the added calcium rather than calcium release.

Although the present study demonstrates a calcium-induced calcium release in sarcoplasmic reticulum vesicles that is similar, in some ways, to that seen in skinned muscle fiber preparations (13–18), the calcium release in the vesicular preparation is much slower than that observed in skinned fibers.

Zusammenfassung

Die Zugabe kleiner Mengen an $CaCl_2$ kann die Ca^{2+}-Freisetzung aus Ca^{2+}-beladenen Vesikeln des sarkoplasmatischen Retikulums induzieren. Bei vesikulären Präparationen ist im Vergleich zu gehäuteten Muskelfasern die Zeit bis zur Ca^{2+}-Freisetzung, nach Erhöhung der Konzentration an ionisiertem Ca^{2+} im Medium von < 1 µM bis 3–5 µM, wesentlich verlängert. Entsprechend ist die Freisetzungsgeschwindigkeit wesentlich verlangsamt.

References

1. *Katz, A. M., D. I. Repke, W. Hasselbach:* Dependence of inophore- and caffeine-induced calcium release from sarcoplasmic reticulum vesicles on external and internal calcium ion concentrations. J. Biol. Chem. **252**, 1938–1949 (1977).
2. *Katz, A. M., D. I. Repke, J. Dunnett, W. Hasselbach:* Dependence of calcium permeability of sarcoplasmic reticulum vesicles on external and internal calcium ion concentrations. J. Biol. Chem. **252**, 1950–1956 (1977).
3. *Louis, C. F., G. Fudyma, P. Nash-Adler, A. M. Katz:* The effect of monovalent cation inophores on calcium uptake by rabbit skeletal muscle sarcoplasmic reticulum vesicles. FEBS Lett. **93**, 61–64 (1978).
4. *Hasselbach, M., M. Makinose:* Über den Mechanismus des Calciumtransportes durch die Membranen des sarkoplasmatischen Reticulum. Biochem. Z. **33**, 94–111 (1963).
5. *Weber, A., R. Herz, I. Reiss:* Study of the kinetics of calcium transport by isolated fragmented sarcoplasmic reticulum. Biochem. Z. **345**, 329–369 (1966).
6. *Hasselbach, W., W. Fiehn, M. Makinose, A. J. Migala:* Calcium fluxes across isolated sarcoplasmic membranes in the presence and absence of ATP. In "The Molecular Basis of Membrane Function" (Tosteson, D.C. ed.) 299–316 (Englewood Cliffs, N.J. 1969).
7. *Makinose, M.:* Possible functional states of the enzyme of the sarcoplasmic calcium pump. FEBS Lett. **37**, 140–143 (1973).
8. *Katz, A. M., D. I. Repke, G. Fudyma, M. Shigekawa:* Control of calcium efflux from sarcoplasmic reticulum vesicles by external calcium. J. Biol. Chem. **252**, 4210–4214 (1977).
9. *Harigaya, S., A. Schwartz:* Rate of calcium binding and uptake in normal animal and failing human cardiac muscle. Circulat. Res. **25**, 781–794 (1969).
10. *Katz, A. M., D. I. Repke, J. E. Upshaw, M. A. Polascik:* Characteristics of dog cardiac microsomes: Use of zonal centifugation to fractionate fragmented sarcoplasmic reticulum, (Na$^+$ + K$^+$) activated ATPase and mitochondrial fragments. Biochim. Biophys. Acta **205**, 473–490 (1970).
11. *Martonosi, A., R. Feretos:* The Uptake of Ca^{++} by sarcoplasmic reticulum fragments. J. Biol. Chem. **239**, 659–668 (1964).
12. *Inesi, G., N. Malan:* Minireview: Mechanisms of calcium release in sarcoplasmic reticulum. Life Sci. **18**, 773–779 (1976).
13. *Endo, M., M. Tanaka, Y. Ogawa:* Calcium induced release of calcium from the sarcoplasmic reticulum of skinned skeletal muscle fibres. Nature **229**, 34–36 (1970).
14. *Ford, L. E., R. J. Podolsky:* Regenerative calcium release within muscle cells. Science **167**, 58–59 (1970).
15. *Endo, M.:* Mechanism of action of caffeine on the sarcoplasmic reticulum of skeletal muscle. Proc. Jap. Acad. **51**, 479–484 (1975).
16. *Endo, M.:* Calcium release from the sarcoplasmic reticulum. Phyiol. Rev. **57**, 71–108 (1977).
17. Fabiato, A., F. Fabiato: Contractions induced by a calcium-triggered release of calcium from the sarcoplasmic reticulum of single skinned cardiac cells. J. Physiol. (London) **249**, 469–495 (1975).
18. *Fabiato, A., F. Fabiato:* Calcium release from the sarcoplasmic reticulum. Circulat. Res. **40**, 119–129 (1977).

Authors' address:

Dr. *A. M. Katz*, Department of Medicine, University of Connecticut Health Center, Farmington CT 06032 (U.S.A.)

Basic Res. Cardiol. **75**, 18–25 (1980)
© 1980 Dr. Dietrich Steinkopff Verlag, Darmstadt
ISSN 0300–8428

Paper, presented at the Erwin Riesch Symposium, Tübingen, April 3–7,1979

Department of Muscle Research, Boston, Biomedical Research Institute;
Department of Neurology, Massachusetts, General Hospital; and Department of
Biological Chemistry, Harvard Medical School, Boston, Massachusetts

Ca²⁺ control of actin-myosin interaction*)

Ca²⁺-Steuerung der Aktin-Myosin-Interaktion

J. Gergely

With 2 figures

Summary

Some aspects of the Ca^{2+}-regulation of actin-myosin interaction are discussed. Emphasis is placed on Ca^{2+}-induced conformational changes in the Ca^{2+}-binding subunit of troponin that leads to deinhibition of the actin-myosin interactions.

Calcium is now widely recognized as one of the cellular messengers that mediate various hormonal and neuro-hormonal effects. In muscle, as it has been clear for about twenty years, calcium plays a crucial role in switching the muscle from rest to activity. This brief review will deal with some aspects of the control calcium exerts on the contraction of striated muscles in higher organisms including cardiac and skeletal muscles, but there will be a brief excursion into muscles of lower organisms as well as smooth muscles of higher organisms. In the latter two, the way by which calcium acts appears to be different.

The current scheme of actin-myosin interaction assumes that there is a cyclic interaction between the myosin heads and actin filaments, this cyclic interaction involving the hydrolysis of an ATP molecule (see e.g. 1). In the virtual absence of calcium ions, which can be produced in vitro by chelators and corresponds to the resting state in vivo brought about the action of the sarcoplasmic reticulum pump, myosin heads cannot bind to actin. This raises the question whether calcium produces a change in the myosin molecule which would then make it impossible for it to undergo some conformational change which would enable it to bind to actin, or whether the cause is in the actin.

Types of regulation

In muscles of higher organisms it appears well established that calcium ions exert an effect on a system located in the thin actin filaments, notably troponin (2). A major part of the talk will deal with thin filament control. At

---

*) The preparation of this manuscript and work in the author's laboratory is supported by grants from NIH (HL-5949), the National Science Foundation and the Muscular Dystrophy Associations of America, Inc.

this point, by way of contrast, I shall briefly discuss those muscles that possess regulatory systems that depend on the direct interaction of calcium with myosin. The existence of this type of control was discovered by *Andrew Szent-Györgyi* and his colleagues in molluscan muscle, and by now it has been shown to be present in many species (3). Over the years many details of this system have been clarified, and it appears that myosin in these muscles possesses a certain type of subunit removable with EDTA treatment, the so-called regulatory light chain (4); when this subunit is removed myosin can combine with actin regardless of the presence of Ca^{2+}. When the light chain is present in myosin interaction takes place only in the presence of calcium.

In all muscle tissues myosin consists of two large subunits, each having a molecular weight of about 200,000 and being associated with two light chains whose molecular weight is of the order of 20,000 (5). It seems that the two light chains associated with a given heavy chain belong to two different classes. In vertebrate muscle one of them can be phosphorylated by an appropriate enzyme (6). The regulatory light chain in molluscan muscle apparently does not undergo phosphorylation, although it can be replaced by the phosphorylatable light chain in skeletal or cardiac muscle (4) which does not exert a regulatory function in its native environment. Only for smooth muscle do the majority of workers believe that calcium control is exerted through the phosphorylation of a myosin light chain (7). Calmodulin, a ubiquitous Ca^{2+}-binding protein, is a cofactor of the enzyme that catalyzes the phosphorylation (8, 9). It seems that after myosin is phosphorylated calcium is no longer required for activation by actin. Recent reports from Ebashi's laboratory question this view and have suggested the participation of yet another protein system, the so-called leiotonin system associated with the thin filaments (10). Future work will have to resolve this.

Perhaps not all speakers at this symposium will agree, but it seems to me that so far no clear evidence has been given that in striated muscles of higher organisms calcium control exerted via myosin has been demonstrated. Recent reports suggest that the interaction between cardiac actin and myosin is inhibited by the light chain that can undergo phosphorylation (7), and perhaps phosphorylation of this light chain will remove this inhibition. The observation may constitute an instance of myosin linked calcium control in a muscle of a higher organism. Earlier reports by *Haselgrove* (11) and *Huxley* (12) indicated that there might be a direct effect of activation of muscle and hence presumably of calcium released in the course of activation on myosin since there appeared indications of changes in the x-ray pattern attributable to the thick myosin filaments. More recent investigations by *Huxley* (13) appear to rule out such direct effect on myosin since in muscles stretched beyond actin-myosin overlap practically no change in the myosin repeat pattern is observed.

Myosin possesses internal flexibility as demonstrated by Morales' group using fluorescence polarization measurements (14) and in our laboratory with the use of electron spin saturation transfer measurements on spin labelled myosin (15). Since movements within the myosin molecule play a crucial role in the myosin crossbridge interaction cycle, undoubtedly efforts will continue to look for effects of calcium on these motions. So far it has not been possible to show the effect of calcium on the motions of myosin but again it may be possible that with more consistent control of the state of phosphorylation of the so-called LC2 light chain to detect calcium dependent changes.

Thin filament control – tropomyosin – troponin

Let me turn to the calcium control in vertebrate striated muscle which is associated with the tropomyosin-troponin system discovered by *Ebashi* and his colleagues. It is well known that rod-like tropomyosin molecules are associated with actin filaments in such a way that two rows of tropomyosin molecules can be visualized in two long-pitched grooves of the doubly helical actin filaments (2). Each tropomyosin spans a stretch of seven actins, and with each tropomyosin molecule there is associated a troponin complex which in turn consists of three subunits. These subunits have been termed TnC, TnI and TnT. The letters affixed to the abbreviations of troponin (Tn) indicate their function. Thus C stands for calcium binding, I for inhibition, T for tropomyosin binding. The currently accepted model is that when calcium binds to troponin C the TnI subunit by which the complex is anchored to actin is released (16, 17), permitting the tropomyosin to change its position on the actin filament in such a way that it no longer blocks the binding of myosin (11, 12) (Fig. 1). This view may be oversimplified and indeed the recent suggestion by *O'Brien* of King's College, London (18) suggests that tropomyosin may be normally in

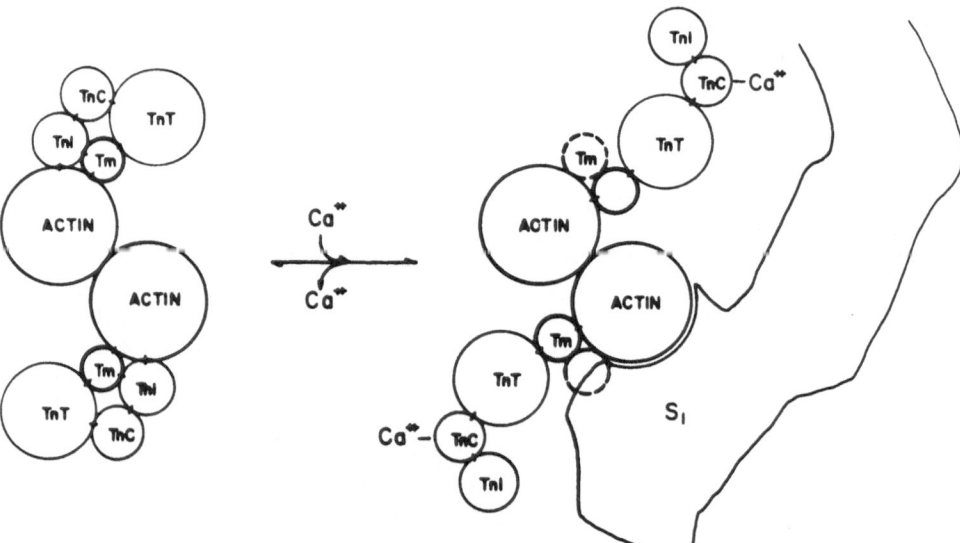

Fig. 1. Scheme of regulation of muscle contraction by troponin and Ca^{2+}. The relative positions of actin, tropomyosin and the head of the myosin molecule (S-1) in the model are essentially as shown. For key see text. Left: relaxation in the absence of Ca^{2+}. Right: activation, $[Ca^{2+}]$ 1 μM. Suggested interactions between proteins are indicated by short connecting lines (based on reference 16).

a position where it could not block the attachment of the myosin head; its change in position induced by calcium binding to troponin would, therefore, act in a more complicated way, perhaps by changing some structural features of actin which in turn would increase the affinity of the latter for myosin.

While the settling of this point would require considerable work by electron microscopists and experts in x-ray diffraction, a number of things concerning the interaction of calcium with troponin are known with a fair degree of certainty as are some details of the structure of the calcium binding unit, troponin C itself. Therefore, in the rest of this paper I should like to focus on some of the questions concerning the interaction of calcium with troponin C and discuss them in terms of some known structural features of troponin C. Finally, I should like to briefly touch upon the problem of how the effect of calcium and troponin C is transmitted to other members of the troponin complex and eventually to tropomyosin and actin, and say something about phosphorylation in the troponin system.

Binding studies on troponin C

Calcium-binding studies on troponin C have revealed the presence of four binding sites (19) falling into two classes differing in their affinity to Ca^{2+} as well as in their specificity. Thus, the sites of higher Ca^{2+} affinity also combine with Mg^{2+} while the sites of lower affinity appear to be specific for Ca^{2+}. There are four regions in the amino acid sequence of TnC (20) that, on the basis of strong homologies with the calcium-binding

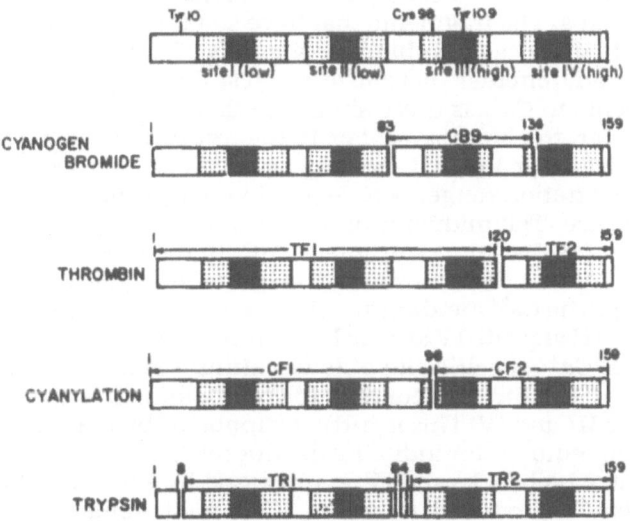

Fig. 2. Schematic diagram of TnC (top) and the fragments isolated for study after digestion with trypsin, thrombin and cyanogen bromide. Isolated fragments are indicated by arrows, the numbers indicating the included residues. Cross-hatched area, calcium-binding loops proper; shaded areas, putative flanking α helices. The four regions are indicating by Roman numerals (reproduced with permission from *Leavis* et al., JBC **253**, 5452, 1978).

protein parvalbumin (21), whose structure has been established by x-ray crystallography, have been identified as the calcium-binding sites. These regions have been numbered I, II, III and IV, starting with the site close to the amino terminus of the peptide chain (fig. 2). Each region, following the pattern of parvalbumin, consists of a so-called calcium-binding loop flanked by two α-helical segments. Region III is perhaps the most interesting one in that it contains a tyrosine residue as well as phenylalanine residues and the only sulfhydryl group of TnC. On the basis of optical changes involving tyrosine, changes in the reactivity of the single sulfhydryl group at Cys 98, and fluorescence and electron spin resonance spectra of probes attached to Cys 98, it appears that site III is one of the Ca-Mg sites (22). The sequence of cardiac troponin C has been determined by *Van Eerd* and *Takahashi* (23), and they concluded on the basis of substitutions in the amino acids at site I that the latter is not functional in cardiac TnC. Cardiac TnC contains two high-affinity sites plus one site of lower affinity (24). If one assumes that site III is a high-affinity site, as is the case in skeletal TnC, and that, apart from substitutions, cardiac site I is homologous to the skeletal site I, one can rule out site I as the other high-affinity Ca-Mg site in skeletal TnC. Thus, the second high-affinity Ca-Mg site must be either site II or IV.

Calcium binding to fragments of troponin C

Properties of the various sites in TnC can be further elucidated and their location in the primary structure pinpointed by the study of fragments produced by chemical (cyanogen bromide) or enzymatic (trypsin, thrombin) means. The fragments that have so far been obtained (see fig. 2) contain one to three calcium-binding sites (25, 26) and changes in tyrosine fluorescence and circular dichroism suggest that the reaction of some of these fragments to Ca^{2+} is quite similar to that of the intact molecule.

In particular, the binding of Ca^{2+} to the tryptic fragment TR2, containing site III – with Tyr 109 in it – as well as site IV, which occurs in the high affinity concentration range, is reflected in changes of circular dichroism and fluorescence. The midpoint of these transitions is at $[Ca^{2+}]$ 5×10^{-8}M, the same value as that found for intact TnC. In the presence of 2 mM Mg^{2+} the value is shifted by an order of magnitude suggesting competitive Mg^{2+}-binding. The Ca^{2+}-binding stoichiometry of two for TR2 supports the view that site III and site IV are the high affinity Ca^{2+}-Mg^{2+} sites. Thus, site II is the other Ca^{2+}-specific site of lower affinity in addition to site I.

The slope of the titration curve at the midpoint indicates an interaction between sites III and IV. This is further supported by the fact that the Ca^{2+} concentration required for inducing the fluorescence change in the thrombin fragment, which lacks site IV, is increased by a factor of 10. Similarly, the cyanogen Br-produced fragment CB9, containing a single site III, shows a Ca^{2+}-induced change in Tyr fluorescence and circular dichroism but at higher Ca^{2+} concentration, indicating a reduced affinity. Fragments produced by either thrombin or trypsin that contain region III (residues 88–119) (TH1 and TR2) bind TnI. Thus, they promise to be useful in the studies of the TnC-TnI interaction which, as we shall see, plays an important role in our thinking about the mechanism of Ca^{2+} regulation.

Mechanism

Previous studies (27) have suggested that binding of calcium to Ca^{2+}-specific sites of TnC is the key event in the regulation of the actin-myosin interaction, while combination with the Ca^{2+}-Mg^{2+} sites is more important for maintaining the conformation of the protein. Thus, the large conformational changes observed on the binding of Ca^{2+} to the high-affinity sites – reflected in changes in circular dichroism – are also produced by Mg^{2+}; but the activation of the actin-myosin system requires Ca^{2+} although Mg^{2+} is present. We found that activation of the actin-myosin interaction occurs whether the Ca^{2+}-Mg^{2+} sites are occupied by Ca^{2+} or Mg^{2+} provided Ca^{2+} is bound to the Ca^{2+}-specific site (19). However, according to other reports, the dependence on Ca^{2+} of ATPase activity and tension development shows antagonism between Ca^{2+} and Mg^{2+} (28). This apparent discrepancy remains to be resolved. The binding of Ca^{2+} to the Ca^{2+}-specific site is accompanied by similar changes in structure which can be monitored by extrinsic probes (22, 29); as well as by NMR spectroscopy (30, 31).

It has been suggested that the activating effect of calcium involves a change in TnI which in turn leads to its release from a binding site on the thin filament permitting the movement of tropomyosin. Changes induced in TnI by the combination of Ca^{2+} with TnC are consistent with this view. In a system consisting of TnC and of TnI carrying a fluorescent label (dansyl) a change occurs when Ca^{2+} binds to TnC (32). This change takes place in a Ca^{2+} concentration range that is characteristic of binding to the calcium-specific sites.

NMR studies have shown that calcium binding to the low affinity specific sites causes some loss of TnC structure (31) rather than a tightening up accompanying calcium binding to the high affinity sites. More recently (33) their loosening up effect has been identified as a moving apart of α-helices in the N-terminal half of TnC which also affects some groups in region III. Kinetic measurements by *Potter* and his colleagues (29) would support the view that *Potter* and I took earlier that the sites involved in regulation are the low affinity sites, since the rate at which calcium binding dissociates from the high affinity sites is far too low to account for actual rates of tension development and relaxation.

Studies with fragments have enabled us (26) and *Perry* (see 6) and his colleagues to conclude that a region close to calcium binding site III is involved in the interactions with TnI. More recently we have been able to pinpoint a short sequence containing negatively charged residues as the interaction site whose counterpart in troponin I, as previously suggested by *Perry* and his colleagues, would be a positively charged peptide sequence. There is a second region both in troponin C and troponin I that interacts and it would seem that while interaction at the negatively charged residues is stable in the absence of calcium, formation of a second link requires calcium binding presumably to the regulatory sites. Details of the interaction of TnT with troponin C remain to be worked out.

There are various sites at which enzymatic phosphorylation (6) can take place in TnI. The precise role of phosphorylation of troponin I has not yet been established, although it seems that in cardiac muscle inotropic effects of adrenaline, say, are accompanied by increased phosphorylation.

A phosphorylation dependent system suggests further avenues for calcium regulation since phosphorylation itself may be subject to complex controls involving other phosphorylation and dephosphorylation steps that may involve regulation by Ca^{2+} (34).

Zusammenfassung

In der vorliegenden Übersicht werden einige Gesichtspunkte der Ca^{2+}-Aktivierung der Aktin-Myosin-Interaktion diskutiert. Besonders betont werden Ca^{2+}-bedingte Konformationsänderungen an der Ca^{2+}-bindenden Untereinheit von Troponin, die zu einer Enthemmung der Aktin-Myosin-Interaktion führen.

References

1. *Huxley, H. E.:* The Mechanism of Muscle Contraction. Science **164**, 1356 (1969).
2. *Ebashi, S.:* Regulatory Mechanism of Muscle, in "Essays in Biochemistry" **10**, P. N. Campbell and F. Dickens, eds., p. 1 (1974).
3. *Lehman, R., A. G. Szent-Györgyi:* Regulation of Muscle Contraction: Distribution of Actin Control and Myosin Control in the Animal Kingdom. J. Gen. Physiol. **66**, 1 (1975).
4. *Kendrick-Jones, J., E. M. Szentkiralyi, A. G. Szent-Györgyi:* Regulatory Light Chains in Myosin. J. Molec. Biol. **104**, 747 (1976).
5. *Lowey, S., H. S. Slayter, A. G. Weeds, H. Baker:* Substructure of the Myosin Molecule I. Subfragments of Myosin by Enzyme Degradation. J. Molec. Biol. **42**, 1 (1969).
6. *Perry, S. V.:* The Regulation of Contractile Activity in Muscle. Biochem. Soc. Trans. **7**, 593 (1979).
7. *Casteels, R., T. Godfraind, J. C. Ruegg,* Eds. "Excitation-Concentration Coupling in Smooth Muscle", Elsevier (Amsterdam 1977).
8. *Dabrowska, R., J. M. F. Sherry, D. K. Aromatorio, D. J. Hartshorne:* Modulator Protein as a Component of the Myosin Light Chain Kinase from Chicken Gizzard. Biochemistry **17**, 253 (1978).
9. *Yagi, K., M. Yazawa, S. Kakiuchi, M. Ohshimia, K. Uenishi:* Identification of an activator protein for myosin light chain kinase as the Ca^{2+} dependent modulator protein. J. Biol. Chem. **253**, 1338 (1978).
10. *Ebashi, S., T. Mikawa, M. Hirata, Y. Nonomura:* The Regulatory Role of Calcium in Muscle. Ann. New York Acad. Sci. **307**, 451 (1978).
11. *Huxley, H. E.:* Structural Changes in the Actin- and Myosin-containing Filaments During Contraction. Cold Spring Harbor Symp. Quant. Biol. **37**, 361 (1972).
12. *Haselgrove, J. C.:* X-Ray Evidence for a Conformational Change in the Actin-containing Filaments of Vertebrate Striated Muscle. Cold Spring Harbor Symp. Quant. Biol. **37**, 341 (1972).
13. *Huxley, H. E.:* Time resolved X-ray Diffraction Studies on Muscle: In Cross-Bridge Mechanism in Muscle Contraction. *H. Sugi* and *G. H. Pollack,* Eds. University of Tokyo Press (1979).
14. *Mendelson, R. A., M. F. Morales, J. Botts:* Segmental Flexibility of the S-1 Moiety of Myosin. Biochemistry **12**, 2250 (1973).
15. *Thomas, D. D., J. C. Seidel, J. S. Hyde, J. Gergely:* Motion of the S-1 Segment in Myosin: Its Proteolytic Fragments and Its Supramolecular Complexes: Saturation Transfer EPR. Proc. Natl. Acad. Sci. (U.S.) **72**, 1729 (1975).
16. *Potter, J. D., J. Gergely:* Troponin, Tropomyosin and Actin Interactions in the Ca^{2+} Regulation of Muscle Contraction. Biochemistry **13**, 2697 (1974).

17. *Hitchcock, S. E., H. E. Huxley, A. G. Szent-Györgyi:* Calcium-sensitive Binding of Troponin to Actin-Tropomyosin; A Two Site Model for Troponin Action. J. Molec. Biol. **80,** 825 (1973).
18. *O'Brien, E. J., E. P. Morris, J. V. Seymour, J. Couch:* Structure of Muscle Thin Filaments. Abstract, VI Internat. Biophysics Congress, Kyoto, p. 311 (1978).
19. *Potter, J. D., J. Gergely:* The Calcium and Magnesium Binding Sites on Troponin and their Role in the Regulation of Myofibrillar ATPase. J. Biol. Chem. **250,** 4628 (1975).
20. *Collins, J. H., J. D. Potter, M. J. Horn, G. Wilshire, N. Jackman:* Structural Studies in Rabbit Skeletal Muscle Troponin C: Evidence for the Replication and Homology with Calcium Binding Proteins from Carp and Hake Muscles. FEBS Lett. **36,** 268 (1973).
21. *Kretsinger, R. E.:* Calcium Binding Protein. Ann. Rev. Biochem. **45,** 239 (1976).
22. *Potter, J. D., J. C. Seidel, P. Leavis, S. S. Lehrer, J. Gergely:* The Effect of Ca^{2+} Binding on Troponin C. Changes in Spin Label Motility, Extrinsic Fluorescence and -SH Reactivity. J. Biol. Chem. **251,** 7551 (1976).
23. *Van Eerd, J.-P., K. Takahashi:* Determination of the Complete Amino Acid Sequence of Bovine Cardiac Troponin C. Biochemistry **15,** 1171 (1976).
24. *Leavis, P. C., E. L. Kraft:* Calcium Binding to Cardiac Troponin C. Arch. Biochem. Biophys. **186,** 411 (1978).
25. *Drabikowski, W., Z. Grabarek, E. Barylko:* Degradation of TnC Component of Troponin by Trypsin. Biochim. Biophys. Acta **490,** 216 (1977).
26. *Leavis, P. C., S. S. Rosenfeld, J. Gergely, Z. Grabarek, W. Drabikowski:* Proteolytic Fragments of Troponin C; Localization of High and Low Affinity Ca^{2+} Binding Sites and Interactions with TnI and TnT. J. Biol. Chem. **253,** 5452 (1978).
27. *Bremel, R. D., A. Weber:* Cooperation within Actin Filaments in Vertebrate Skeletal Muscle. Nature **238,** 97 (1972).
28. *Donaldson, S. K., J. Kerrick:* Characterization of the Effects of Mg^{2+} on Ca^{2+} + Sr^{2+} Activated Tension Generation of Skinned Skeletal Muscle Fibers. J. Gen. Physiol. **66,** 427 (1975).
29. *Johnson, J. D., S. C. Charlton, J. D. Potter:* A Fluorescence Stopped Flow Analysis of Ca^{2+} Exchange with Troponin C. J. Biol. Chem. **254,** 3497 (1979).
30. *Seamon, K. B., D. J. Hartshorne, A. A. Bothner-By:* Ca^{2+} and Mg^{2+} Dependent Conformations of Troponin C as determined by ^{1}H and ^{19}F NMR. Biochemistry **16,** 4039 (1977).
31. *Levine, B. A., D. Mercola, J. M. Thornton, D. Coffman:* Calcium Binding by Troponin C. A Proton Magnetic Resonance Study. J. Molec. Biol. **115,** 743 (1977).
32. *Leavis, P. C.:* A Fluorescence Change in the Troponin C-Troponin I Complex Upon Calcium Binding to the Calcium-specific Binding Sites. Fed. Proc. **35,** 1746 (1976).
33. *Evans, J. S., B. A. Levine, P. C. Leavis, J. Gergely, Z. Grabarek, W. Drabikowski:* Proton Magnetic Resonance Studies in Proteolytic Fragments of TnC: Structural Homology with the Native Molecule Biochim. Biophys. Acta (in press).
34. *Cohen, P.:* The Role of Cyclic AMP-dependent Protein Kinase in the Regulation of Glycogen Metabolism in Mammalian Skeletal Muscle. Current Topics in Cellular Regulation **14,** 117, *B. L. Horecker* and *E. R. Stadtman,* Eds., Academic Press (1978).

Authors' address:

Dr. *J. Gergely,* Dept. of Muscle Research, Boston Biomedical Research Institute, Boston, Massachusetts (USA) 02114

Basic Res. Cardiol. **75**, 26–33 (1980)
© 1980 Dr. Dietrich Steinkopff Verlag, Darmstadt
ISSN 0300–8428

Paper, presented at the Erwin Riesch Symposium, Tübingen, April 3–7, 1979

II. Physiologisches Institut der Universität Heidelberg

Investigations on glycerinated cardiac muscle fibres in relation to the problem of regulation of cardiac contractility – effects of Ca^{++} and c-AMP*)

Untersuchungen zur Regulation der Kontraktilität in glyzerinextrahierten Herzmuskelpräparaten – Einflüsse von Ca^{++} und c-AMP

J. W. Herzig and *J. C. Rüegg*

With 3 figures

Summary

Alterations in myocardial contractile force and maximum unloaded shortening velocity (V_{max}) occurring in the course of isometric twitch contraction and with changes in inotropism are assumed to be mediated by changes in intracellular Ca^{++} and/or c-AMP concentration. In the present study, the influences of Ca^{++} and cyclic AMP upon the contractility of briefly glycerinated myocardial preparations are described. It is shown that Ca^{++} ions affect tension and V_{max}, as measured by rectangular releases in length, in different concentration ranges. This suggests that, besides the number of attached crossbridges regulated by Ca^{++} binding to troponin C, a Ca^{++}-dependent phosphorylation of the P-light chain of myocardial myosin may be involved in the regulation of V_{max}. Cyclic AMP, on the other hand, induces phosphorylation of troponin I, thereby reducing the sensitivity of tension to Ca^{++}.

It is concluded that the positive inotropic effect of catecholamines may be mediated by the described actions of intracellular Ca^{++} and c-AMP upon the contractile structures where c-AMP-dependent troponin phosphorylation could account for the acceleration of relaxation.

In glycerol-extracted cardiac preparations (2, 12), single disrupted myocardial cells (5), and electrically stimulated papillary muscle (3), tension and maximum unloaded velocity of shortening (V_{max}) have been demonstrated to be sensitive to changes in Ca^{++} concentration.

It has been shown (11) that the increase in peak tension under positive inotropic conditions induced by catecholamines or high extracellular Ca^{++} is always associated with a corresponding increase in the number of cross bridges attached to actin at any one moment. This new contractility parameter was derived from very rapid measurements of immediate stiffness, according to *Huxley* and *Simmons* (14). Experiments with glycerol-extracted cardiac muscle have shown that, during Ca^{++} activation, tension and the number of attached cross bridges always change proportionally

---

*) Supported by the Deutsche Forschungsgemeinschaft (SFB 90)

(13) while V_{max}, measured during rectangular releases in length (cf. Methods), requires a higher Ca^{++} concentration for half maximal activation than tension (12).

In the present study, the influence of Ca^{++}, c-AMP, inorganic phosphate and changes in the ratio of ATP to ADP upon cardiac tension development and V_{max} have been investigated in glycerol-extracted porcine trabecula septo-marginalis. The results show that the Ca^{++} sensitivities of tension and V_{max} can be changed independently from one another. It is suggested that Ca^{++}- and c-AMP-dependent phosphorylation of myocardial contractile proteins may, besides the Ca^{++} control of troponin, play an important role in the regulation of myocardial contractility and inotropism.

Methods

Immediately subendocardial fibre bundles from the trabecula septo-marginalis were prepared from fresh pig hearts. The bundles were divided by means of fine forceps into preparations with a length of ca. 5 mm and diameters between 0.1 and 0.25 mm. The preparations were then shaken 2 × 24 hours at 4 °C in a solution containing 50 vol.% glycerol, 20 mM histidine, 10 mM NaN_3 and 0.5% of the detergent Lubrol WX, pH 7.3. After that, the preparations were transferred into fresh glycerol solution at pH 7.0 without Lubrol WX and stored at –18 °C.

After mounting the fibre bundles on the mechanical apparatus (see below) the glycerol was washed out with a solution containing $MgCl_2$ 10 mM; EGTA 5 mM; KCl 15 mM; histidine 20 mM; NaN_3 5 mM; pH 6.7; free Ca^{++} concentration: $\sim 10^{-8}$ M.

The preparations were then relaxed in the relaxation solution containing ATP 10 mM; $MgCl_2$ 10 mM; EGTA 5 mM; histidine 20 mM; NaN_3 5 mM; NaCl 10 mM; creatine phosphate 10 mM; creatine kinase (CPK) 25 u/ml; pH 6.7; free Ca^{++} concentration: $\sim 10^{-8}$ M.

Isometric contraction was induced in the contraction solution which was identical to the relaxation solution with the exception that it additionally contained 5 mM $CaCl_2$, resulting in a free Ca^{++} concentration of 1.2×10^{-5} M. For intermediate Ca^{++} concentrations, mixtures of relaxing and contraction solutions were used. For some experiments, 10 mM NaF instead of NaCl, 10^{-4} M Theophylline and c-AMP in the range between 10^{-5} and 10^{-3} M were added. In some cases, the ATP reconstituting system (CPK and creatine phosphate) was left out adjusting ionic strength by addition of KCl.

The preparations were mounted with a fast setting glue between an AME AE 801 force transducer (natural frequency ~ 15 kHz) and a Ling Dynamics 101 vibrator which for stiffness measurements was driven by a velocity-dependent servo-amplifier allowing rectangular length changes to be performed within 0.5 ms (cf. 9). For measurements of V_{max} releases performed within 5 ms were applied to the preparation thereby releasing it by different amplitudes below slack length. The time interval from the onset of release to the onset of tension redevelopment was plotted against shortening. The slope of the resulting straight line provided a measure of the shortening velocity at zero load (V_{max}) (cf. also 6).

At the beginning of every experiment, the sarcomere length in relaxation solution, as measured by laser diffraction, was adjusted to values between 2.4 and 2.5 μm at which sarcomere length resting tension was negligible. Temperature was kept constant at 22 °C.

Results

Glycerol-extracted preparations from the porcine trabecula septo-marginalis were immersed in a Mg-ATP-containing medium (cf. Methods) and

activated by Ca^{++} in the concentration range between 10^{-8} and 10^{-5} M.
Isometric tension and actomyosin ATPase activity showed the well-
known sigmoidal dependence on pCa, with half maximal activation at
$\sim 7 \times 10^{-7}$ M Ca^{++} (fig. 1A). Immediate stiffness, measured according to
Huxley and *Simons* (14) by quick rectangular changes in length, also
showed the same Ca^{++} dependence (fig. 1A).

Ca^{++} regulation of unloaded shortening velocity

In order to determine the Ca^{++} dependence of unloaded shortening
velocity, glycerol-extracted myocardial preparations were isometrically
contracted at various Ca^{++} concentrations in the presence of an ATP-
reconstituting system (CPK and creatine phosphate). At several states of
Ca^{++} activation, the preparations were rapidly released below slack length
by various amplitudes (fig. 2, inset). Thereby, the isometric tension
developed by the preparation before the release dropped down to zero but
started to reappear at the moment at which the preparation had shortened
by the amplitude of the release and was no longer slack.

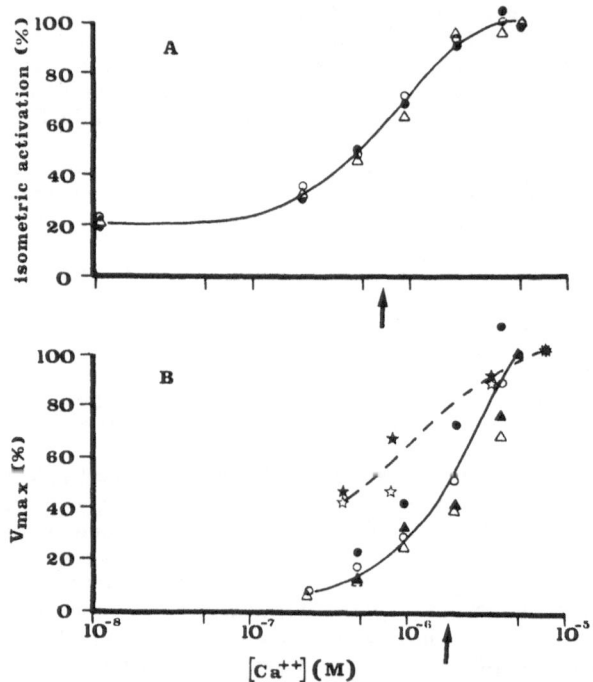

Fig. 1. Ca^{++} activation of contractility. In A, measurements of tension (○), immediate stiffness (●) and actomyosin ATPase (▲) are shown. B shows measurements of
V_{max} in the presence (solid line, ○, ●, △, ▲) and absence (dashed line, star symbols)
of an ATP-reconstituting system (CPK and creatine phosphate). Different symbols
signify experiments in different preparations. Arrows indicate Ca^{++} concentration
required for half maximal effect, both in the presence of CPK and creatine phosphate. Note that in the absence of an ATP-reconstituting system V_{max} is a factor of
5–10 slower than in its presence. For experimental conditions, cf. Methods and
figure 2.

Plotting the release amplitude versus the elapsed time which passed between the release and the moment at which the tension started to redevelop resulted in diagrams as shown in figure 2. At various Ca^{++} concentrations, different shortening-time relations were obtained, the slopes of which represent the velocity of shortening, given as shortening amplitude over time. It is shown that, after an instantaneous (Ca^{++}-independent) shortening, the resulting shortening-time relations during the first ca. 5% of shortening fit a straight line (cf. 6) deviating from the linear function in the range of larger shortenings, where the decreasing slope indicates a deceleration of shortening.

Taking the slopes of the linear portions of the shortening-time relations as a measure of maximum unloaded shortening velocity (V_{max}), it is shown that with increasing Ca^{++} concentration between 2×10^{-7}M and 9×10^{-6} M, V_{max} increased more than tenfold from 0.07 to 0.9 lengths/sec (fig. 1B). The half maximal effect was observed at 1.7×10^{-6} M Ca^{++}.

In figure 1B, V_{max} measured in experiments as described above is plotted versus the Ca^{++} concentration. It is shown that the Ca^{++} sensitivity of V_{max} is lower than that of tension and stiffness (cf. fig. 1A) when it is considered that the Ca^{++} concentration required for the half maximal effect upon V_{max} (2×10^{-6} M) is a factor of about 3 higher than in the case of the other parameters, where half maximal activation is reached near 7×10^{-7} M Ca^{++}.

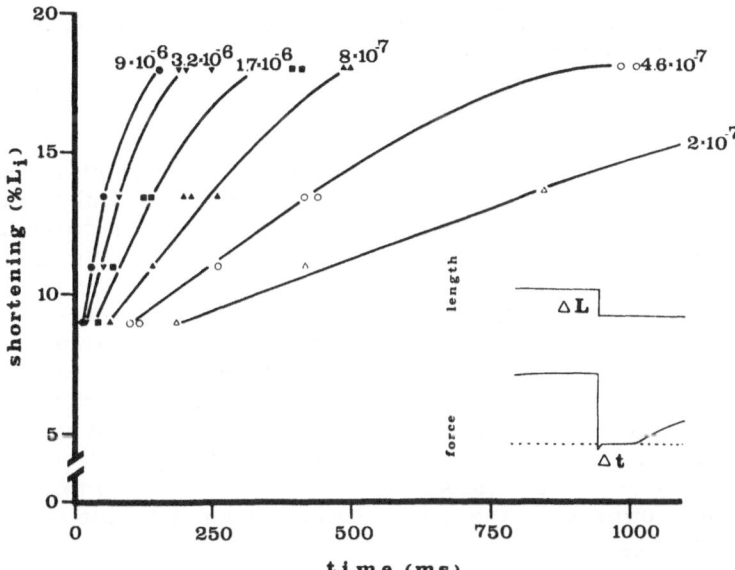

Fig. 2. Measurements of unloaded shortening velocity at different Ca^{++} concentrations. Inset shows method. The release amplitude $\triangle$ L (shortening) is plotted versus the time interval $\triangle$ t between the release and the onset of tension redevelopment. The slopes of the straight portions of the resulting shortening-time relations are taken as a measure of V_{max}. Numbers signify Ca^{++} concentrations in moles/litre. For experimental conditions, cf. Methods.

Addition of 10 mM inorganic phosphate reduced both tension and V_{max} by about 20% without changing the Ca^{++} sensitivity of both parameters.

In another series of similar experiments, V_{max} was measured in the absence of an ATP-reconstituting system. V_{max} at 10^{-5} M Ca^{++} was found to be a factor of 5–10 smaller than in the presence of CPK and creatine phosphate. While the Ca^{++} sensitivity of tension was not significantly altered, the Ca^{++} dependence of V_{max} in the absence of the ATP-reconstituting system was shifted to lower Ca^{++} concentrations (with respect to the results obtained in the presence of CPK and creatine phosphate (fig. 1B)) thereby approximating the Ca^{++} dependence of tension.

Influence of c-AMP on myocardial contractility

Glycerol-extracted myocardial preparations were isometrically contracted by Ca^{++}. Addition of 10 mM NaF and 10^{-4} M theophylline did not influence the Ca^{++} sensitivity of tension and V_{max} as measured in the presence of an ATP-reconstituting system. Further addition of 10^{-5} M–10^{-3} M c-AMP only slightly reduced the isometric tension at 10^{-5} M Ca^{++} but markedly reduced the tension developed at 7×10^{-7} M Ca^{++} (fig. 3) while the Ca^{++} sensitivity of V_{max} was much less influenced. With 10^{-5} M c-AMP, the reduction in tension at 7×10^{-7} M Ca^{++} was between 40 and 50%. With increasing c-AMP concentration up to 10^{-3} M no further tension reduction could be observed. In any case, application of c-AMP resulted in a shift of the Ca^{++} sensitivity of tension to higher Ca^{++} concentrations. Stiffness measurements obtained by rapid rectangular changes in length showed that also in the presence of c-AMP the proportionality between immediate stiffness and tension (fig. 3) was maintained.

Discussion

As measurements of immediate stiffness (cf. 14) in various myocardial preparations have shown, changes in isometric tension are always associated with corresponding alterations of the number of cross bridges attached to actin at any one moment (11, 13). This can be mimicked in experiments with glycerol-extracted myocardial preparations by changes in the "intracellular" Ca^{++} concentration. During shortening, even under zero external load, the myofilaments have to move against internal shearing forces. With a Ca^{++}-induced increase in the number of cross bridges, the ratio of contractile force to internal shortening resistence would increase, thereby facilitating shortening and increasing its velocity (cf. also 2). Since V_{max}, as shown in the present study, may also be altered independently of tension and stiffness (cf. also 10), the number of cross-bridges interacting with the actin filaments cannot be the only factor determining V_{max}.

Ca^{++} regulation of contractility

As shown in figure 1, the Ca^{++} concentration required for half maximal activation of V_{max} is about three times higher than the respective concentration for tension. This finding is in contrast with the observation reported by *Brenner* and *Jacob* (2) that the apparent velocity of unloaded shortening as measured during isotonic releases shows the same Ca^{++} sensitivity as tension. On the other hand, experiments carried out in living papillary muscles (3) and disrupted myocardial cells (5) have demonstrated that V_{max} is accelerated with increasing Ca^{++} concentration but does not necessarily correspond to the level of activation reached during the twitch (10, cf. also 4), while other authors report an increase in V_{max} with increasing force on the ascending limb of the length-tension diagram (8). A lowering of the ratio ATP/ADP, as supposed to occur in the absence of an ATP-reconstituting system, alters the Ca^{++} sensitivity of V_{max}, thereby bringing the Ca^{++} sensitivities of tension and V_{max} close together (fig. 1B). On the other hand, in the presence of c-AMP the Ca^{++} sensitivity of tension is shifted to higher Ca^{++} concentrations (fig. 3) whereas V_{max} is barely affected (unpublished experiments).

The observed differences in the Ca^{++} sensitivities of tension and V_{max} suggest that the Ca^{++} regulations of tension and V_{max} occur at different sites within the contractile structures of the heart. This is supported by the observation that in glycerol-extracted myocardial preparations desensitized by aging, isometric tension and stiffness are Ca^{++}-independent but V_{max} is still accelerated with increasing Ca^{++} concentration although much less than in the presence of a functionable Ca^{++}-troponin regulation of tension (unpublished observation). As *Bárány* and *Bárány* (11) point out, during tetanic activation the 18,000 dalton light chain of skeletal myosin is phosphorylated, presumably by a Ca^{++}-dependent protein kinase. Analogously, a Ca^{++}-dependent phosphorylation of the myocardial P-light chain may be involved in the regulation of V_{max} via alterations in cross-bridge kinetics (12). This is supported by the fact that the Ca^{++} concentration required for the half maximal effect upon V_{max} coincides with the Ca^{++} concentration for half maximal activation of the modulator regulated cardiac light chain kinase which is near 2×10^{-6} M *(Yagi, personal communication)*.

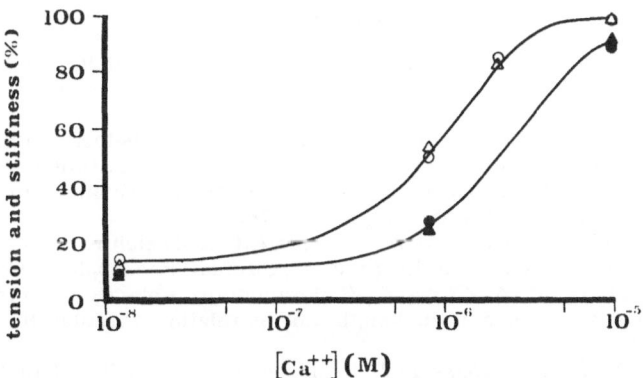

Fig. 3. Reduction of the Ca^{++} sensitivity of tension (○) and stiffness (△) by 10^{-4} M c-AMP in the presence of NaF and theophylline. Note that in the presence of c-AMP (filled symbols) the relation between tension and stiffness and Ca^{++} is shifted to higher concentrations, with little effect upon maximal activation. Tension and stiffness are expressed as percentage of the values obtained at 10^{-5} M Ca^{++} in the absence of c-AMP. For experimental conditions, cf. Methods.

The observed decrease in Ca^{++} sensitivity of tension in the presence of c-AMP is consistent with the observation that in cardiac myofibrils the Actomyosin ATPase activity is decreased by phosphorylation of troponin I by means of a c-AMP-dependent protein kinase (15). A c-AMP-dependent troponin I phosphorylation has also been shown in glycerinated myocardial preparations (15). It is therefore assumed that briefly glycerinated myocardial preparations contain endogenous protein kinases (cf. also 16) which are activated by c-AMP and Ca^{++} ions respectively. The c-AMP-induced decrease in isometric force at a given Ca^{++} concentration could account for the acceleration of the relaxation phase observed under positive inotropic conditions mediated by catecholamines (cf. also 7).

Zusammenfassung

Es wird vermutet, daß Veränderungen der kontraktilen Kraft des Myokards und der maximalen lastfreien Verkürzungsgeschwindigkeit (V_{max}) während der isometrischen Zuckung und bei inotropen Interventionen durch Änderungen der intrazellulären Ca^{++}- und c-AMP-Konzentrationen mediiert werden. In der vorliegenden Arbeit werden Einflüsse von Ca^{++}-Ionen und c-AMP auf die Kontraktilität kurz glyzerinierter Herzmuskelpräparate beschrieben. Ca^{++}-Ionen beeinflussen Kraft und V_{max}, gemessen durch rechteckförmiges release der Länge, in unterschiedlichen Konzentrationsbereichen. Dies deutet darauf hin, daß, neben der durch Ca^{++}-Bindung an Troponin C regulierten Anzahl angehefteter Querbrücken, eine Ca^{++}-abhängige Phosphorylierung der P leichten Kette des myokardialen Myosins an der Regulation von V_{max} beteiligt sein könnte. c-AMP-abhängige Phosphorylierung des Troponin I dagegen erniedrigt die Ca^{++}-Empfindlichkeit der Kraft.

Es wird postuliert, daß positiv inotrope Effekte nach Gabe von Katecholaminen durch die beschriebenen Einflüsse von intrazellulärem Ca^{++} und c-AMP auf die kontraktilen Strukturen selbst mediiert werden könnten, wobei die c-AMP-abhängige Troponin-Phosphorylierung für die Beschleunigung der Relaxation bedeutsam sein könnte.

References

1. *Bárány, K., M. Bárány:* Phosphorylation of the 18,000-dalton light chain of myosin during a single tetanus of frog muscle. J. Diol. Chem. 252, 4752–4754 (1977).
2. *Brenner, B., R. Jacob:* Maximum unloaded shortening velocity of mammalian cardiac and skeletal muscle as a function of free Ca^{++}-concentration and filament overlap. Significance of investigations in glycerinated muscle fibres. Pflügers Arch. Eur. J. Physiol. **373,** R 14 (1978).
3. *Brutsaert, D. L., V. A. Claes, M. A. Goethals:* Effect of calcium on force-velocity-length relations of heart muscle of the cat. Circulat. Res. **32,** 385–392 (1973).
4. *Brutsaert, D. L., V. A. Claes, E. H. Sonneblick:* Velocity of shortening of unloaded heart muscle and the length-tension relation. Circulat. Res. **29,** 63–75 (1971).
5. *De Clerck, N. M., V. A. Claes, D. L. Brutsaert:* Force velocity relations of single cardiac muscle cells. J. Gen. Physiol. **69,** 221–241 (1977).
6. *Edman, K. A. P.:* Maximum velocity of shortening in relation to sarcomere length and degree of activation of frog muscle fibres. J. Physiol. **278,** 9–10 P (1978).
7. *Fabiato, A., F. Fabiato:* Relaxing and inotropic effects of cyclic AMP on skinned cardiac cells. Nature **253,** 556–558 (1975).

8. *Gülch, R. W., R. Jacob:* Length-tension diagram and force-velocity relations of mammalian cardiac muscle under steady state conditions. Pflügers Arch. Eur. J. Physiol. **355,** 331–346 (1975).
9. *Güth, K., H. J. Kuhn:* Stiffness and tension during and after sudden length changes of glycerinated rabbit psoas muscle fibres. Biophys. Struct. Mechanism **4,** 223–236 (1978).
10. *Hamrell, B. B.:* Unloaded shortening (V_{max}) and maximal force (P_o): interaction with time and Ca^{++}. Fed. Proc. **37,** 461 (1978).
11. *Herzig, J. W.:* A cross-bridge model for inotropism as revealed by stiffness measurements in cardiac muscle. Basic Res. Cardiol. **73,** 273–286 (1978).
12. *Herzig, J. W.:* Ca^{++} activation of unloaded shortening velocity and cross-bridge kinetics in glycerol extracted mammalian cardiac muscle. Pflügers Arch. Eur. J. Physiol. **377,** R 2 (1978).
13. *Herzig, J. W., J. C. Rüegg:* Myocardial cross-bridge activity and its regulation by Ca^{++}, phosphate and stretch. In: Myocardial Failure, pp. 41–51, Eds.: *G. Riecker* et al. (Berlin–Heidelberg–New York 1977).
14. *Huxley, A. F., R. M. Simmons:* Proposed mechanism of force generation in striated muscle. Nature **233,** 533–538 (1971).
15. *Köhler, G., J. W. Herzig, R. Achazi, J. C. Rüegg:* Phosphorylation of regulatory proteins and Ca^{++} activated ATPase activity in cardiac natural actomyosin, myofibrils and glycerinated muscle fibres. Hoppe-Seyler's Z. Physiol. Chem. **360,** 305 (1979).
16. *McClellan, G. B., S. Winegrad:* The regulation of the calcium sensitivity of the contractile system in mammalian cardiac muscle. J. Gen. Physiol. **72,** 737–764 (1978).

Authors' address:

Dr. *J. W. Herzig*, II. Physiologisches Institut der Universität Heidelberg, Im Neuenheimer Feld 326, D-6900 Heidelberg (Germany)

Basic Res. Cardiol. **75**, 34–39 (1980)
© 1980 Dr. Dietrich Steinkopff Verlag, Darmstadt
ISSN 0300–8428

Paper, presented at the Erwin Riesch Symposium, Tübingen, April 3–7, 1979

Laboratory of Physical Biology, National Institute of Arthritis, Metabolism, and Digestive Diseases, National Institutes of Health, Bethesda, Maryland, U.S.A.

The rate-limiting step in muscle contraction

Der geschwindigkeitsbegrenzende Schritt bei der Muskelkontraktion

R. J. Podolsky

With 3 figures

Summary

The motion of skinned muscle fibers in chemically controlled bathing solutions is examined to obtain information about the cross bridge cycle. The effects of an ATP regenerating system and ionic strength on both the transient and the steady response to step changes in load are compared. The transient is changed in characteristic ways by these factors, but the steady motion is unaffected. If changes in the transient reflect changes in the rates of "making" and "breaking" cross bridges, these results suggest that the rate of physiological contraction is limited by a slow transition in the unattached myosin molecule rather than the making and breaking of cross bridges *per se.*

In the present paper I shall describe the effect of several chemical factors on the steady-state force-velocity relation and the mechanical transients that appear when a fiber is subjected to sudden changes in load. The main result is that factors that modulate the interaction of myosin and actin during ATP hydrolysis in solution change the transients but not the steady contraction velocity. This suggests that the rate-limiting step in the cross bridge cycle in the fiber may be an intramolecular transition in the myosin molecule rather than the "making" or "breaking" of the cross bridge *per se.*

Methods

The experiments were made with mechanically skinned muscle fibers from the frog. The fiber was perfused with various solutions of known chemical composition using a temperature-controlled solution changer. The general procedure was to perfuse the fiber first in a relaxing solution (pCa 9) and then to fully activate the fiber by raising the calcium level to at least pCa 5. After steady isometric force was developed, the lever was released and the fiber motion under constant load was recorded.

Results

Skinned fiber response

Typical responses of a skinned fiber segment are shown in figure 1 (1). The motion that takes place immediately after the lever is released, when the force changes quickly from P_0 to P, characterizes the "series elastic element" (2). We shall focus primarily on the subsequent isotonic motion, that is, the motion that takes place after the load has reached the final steady value. This consists typically of a transient phase followed by a phase of steady shortening.

The steady force and velocity of the skinned fiber in a simple bathing solution (see legend for fig. 1) is close to that of an intact muscle fiber in Ringer solution (3). The transient response has the same general shape in the two preparations, but its duration is about two times longer in the skinned fiber. The fact that the transient is prolonged but the steady motion is unchanged when a fiber is skinned and then allowed to shorten in a simple bathing solution indicates that the kinetic parameters that

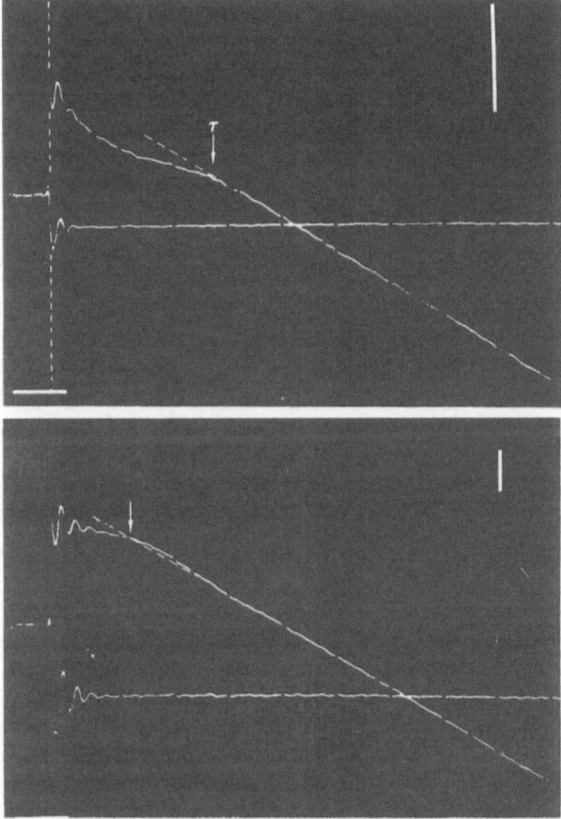

Fig. 1. Response of a skinned muscle fiber to step changes in load. Top trace, displacement; middle trace, force; bottom trace, zero of force. The steady isometric force is 72 mg weight. The back extrapolation of the steady motion is indicated by a fine *dashed line;* the *arrow* marks the null time. The steady velocities at the two relative loads are close to those found in intact fibers. Bathing solution, 140 mM KCl, 5 mM ATP, 1 mM $MgCl_2$, 10 mM imidazole, 2.94 mM CaEGTA, 0.06 mM EGTA (pCa 5.0, pH 7.0, 3 °C). Segment length, 3.9 mm; *vertical scale bar,* 50 Å/half sarcomere; *horizontal scale bar,* 20 ms. From *Podolsky, Gulati,* and *Nolan* (1974).

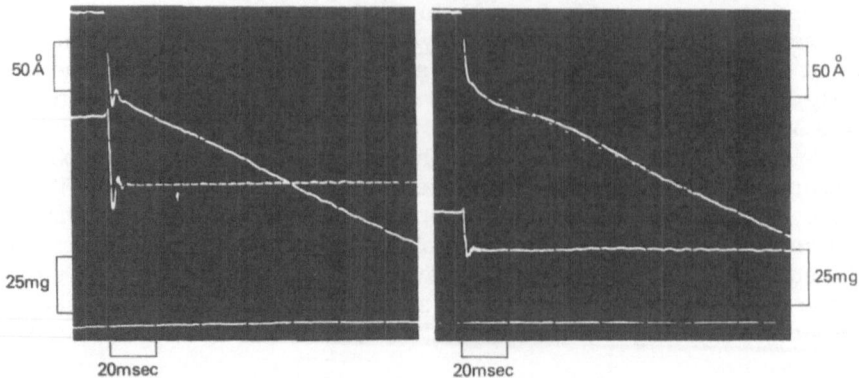

Fig. 2. Influence of ionic strength on the motion of a skinned muscle fiber. Same display as figure 1. The ionic strength on the left is 190 mM, and on the right it is 260 mM. The steady velocity and null time are the same at the two ionic strengths; the amplitude of the transient is about 3 times greater at the higher ionic strength. Temperature, 5–6 °C. From *Gulati* and *Podolsky* (1978).

determine the time course of the presteady motion may be different from those that control the steady motion.

Effect of an ATP-regenerating system

The approach to the steady state can be accelerated in skinned fibers by adding an ATP regenerating system to the simple bathing solution. Specifically, addition of 10 mM creatine phosphate (CP) and 300 units/ml creatine phosphokinase (CPK, Sigma Chemical Company), and an increase in the $MgCl_2$ concentration from 1 to 5 mM, causes the null times to decrease twofold (*Tawada & Podolsky,* unpublished experiments). Under these conditions the skinned fiber responds to both calcium activation and step changes in load in ways that closely resemble the intact fiber.

Effect of ionic strength

The influence of ionic strength on the contractile properties of skinned muscle fibers is of interest because this parameters is known to affect the association of actin and myosin in solution (4), and would therefore be expected to influence the rates of cross bridge making and breaking in the fiber. The experimental results are shown in figure 2 (5). Increasing the ionic strength from 190 mM to 260 mM causes the steady isometric force to decrease about twofold but does not affect the steady motion at a given relative load. The transients have the same null time but the amplitude in the higher ionic strength solution is about twice that in the control solution.

Discussion

The results can be summarized by saying that the steady state contraction velocity remains constant under several conditions that cause the transient to change markedly.

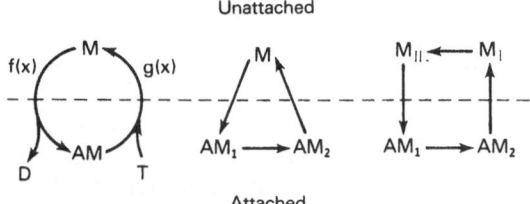

Fig. 3. Diagrams of cross bridge cycles with different numbers of states. In a two-state cycle (left) myosin M is either attached to actin A, forming a cross bridge AM, or unattached. The three-state cycle (center) has two attached states, AM_1 and AM_2; the four-state cycle (right) has, in addition, two unattached states, M_I and M_{II}, of which only M_{II} can form a cross bridge.

The increased null time seen in skinned fibers in simple bathing solutions, relative to intact fibers, appears to be due to the loss of CPK activity in the skinned fibers, since the null time can be brought back to the intact fiber value by adding CPK, CP, and $MgCl_2$ to the bathing solution. The mechanism of the CPK effect is not known, but preliminary studies (*Tawada & Podolsky,* unpublished experiments) indicate that, by catalyzing the transfer to phosphate from CP to ADP, CPK reduces the concentration of ADP within the fiber volume. This implies that the transient is prolonged in the simple bathing solution because ADP inhibits a step in the cross bridge cycle.

Ionic strength changes the amplitude rather than the null time of the transient, which is qualitatively different from the CPK effect. This is not surprising since the two factors clearly act through different mechanisms: CPK has little effect on the steady isometric force, while increasing the ionic strength reduces this force.

The cross bridge cycle

These results have implications regarding the number of kinetically significant steps in the cross bridge cycle. The diagram on the left of figure 3 shows the two-state cycle (6). The myosin molecule, M, is either attached to the actin filament, forming a force generating cross bridge, AM, or unattached. Model calculations (3, 7) show that in this scheme both the velocity for a given force and the time course of the isotonic transient depend on the magnitudes and spatial distribution of f and g, the rate functions for making and breaking cross bridges, respectively (6). The sensitivity of the velocity to f and g may depend on the load, but, in general, there will be certain loads for which the velocity will vary when f and/or g are varied. Therefore if we take the effects of CPK and ionic strength on the null time and amplitude of the transient as evidence that f and g depend on both the ADP concentration and ionic strength of the bathing solution, the insensitivity of the steady velocity to these parameters cannot be explained in a straightforward way by a two-state cycle for cross bridge action.

In the center diagram of figure 3 the activity cycle contains two attached states, AM_1 and AM_2, and one unattached state. AM_1 represents a low force configuration of the cross bridge, and $AM_1 \rightarrow AM_2$ represents a transition to a high force state. *Huxley* and *Simmons* (8) associated this type of transition with the very rapid force transient seen on the 2–4 millisecond time scale after a quick length step is imposed on the activated fiber. The cross bridge making $(M \rightarrow AM_1)$ and breaking $(AM_2 \rightarrow M)$ processes are supposed to take place on a time scale that is considerably slower than the force generating transition. The center diagram in this case collapses into a two state cycle which, as mentioned above, is inconsistent with the present results since changes in the relatively slow transients seen in figures 1 and 2 would then be expected to be associated with changes in the force-velocity relation.

The diagram on the right of figure 3 is the next stage of complexity for the cross bridge cycle. In this four-state cycle (9), only one of the unattached states, M_{II}, can react with A to form a cross bridge. If the transition M_I to M_{II} is the slowest step in the cycle, it will limit the turnover rate and therefore the contraction velocity. If, in addition, the $AM_1 \rightarrow AM_2$ transition is taken to be very fast, as in the three-state cycle, the f and g transitions would occur in the time domain defined by the duration of the isotonic transients. In this case changes in f and/or g could produce changes in the transients but would not be expected to change the force-velocity relation, which is consistent with the present data.

The discussion thus far has not taken into account the dependence of f and g on x, the relative position of the myosin and actin molecules on the two types of filaments. This can be done approximately by considering the spatially averaged value of the rate function and the transit time for the two molecules (10). However, for rigorous treatment the model must be defined in mathematical terms and calculations carried out in detail (see, for example, *Huxley* [6]; *Podolsky, Nolan & Zaveler* [7]; *Hill* [11]).

Relation to actomyosin ATPase in solution

During the actin-activated hydrolysis of ATP by heavy meromyosin (HMM) or subfragment-1 (S-1) in solution, at low temperature and low ionic strength, myosin seems to exist in two states, one which is able to bind to actin and another which is unable to bind to actin (12). The present analysis suggests that similar myosin states exist during the cross bridge cycle in the organized system, since two unattached states may be needed to account for the pattern of responses described here, and that the transition between these states controls the contraction velocity.

Zusammenfassung

In Badelösungen bekannter Zusammensetzung wurde die Verkürzung gehäuteter Muskelfasern untersucht, mit dem Ziel, Informationen über den Querbrückenzyklus zu erhalten. Die Effekte eines ATP-regenerierenden Systems und der Ionenstärke auf die transitorische Phase nach stufenweiser Änderung der Last und auf die Verkürzungsgeschwindigkeit nach Erreichen eines Gleichgewichtszustandes werden verglichen. Die Übergangsphase wird durch diese Faktoren in charakteristischer Weise verändert, während der anschließende Verkürzungsprozeß unbeeinflußt bleibt. Sofern Änderungen in der transitorischen Phase Veränderungen in der Geschwindigkeit der Bildung und Ablösung der Querbrücken widerspiegeln, lassen diese Ergebnisse vermuten, daß die Geschwindigkeit der physiologischen Kontraktion durch eine langsame Veränderung am Myosinmolekül im nicht angehefteten Zustand begrenzt wird und nicht durch die Bildung und das Ablösen der Querbrücken per se.

Acknowledgement

I am grateful to *Katsuhisa Tawada* for permission to cite unpublished experiments and to *Evan Eisenberg* for helpful discussion.

References

1. *Podolsky, R. J., J. Gulati, A. C. Nolan:* Contraction transients of skinned muscle fibers. Proc. Natl. Acad. Sci. U.S.A. **71**, 1516 (1974).
2. *Ford, L., E., A. F. Huxley, R. M. Simmons:* Tension responses to sudden length change in stimulated frog muscle fibers near slack length. J. Physiol. (Lond.) **269**, 441 (1977).
3. *Civan, M. M., R. J. Podolsky:* Contraction kinetics of striated muscle fibers following quick changes in load. J. Physiol. (Lond.) **184**, 511 (1966).
4. *Rizzino, A. A., W. W. Barouch, E. Eisenberg, C. Moos:* Actin-heavy meromyosin binding: determination of binding stoichiometry from ATPase kinetic measurements. Biochemistry 9, 2402 (1970).
5. *Gulati, J., R. J. Podolsky:* Contraction transients of skinned muscle fibers: effects of calcium and ionic strength. J. Gen. Physiol. **72**, 701 (1978).
6. *Huxley, A. F.:* Molecular structure and theories of contraction. Prog. Biophys. Biophys. Chem. **7**, 255 (1957).
7. *Podolsky, R. J., A. C. Nolan, S. A. Zaveler:* Cross-bridge properties derived from muscle isotonic velocity transients. Proc. Natl. Acad. Sci. U.S.A. **64**, 504 (1969).
8. *Huxley, A. F., R. M. Simmons:* Proposed mechanism of force generation in striated muscle. Nature **233**, 533 (1971).
9. *Eisenberg, E., T. L. Hill:* A cross-bridge model of muscle contraction. Prog. Biophys. Molec. Biol. **33**, 55 (1978).
10. *Podolsky, R. J.:* The nature of the contractile mechanism in muscle. In Biophys. Physiol. Pharm. Actions, *A. M. Shanes* (ed.), American Association for the Advancement of Science pg. 461 (Washington D. C. 1961).
11. *Hill, T. L.:* Theoretical formalism for the sliding filament model of contraction of striated muscle. Part I. Prog. Biophys. Mol. Biol. **23**, 267 (1974).
12. *Eisenberg, E., W. W. Kielley:* Evidence for a refractory state of heavy meromyosin and subfragment-1 unable to bind to actin in the presence of ATP. Cold Spring Harbor Symp. Quant. Biol. **37**, 145 (1973).

Author's address:

Dr. *R. J. Podolsky,* Building 6, Room 110, National Institutes of Health, Bethesda, Maryland 20205, U.S.A.

Basic Res. Cardiol. **75**, 40–46 (1980)
© 1980 Dr. Dietrich Steinkopff Verlag, Darmstadt
ISSN 0300-8428

Paper, presented at the Erwin Riesch Symposium, Tübingen, April 3–7, 1979

Physiologisches Institut II, Universität Tübingen

Calcium activation and maximum unloaded shortening velocity. Investigations on glycerinated skeletal and heart muscle preparations*)

Calcium-Aktivierung und maximale lastfreie Verkürzungsgeschwindigkeit. Untersuchungen an glycerinisierten Skelett- und Herzmuskelpräparaten

B. Brenner and *R. Jacob*

With 3 figures

Summary

In the present paper a method is described which allows differentiation of direct and indirect, shortening-induced effects of any parameter on maximum unloaded shortening velocity. It is shown that curvature of the length trace in isotonic quick releases should be attributed to shortening-induced changes in the afterload per cross bridge during such a quick release, caused, for example, by either a shortening-induced, internal load or a deactivation of the contractile system.

To evaluate shortening behaviour throughout the total course of isotonic quick releases, shortening velocity was plotted against the momentary length during the releases. These length-velocity relations yield straight lines when graphed on a floating-point scale, i.e., shortening velocity decreases exponentially with increasing amount of shortening during an isotonic release. Extrapolation of the length-velocity plots to the initial length of the releases allows determination of shortening velocity without alteration by shortening-induced increase in cross-bridge afterload.

Using this method, it is shown that sarcoplasmic Ca^{++} concentration neither has an effect on maximum unloaded shortening velocity in skeletal muscle, nor in cat myocardium. Furthermore, it is demonstrated that the described shortening-induced changes in cross-bridge afterload resulting in a decrease in shortening velocity may be the source of the Ca^{++} dependence of V_{max} published by different authors.

A question of fundamental importance in hypertrophy research is the extent to which alterations of the mechanical parameters isometric tension (p_o) and isotonic shortening velocity at zero load (V_{max}) should be attributed to either changes in electromechanical coupling conditions or alterations of the contractile system itself.

On the level of the contractile system, any alteration induced by hypertrophy could in principle be traced either to changes in the Ca^{++} sensitivity of the contractile system, or alterations of the elementary process itself.

---

*) Supported by the Deutsche Forschungsgemeinschaft.

The first possibility may only be of importance in the case of actual Ca^{++} dependence of both mechanical parameters p_o and V_{max}. Such a Ca^{++} effect has been proven for isometric tension development. There is still disagreement, however, concerning the Ca^{++} dependence of unloaded shortening velocity (2; 3; 4; 5; 7). To overcome the discrepancy in views on the question of any effect of sarcoplasmic (Ca^{++}) on V_{max} we reexamined this problem. Particular attention was paid to consideration of changes in cross-bridge afterload during shortening, which could feign an effect of (Ca^{++}) on unloaded shortening velocity.

Suitable experimental objects are provided by chemically isolated contractile systems (3; 6) since the biochemical milieu surrounding the myofibrils can easily be controlled. This means that the isolated contractile system allows characterization of the contractile behaviour without complication by other cell functions.

Because of the smaller complexity of the single-fiber preparation of skeletal muscle, we used this technique to develop a method which differentiates between immediate effects of any parameter on V_{max}, and those effects indirectly brought about by shortening-induced changes in cross-bridge afterload during shortening.

Methods

The experiments were carried out using single glycerinated rabbit psoas muscle fibers as well as cat papillary muscles of the right ventricle. At first the preparations were incubated in relaxation solution (pCa about 9). Afterwards they were activated in a step-wise manner by exchanging the relaxation solution for activation solutions of various pCa values. After isometric tension had reached a steady state, isotonic shortening velocity was measured by the use of tension-controlled quick release. For further details see *Brenner* (1).

Results and discussion

Length-velocity relations

In a tension-controlled quick release, skeletal and heart muscle show basically the same shortening behaviour (fig. 1a/b). An initial, sudden shortening is followed by the "steady state" of shortening. To evaluate the shortening behaviour of this second phase more comprehensively than by determination of the shortening velocity at a given time or a defined momentary length, shortening velocity was analyzed as a function of the corresponding sarcomere length. These length-velocity relations yield straight lines when graphed on a floating-point scale (fig. 1c). I.e., shortening velocity decreases exponentially with progressive shortening.

Effect of (Ca^{++}) on length-velocity relations

Variation in free sarcoplasmic Ca^{++} concentration causes a change in the slope of the length-velocity relations (fig 2a), whereby a higher (Ca^{++}) is accompanied by a smaller decrease in velocity during the release. Furthermore, all straight-line plots obtained at different (Ca^{++}) converge in a field around the starting length (l_s) of all quick releases.

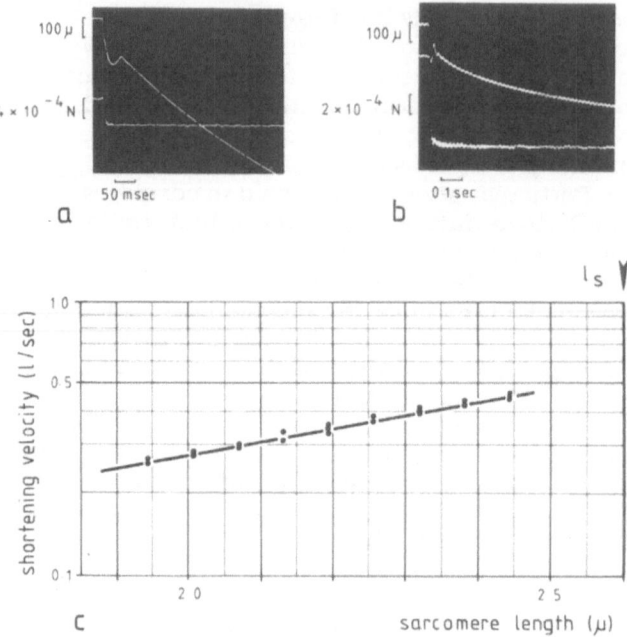

Fig. 1 Characterization of the shortening behaviour in isotonic quick releases. a) Original registration: Single fiber of rabbit psoas muscle ($\emptyset$ 55 × 70 μ, $l_s \triangleq 3.2$ mm = 2.45 μ/sarcomere, T = 3°C). b) Original registration: Cat papillary muscle ($\emptyset$ 180 × 200 μ, l_s = 1.8 mm, T = 13 °C, (Ca^{++}) = 0.38 μmole/l). c) Length-velocity plot, obtained by correlating shortening velocity with the corresponding sarcomere length throughout an isotonic quick release (experimental conditions as described in (a)).

Effect of external afterload on length-velocity relations

Additional afterload of the contractile system during an isotonic quick release causes a parallel shift of the length-velocity relations to smaller velocity values (fig. 2b). At different Ca^{++} concentrations the amount of this parallel shift is determined by the absolute value of the external afterload, but is independent of the sarcoplasmic Ca^{++} concentraion (fig. 2c), provided that quantification of the effect of an external load on the length-velocity relation is based on the horizontal shift to the right.

The effect of the initial sarcomere length on length-velocity relations

An alteration of the initial sarcomere length (l_s) induces a parallel shift of the length-velocity relation (fig. 2d), the degree of which is independent of the Ca^{++} concentration, but corresponds to the variation in the starting sarcomere length.

Comparison of the effects of external afterload and variation of the starting sarcomere length on length-velocity relations

In the experiment, illustrated by figure 2e, three unloaded quick releases (Nos. 1–3) were started at sarcomere lengths of 2.3, 2.5 and 2.7 μ.

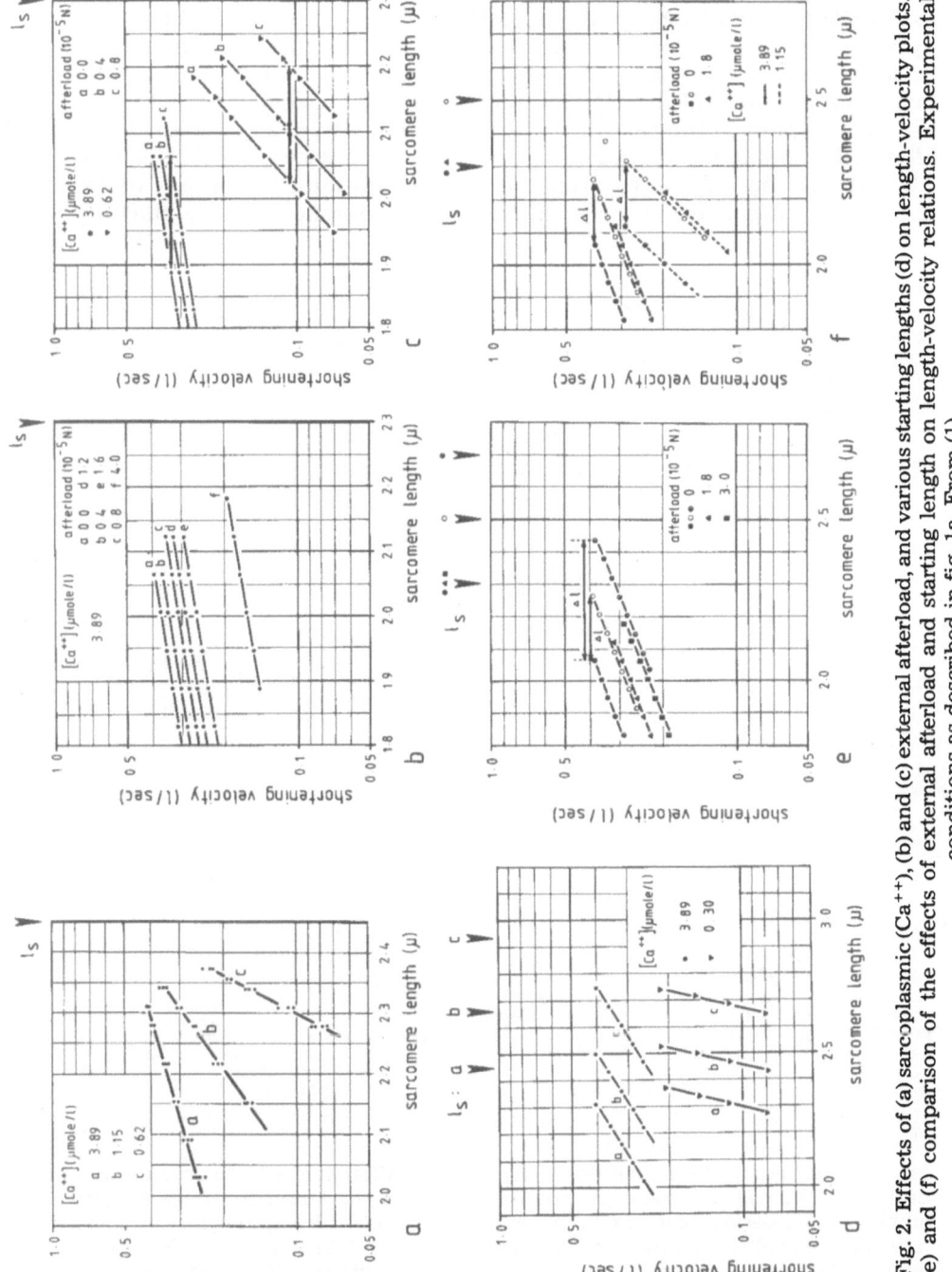

Fig. 2. Effects of (a) sarcoplasmic (Ca⁺⁺), (b) and (c) external afterload, and various starting lengths (d) on length-velocity plots. (e) and (f) comparison of the effects of external afterload and starting length on length-velocity relations. Experimental conditions as described in fig. 1a. From (1)

Furthermore, two other releases (Nos. 4, 5) were studied (starting sarcomere length 2.3 µ), during which the contractile system was loaded by an external afterload of 1.8 (3.0) 10^{-5} N. Below 2.2 µ, the shortening behaviour (represented by the length-velocity relations) of quick release No. 2 (l_s = 2.5 µ, no external afterload) is approximately identical with the shortening behaviour of quick release No. 4 (l_s = 2.3 µ, external afterload 1.8 × 10^{-5} N). This also applies in the case of quick release No. 3 (l_s = 2.7 µ, no external afterload) compared with quick release No. 5 (l_s = 2.3 µ, external afterload 3.0 × 10^{-5} N). In other words, the effect of an additional shortening of 0.2 (0.4) µ per sarcomere, corresponding to the differences in the starting

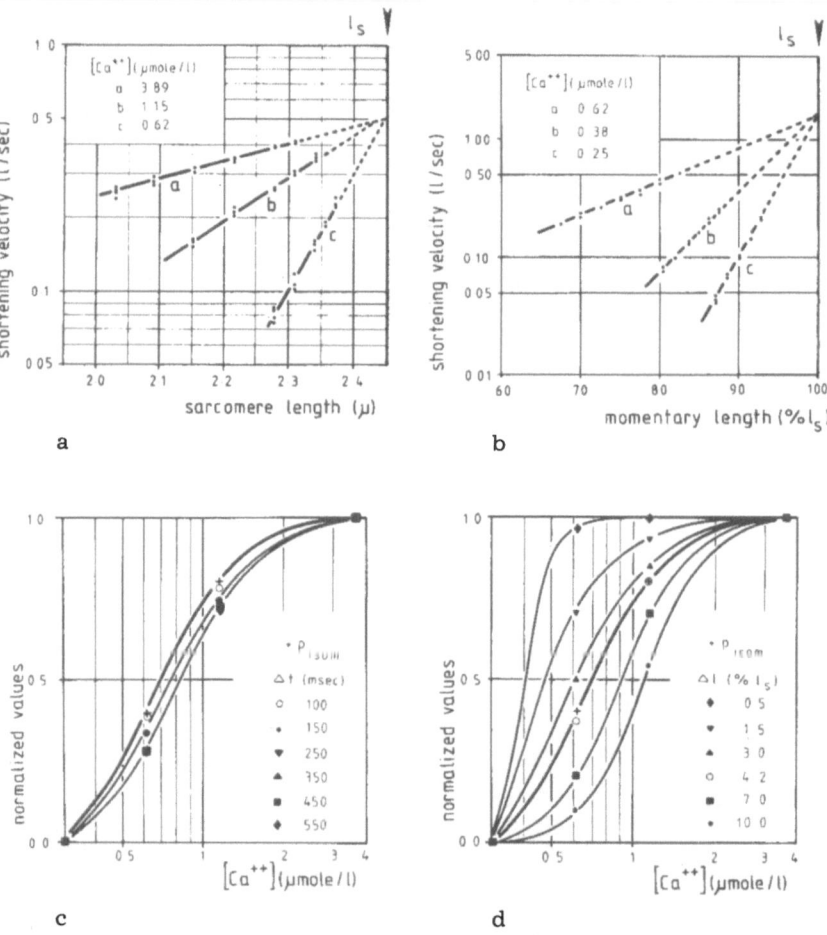

Fig. 3 Extrapolation of the length-velocity plots at different (Ca^{++}), to account for shortening induced alteration of cross-bridge afterload during the releases. (a) Rabbit psoas fiber, (b) cat papillary muscle. Note that all length-velocity plots converge in a field around the starting lengths (l_s). (c) Ca^{++} dose-response curves for isometric tension (+) and shortening velocity, read at different times, Δt, after the start of the unloaded releases (apparent V_{max}). (d) Ca^{++} dose-response curves for isometric tension (+) and shortening velocity, read after various amounts of shortening, Δl, during unloaded isotonic quick releases.

sarcomere lengths of the compared quick releases, can be simulated by an external afterload of about 1.8 (3.0) $\times$ 10^{-5} N. The required external afterload for simulating the effects of a given amount of shortening Δl is not affected by the sarcoplasmic Ca^{++} concentration (fig. 2f). This means that during an isotonic quick release any amount of shortening has an effect on further shortening which could be mimicked by an external afterload imposed on the contractile system instead of the preceding shortening. Both of the mentioned factors cause a reduction in shortening velocity. Thus, the decrease in shortening velocity during a quick release could be traced to an "internal afterload" due to shortening. The *total amount* of this shortening-induced, "internal afterload" is determined by the degree of shortening up to the actual length at which velocity is determined, but is not affected by the free sarcoplasmic Ca^{++} concentration (fig. 2e, f). Therefore, after a given shortening Δl the increase in afterload *per cross bridge* due to this shortening-induced "internal afterload" should be inversely proportional to the degree of activation of the contractile system. This may explain the steeper slope of the length-velocity relations at lower (Ca^{++}).

To reveal a direct effect of Ca^{++} concentration on isotonic shortening velocity, this shortening-induced change in afterload per cross bridge should be taken into account, because the velocity should be determined at a total afterload of zero (V_{max}), or at least at an identical cross-bridge afterload at all degrees of activation.

The simplest way to overcome complications due to shortening-induced changes in cross-bridge afterload, when analyzing effects of Ca^{++} on isotonic shortening, may be given by the extrapolation of the length-velocity plots to the starting length of all quick releases, a point at which a Δl-induced alteration in cross-bridge afterload does not occur.

All length-velocity plots obtained at different (Ca^{++}) converge in a field around the starting length of the corresponding quick releases (fig. 3a/b). Thus one has to conclude that the sarcoplasmic free Ca^{++} concentration neither has any effect on maximum unloaded shortening velocity in skeletal muscle, nor in cat myocardium, provided the shortening-induced changes in cross-bridge afterload mentioned above are taken into account.

In a quick release at zero external afterload, shortening velocity which is read at a defined point in time (Δt) after the start of the release (fig. 3c) or, determined after a given amount of shortening Δl (fig. 3d), i.e., the "apparent" V_{max}, shows a clear Ca^{++} dependence which should be traced to the shortening-induced changes in cross-bridge afterload during the releases.

Zusammenfassung

In der vorliegenden Arbeit wird eine Methode beschrieben, die eine Unterscheidung zwischen direkten und indirekten (verkürzungsinduzierten) Effekten verschiedener Parameter auf die lastfreie Verkürzungsgeschwindigkeit erlaubt. Es wird gezeigt, daß die Krümmung des Längensignals in isotonischen „quick releases" auf verkürzungsinduzierte Änderungen der Nachbelastung der einzelnen Querbrücke zurückgeführt werden kann. Diese Änderung der Nachbelastung könnte beispielsweise durch eine von der Verkürzung selbst hervorgerufene „innere Last" oder Deaktivierung des kontraktilen Systems verursacht werden.

Um das Verkürzungsverhalten während des gesamten isotonischen „quick release" beurteilen zu können, wurde die Verkürzungsgeschwindigkeit als Funktion der Momentanlänge aufgetragen. Bei halblogarithmischer Darstellung entsprechen diese Längen-Geschwindigkeits-Beziehungen Geraden, was bedeutet, daß die Verkürzungsgeschwindigkeit in jedem einzelnen „quick release" mit fortschreitender Verkürzung exponentiell abfällt. Eine Extrapolation der Längen-Geschwindigkeits-Beziehungen zur Ausgangslänge aller „quick releases" ermöglicht eine Bestimmung der Verkürzungsgeschwindigkeit an einem Punkt, wo noch keine verkürzungsinduzierte Änderung der Querbrückenbelastung zu berücksichtigen ist.

Bei Anwendung dieser Methode läßt sich weder beim Skelettmuskel noch beim Katzenmyokard ein Effekt der sarkoplasmatischen Ca^{++}-Konzentration auf die lastfreie Verkürzungsgeschwindigkeit nachweisen. Weiterhin wird demonstriert, daß die von verschiedenen Autoren beschriebene Calcium-Abhängigkeit von V_{max} auf die erwähnte Änderung der Querbrückenbelastung unter der Verkürzung zurückgeführt werden kann.

References

1. *Brenner, B.:* Effect of free sarcoplasmic Ca^{++} concentration on maximum unloaded shortening velocity. Measurement on single glycerinated rabbit psoas muscle fibers (in preparation).
2. *Gulati, J., R.J. Podolsky:* Contraction transients of skinned muscle fibers: effects of calcium and ionic strength. J. Gen. Physiol. **72**, 701–716 (1978).
3. *Julian, F.J.:* The effect of calcium on the force-velocity relation of briefly glycerinated frog muscle fibres. J. Physiol. **218**, 117–145 (1971).
4. *Maughan, D.W., E.S. Low, N.R. Alpert:* Isometric force development, isotonic shortening, and elasticity measurements from Ca^{++}-activated ventricular muscle of the guinea pig. J. Gen. Physiol. **71**, 431–451 (1978).
5. *Podolsky, R.J., L.E. Teichholz:* The relation between calcium and contraction kinetics in skinned muscle fibres. J. Physiol. **211**, 19–35 (1970).
6. *Szent-Györgyi, A.:* Free-energy relations and contractions of actomyosin. Biol. Bull. **96**, 140–161 (1949).
7. *Wise, R.M., J.F. Rondinone, F.N. Briggs:* Effect of calcium on force velocity characteristics of glycerinated skeletal muscle. Amer. J. Physiol. **221**, 973–979 (1971).

For reprints:

Dr. *B. Brenner*, Physiol. Institut II der Univ. Tübingen, Gmelinstraße 5,
7400 Tübingen

Basic Res. Cardiol. **75**, 47–56 (1980)
© 1980 Dr. Dietrich Steinkopff Verlag, Darmstadt
ISSN 0300–8428

Paper, presented at the Erwin Riesch Symposium, Tübingen, April 3–7, 1979

Pharmakologisches Institut der Universität Tübingen

Some aspects on the regulation of carbohydrate and lipid metabolism in cardiac tissue

Einige Gesichtspunkte zur Regulation des Kohlenhydrat- und Fettstoffwechsels im Herzen

M. Siess

With 3 figures

Summary

FFA are the main substrate of biological oxidation in cardiac muscle under normal conditions. But it could be shown in man and animal that during heavy exercise there is a shift to preferential oxidation of lactate.

During oxygen deficiency in hypoxic or ischemic situations which may occur lightly in distinct areas of hypertrophic hearts after exercise, lactate, α-glycerol phosphate and acyl-CoA as well as triglyceride levels in cardiac tissue may increase, whereas FFA are less oxidized. Unoxidized intracellular FFA and acyl-CoA, which are not esterified in a sufficient way to triglycerides, may impair oxidative phosphorylation in mitochondria, the P/O quotient as well as cardiac function perhaps by an interference with Ca^{++} movements during the contraction cycle. With the examples of anoxia and complete ischemia as the two extreme situations of O_2 deficiency some principles of the alteration of cardiac metabolism are pointed out, and furthermore attempts to improve anoxic tolerance of cardiac tissue.

The energy supply needed for the contractile activity of the heart muscle cell depends on a sufficient transfer of oxygen to the respiratory chain in the mitochondria as well as on substrates available from endogenous or exogenous sources mobilized, metabolized and mutually competing in the various steps of biological oxidation.

FFA and carbohydrates are important cardiac fuels and many scientists have studied the regulation of carbohydrate and lipid metabolism in cardiac muscle. An excellent general view on this field has been given by *Neely* and *Morgan* (1964).

There are some differences between the animal species and man in regard to the participation of long-chain FFA in the total O_2 consumption: It amounts in rats to 90 %, in dogs to 35–75 %, in guinea pigs to 30–40 % and in man it ranges between 20 and 70 %. It is now well established (*Keul* et al., 1965) that during heavy exercise in man lactate is preferentially oxidized whereas the participation of FFA in the increased total O_2 consumption decreases. Similar effects could be observed in isolated atria of guinea pigs at a combined incubation with palmitate and glucose during β-adrenergic stimulation (*Siess* 1977). These variations can be explained by the fact that in *well oxygenated* hearts the participation of carbohydrates and lipids in the biological oxidation depends on substrate concentrations, transport through the cell-membrane as well as flux through the various steps of metabolism in the *glycolysis pathway for carbohydrates and the β-oxidation pathway for FFA,* both reaching at the acetyl-CoA level the entry into the Krebs-cycle in which CO_2 is produced and H_2 moved to the respiratory chain.

The flux of electrons in the respiratory chain is determined in well-oxygenated hearts by the ATP/ADP ratio connected with the NADH/NAD quotient. At higher requirements of ATP, the electron flux increases due to an increased work producing a shift to ADP and it depends now on the *activation of the key enzymes* in both systems if FFA or carbohydrates are oxidized preferentially. According to the mass action order, the concentration of substrates and products, the feedback of metabolites in the single step reactions as well as the ATP-, ADP-, NAD-, NADH- and P_i-concentrations determine the speed of the flux. The enzyme activities are also regulated by hormones or second messengers like c-AMP, or the pH and the O_2 pressure.

Since substrates are easily available from exogenous or endogenous sources, the *main restraint* in *cardiac energy supply is oxygen. In hypertrophic hearts an imbalance between energy supply and energy demand may occur during an increased cardiac work due to circulation problems especially in subendocardial areas* and probably also due to an impaired penetration of O_2 and substrates through the cell- and mitochondrial membranes. The consequences can be observed as *hypoxic* or *ischemic* situations (*Büchner* 1973) with alterations of the contractile activity and efficiency as well as of the *carbohydrate-* and *lipid metabolism.* Under experimental conditions in vivo and in vitro it can be easily shown that hypoxia decreases the contractile activity which can be reversed very quickly by an increase of the O_2 pressure. This can be observed, for example, in patients during an attack of angina pectoris. If this attack is treated with nitrates, the energetically depressed contractile activity increases not as a direct positive inotropic effect of this drug but by an restituted energy- and O_2-supply after the improvement of the cardiac microcirculation due to a decreased enddiastolic ventricular pressure. This once more is the consequence of the decreased arterial resistance and the venous pooling in the periphery caused by nitroglycerin.

Since hypoxia and ischemia, as most common situations, influence the carbohydrate- and lipid metabolism in a different way, I would like to point out some observations which may be important also for cardiac function.

In contrast to hypoxia or anoxia, where only the oxygen supply is inhibited, ischemia of the myocardium has two more important consequences; firstly a reduction not only in oxygen supply, but also in substrates, and secondly a retention of the products of metabolism by the restricted blood flow. Therefore detrimental effects of ischemia on the survival of the myocardial cell are more expressed under these circumstances than during hypoxia or anoxia with an unlimited exchange of substrates and metabolites between the myocardium and an unrestrained blood flow.

I. Carbohydrate metabolism

A) Aerobic conditions

Glucose penetrates the cell membrane with a carrier, which requires no energy and leads to an equilibrium of sugar concentrations inside and outside the cell. At physiological blood concentrations of 5 mM glucose, insulin activates this transport, at 10 or 15 mM the transport is no more insulin-dependent. Via hexokinase- and phosphofructokinase reactions the glycolytic pathway is reached or glucose is stored as glycogen.

B) Anaerobic conditions

1. Hypoxia

During hypoxia as a consequence of O_2-deficiency, the electron flux in the respiratory chain is retarded and NADH concentration increases, and enzyme reactions which depend on the NADH/NAD quotient change flux and direction in carbohydrate metabolism for production of lactate and α-glycerolphosphate:

1. Transport of glucose is increased.
2. Hexokinase reaction and glycogen degradation is activated.
3. Phosphofructokinase activity increases also (fig. 1).

Therefore glucose utilization and glycogen degradation is strongly enhanced related to aerobic conditions and the glycolytic flux is accelerated (Pasteur-effect). Since glycolysis is the only source of energy supply during anoxia and ischemia, which produces stoichiometrically only 5 % ATP related to the amount of one oxidized glucose molecule, it is important for survival of the cardiac cell to maintain the increased glycolytic flux. This, however, is only possible

1. with a sufficient lactate washout from the intra- and extracellular space into the blood
2. an optimal supply of glucose from exogenous or endogenous sources and
3. a high NAD pool.

2. Anoxia

During strict anoxic conditions with an unlimited lactate washout and a sufficient glucose supply, it could be shown a long lasting strongly reduced contractile activity in isolated atria of guinea pigs stimulated with a low frequency (*Siess* and *Seifart*, 1979). Energy consumption measured as reduced contractile work and anoxic energy supply determined as lactate production rate have been here in an equilibrium for about 6 hours. Glucose utilization increased about 6-fold related to aerobic conditions (Pasteur-effect), and the ATP production reached a level of 50 % related to the strongly reduced aerobic work (5 % of the maximum). In this "anoxia test" lactate could leave the intracellular space, and the increased NADH/NAD turnover could keep the glycolytic flux running as only source of energy. The Pasteur-effect provided here not only the anoxic survival of the myocardial cell, but during about 6 hours also a minimum of contractile activity. It is of interest that the lactate production rate reaches the maximum after about 30 minutes and is correlated with an improvement

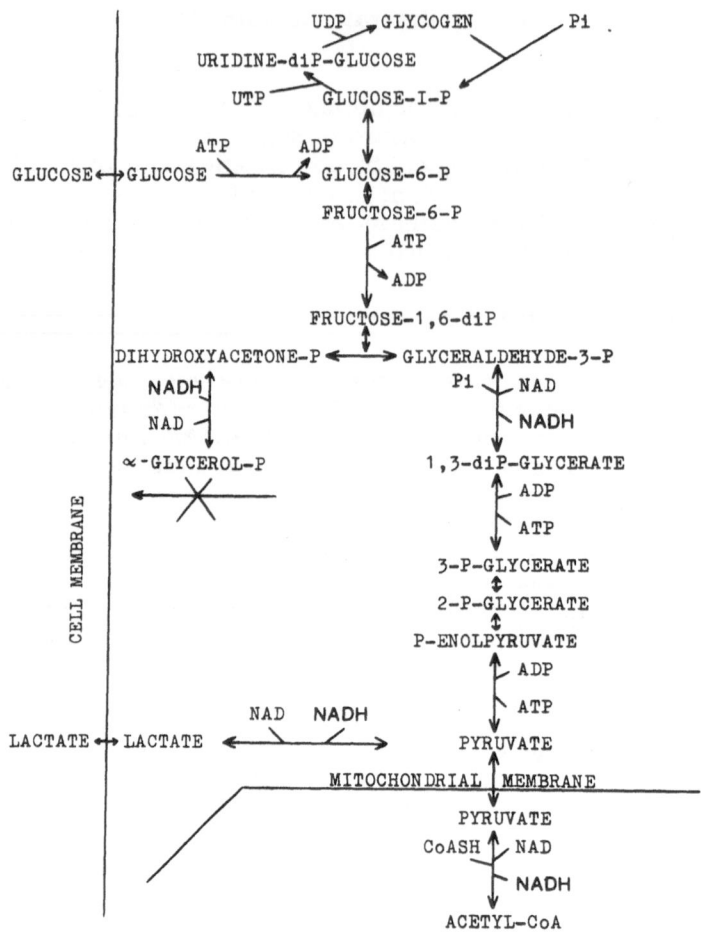

Fig. 1. Pathway of glucose and glycogen metabolism (*Neely* and *Morgan* 1974, modified).

of the anoxic contractile activity. The intracellular ATP level amounted to 70 %, CP only to 9 % after 2 hours anoxia.

This difference in the behaviour of both energy-rich phosphates during O_2-deficiency is well established (*Gudbjarnasson* et al., 1971) and can be explained: Creatinkinase I, located in the mitochondrial membrane, transfers the $\sim$ P from mitochondrial ATP to creatine producing CP (fig. 2).

In anoxia this transfer will be reduced due to an inhibition of creatinkinase I by lactate and decrease of pH. Also the adenine nucleotide translocase will be inhibited by an increased acyl-CoA. The small amount of ATP bound in the actomyosin compartment (1–5 %) can be regenerated solely from the cytosolic CP-pool by creatinkinase II, which is exhausted quickly, dependent on the frequency of contraction cycles and the initial aerobic contractile force. Therefore negative inotropic action follows. With increasing glycolytic ATP production in the cytosol after 30 minutes anoxia more energy-rich phosphate is transferred by creatinkinase III to creatine providing at a low CP level a reduced ~ P transfer to regenerate the actomyosin-ATP causing an improved but still reduced anoxic contractility.

3. Ischemia

The other extreme condition of O_2 deficiency, ischemia by complete coronary arterial occlusion has been demonstrated by *Gudbjarnasson* and coworkers (1971). Here the maximal rate of lactate production is reached in the first minute after occlusion.

This then decreases rapidly during 3 minutes. The lactate/pyruvate quotient therefore increases during the first minutes to a level kept constant during more than 10 minutes. Here the lactate washout was restricted and therefore the initially increased glycolysis as well, presumably by a strongly decreased intracellular pH. The intracellular metabolites lactate as well as DHA-P, G-3-P- and to highest degree α-glycerol-P were accumulated. The energy supply was stopped and the first stage of infarction reached.

Recently *Achs* and *Garfinkel* (1979) presented a computer model of glycolysis, the Krebs-cycle and related metabolism in an acutely ischemic dog heart after complete occlusion involving 122 metabolites, 65 enzymes and 406 chemical reactions, using their own experimental data and also studies of *Wollenberger* and *Krause* (1968), *Kübler* and *Spieckermann* (1970) and other authors demonstrating this most complicated oscillating

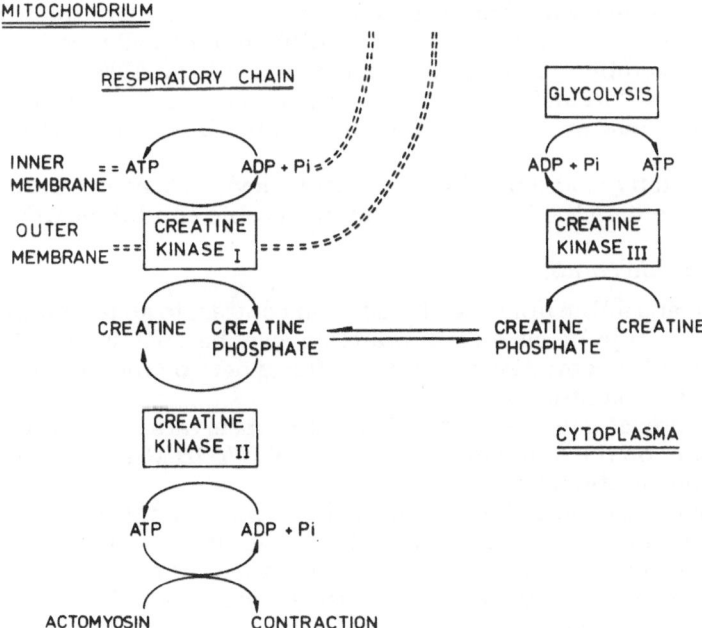

Fig. 2. Transfer of energy-rich phosphate to actomyosin in the heart (*Gudbjarnasson* et al. 1970, modified).

alteration of metabolism. They reported that in the first two minutes cytosolic pH decreases from 7.1 to 6.6, mitochondrial pH from 7.3 to 6.9, CP from 100 to 36 % whereas ATP only to 90 %.

The increased concentration of lactate and the strongly decreased pH inhibit creatinkinase I in mitochondria (fig. 2) leading to a decreased transfer of ~ P to creatine in the cytosol. Since the lactate production rate is reduced in the first minutes, the NADH/NAD ratio increases much more than in the case of lactate washout and at the triosephosphate level α-glycerol phosphate concentration increases which cannot penetrate the cell and will be synthesized with the increasing acyl-CoA to triglycerides.

These both extreme experimental situations of oxygen deficiency as anoxia and ischemia after complete arterial occlusion show clearly the important points of cardiac cell survival. We have to consider, however, that under hypoxia or ischemia in *patients* with hypertrophic hearts or coronary heart disease the Krebs-cycle with the remaining oxidative phosphorylation is still the main energy supply, but on a reduced level in a wide range of variations. Here the retention of metabolites has consequences on the pH, the enzymes activities, membrane structures and the P/O quotient. Metabolites stemming not only from carbohydrate but more from lipid metabolism are here of special interest.

II. Lipid metabolism

A) Aerobic conditions

The water-insoluble long-chain fatty acids are bound to albumin and cross the capillary membrane bound to the extracellular protein and reach the cell membrane. FFA permeate by diffusion the cell membrane. Inside the cell at aerobic conditions FFA are bound with an ATP requiring step to CoA as acyl-CoA and are then normally transferred via acylcarnitin in the acyl-transferase system from the outer to the inner mitochondrial membrane.

In the fatty acid oxidation spiral from acyl-CoA, acetyl-CoA is cleaved off which enters the Krebs-cycle under aerobic conditions (fig. 3).

B) Anaerobic conditions

From anaerobic lipid metabolism – in contrast to anaerobic glycolysis – no energy supply by ATP production can be sustained. FFA and its metabolite concentrations may have effects here on membranes in regard to function and structure.

In hypoxia or ischemia the following observations have been made, depending on the quotient and turnover of NADH/NAD and the FFA and ATP concentrations:

1. An increase of acyl-CoA has been observed since the cleavage of acetyl-CoA is reversed. Long-chain fatty acids are synthesized parallel to lactate- and α-glycerol-P-production with NADH and NADPH as reducing equivalents. New FFA may also be synthesized from amino-acid-carbon skeletons.
2. Therefore cardiac acetyl-CoA decreases and triglycerides (TG) may increase in dependence of the lactate washout and the α-glycerol-P-

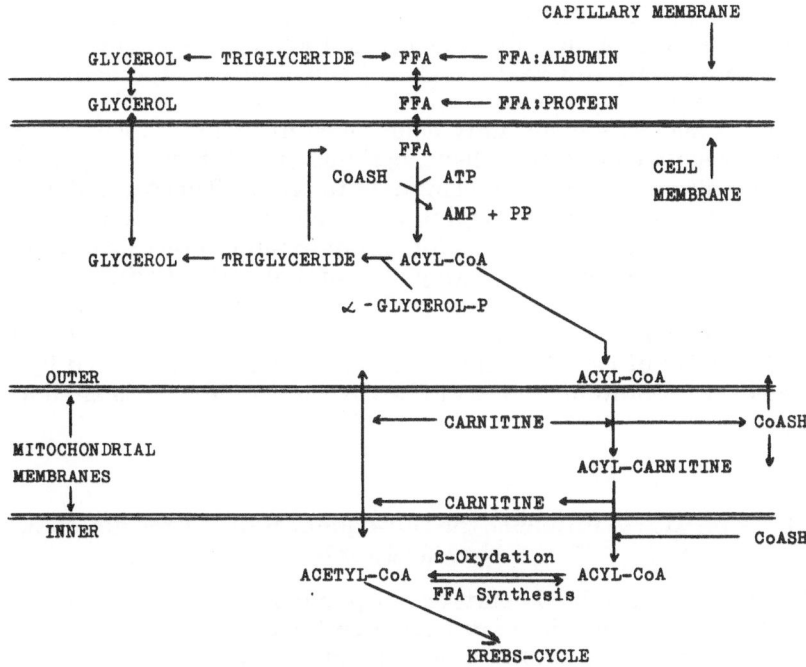

Fig. 3. Pathway of fatty acid metabolism in the heart (*Neely* and *Morgan* 1974, modified).

production, and the degree of O_2 deficiency. α-Glycerol-P and acyl-CoA will be composed to TG, which cannot leave the cell. Triclyceride concentrations increased to fat droplets in the myocardial cell may impair the contractile force mechanically.

3. The oxidation of FFA will therefore decrease and the inhibition of glucose utilization by FFA is abolished.
4. Acyl-CoA has uncoupling effects on the oxidative phosphorylation in hypoxia and ischemia and the P/O quotient decreases in mitochondria.
5. The adenine nucleotide translocation in mitochondria is inhibited by FFA and acyl-CoA.
6. The question if under special conditions FFA – not bound to acyl-CoA-interfere in the cytosol or in the cell membrane with Ca^{++} fluxes during the contraction cycle is up to now not clear. Endogenously liberated FFA from cardiac lipids by adrenergic lipolysis are unlikely since here lipolysis by catecholamines in hypoxia or anoxia never was observed and triglyceride synthesis is increased.

Exogenous FFA in the coronary blood increased after adrenergic liberation from adipose tissue may enter the cardiac cell in dependence of concentration and flow rate. If these FFA are not bound as acyl-CoA by lack of reaction with ATP and if they are not oxidized or esterified, it could be possible that FFA may interact with Ca^{++} fluxes during the contraction cycle. *Oliver* and coworkers (1968) observed that arrhythmias in infarction in man have been associated with very high plasma levels of FFA. We have seen in our studies with isolated atria that FFA uptake and oxidation rate is concentration dependent (*Siess* et al., 1970). We have observed like other authors that under aerobic conditions as well as in the mentioned "anoxia test" short- and long-chain fatty acids have in higher concentrations at 0.5–2 mM negative inotropic effects, perhaps more effective at pH 7.1 than pH 7.4 and also at an increasing length of the chain. This cardiodepressive effect can be antagonized by cardiac glycosides or an increased Ca^{++} concentration. But this is no absolute proof for an interaction of FFA with Ca^{++} fluxes. Spontaneously beating atria and electrically driven left atria sometimes develop in normoxia under FFA arrhythmias, especially at higher frequencies and temperatures. It seems possible that arrhythmogenic effects of catecholamines during anoxia are enhanced by FFA. But the exact conditions to get FFA arrhythmogenic in atria are not clear yet.

III. Possibilities to influence the consequences of oxygen deficiency in cardiac muscle

Since in hypertrophied hearts as morphological equivalents of hypoxia or ischemia "multiple single cell necrosis" could be observed (*Büchner* 1973), improvement of anoxic tolerance of the myocardial cell seems of special interest.

A) Attempts to improve anoxic tolerance of the myocardial cell

1. Protection of the energy-rich phosphate pool (ATP + CP) and adenine nucleotides (AN).
2. Protection of the NAD- + NADH-pool as main restraint of anaerobic glycolysis.
   This can be tried:
   a) by attempts to adapt cardiac performance to the restricted energy supply or to improve the energy supply *during coronary artery* diseases by antianginal drugs;
   b) by improvement of the *efficiency* of the total cardiac work *at heart failure* with carefully dosed cardiac glycosides lowering an increased heart rate and improving the contraction force of the single beat, which needs less O_2 than the same contractile work due to an increased heart rate (*Siess*, 1977);
   c) as possible aspects for the future, by addition of precursors of energy-rich phosphates or pyridine nucleotides to infusion fluids to preserve the pools of energetic important compounds in the myocardial cell. This could be important for cardioplegic solutions (*Siess* and *Seifart*, 1979); *Delabar* et al., 1979, *Seifart* et al., 1979).
3. The maintenance of glycolytic flux (Pasteur-effect) by glucose supply and lactate washout avoiding detrimental decrease of pH seems the most crucial point in ischemia. Many authors have reported that the cardiac glycogen storage as well as glucose supply together with insulin may improve anoxic tolerance.

B) Attempts to avoid an increase of intracellular unoxidized FFA and acyl-CoA

1. Avoidance of an increased FFA level in the blood after adrenergic induced lipolysis of adipose tissue by drugs.
2. Inhibition of penetration of FFA into the myocardial cell by drugs? (*Schraven*, 1978; *Süßkand* et al., 1979).
3. An intracellular decrease of the detrimental effects of accumulated unoxidized FFA and acyl-CoA could be expected by an increased triglyceride production from acyl-CoA and α-glycerol phosphate. But fat droplets may impair contractile force.

C) Attempts to inhibit effects of liberated biogenic amines by drugs

D) Attempts to stabilize lysosomes in the cardiac muscle by drugs

All attempts to avoid hypoxic or ischemic alterations of the cardiac energy metabolism in hypertrophied hearts are symptomatic and therefore doubtful.

To avoid excessive cardiac hypertrophy with hypoxic and ischemic consequences would be the better way.

Zusammenfassung

FFA sind das bevorzugte Substrat der biologischen Oxidation im Herzmuskel unter normalen Bedingungen. Es konnte bei Mensch und Tier gezeigt werden, daß während schwerer körperlicher Belastung Laktat bevorzugt verbrannt wird.

Während eines O_2-Mangels in hypoxischen oder ischämischen Situationen, welche leicht in bestimmten Arealen hypertrophischer Herzen unter körperlicher Belastung entstehen, nimmt die Konzentration von Laktat, α-Glycerophosphat, Acyl-CoA und Triglyceriden im Herzmuskel zu, wohingegen die Oxidation von FFA abnimmt.

Nicht oxidierte intrazelluläre FFA und Acyl-CoA, welche nicht in genügendem Ausmaß zu Triglyzeriden verestert werden, können die oxidative Phosphorylierung in Mitochondrien, den P/O-Quotient und die Herzfunktion vielleicht über eine Beeinflussung der Ca^{++}-Fluxe während des Kontraktionszyklus beeinträchtigen. Am Beispiel von zwei extremen Situationen des O_2-Mangels, Anoxie und vollständiger Ischämie werden einige Grundzüge der Änderungen des Herzstoffwechsels dargelegt sowie Ansätze zu einer Verbesserung der Anoxietoleranz im Herzmuskel.

References

1. *Achs, J., D. Garfinkel:* Metabolism of the Acutely Ischemic Dog Heart, I+II, Amer. J. Physiol. **236** (1), R 21–R 39 (1979).
2. *Büchner, F.:* Zur Bedeutung der Hypoxie für die Insuffizienz des hypertrophierten Herzmuskels S. 103–106. „Das chronisch kranke Herz", *Ed. Roskamm.; Reindell, H.,* (Stuttgart 1973).
3. *Delabar, U., M. Siess:* Synthesis and Degradation of NAD in Guinea Pig Cardiac Muscle. I. Bas. Res. Cardiol. **74**, 528–544 (1979), II. Bas. Res. Cardiol. **74**, 571–593 (1979).
4. *Gudbjarnasson, S., P. Mathes, R. G. Ravens:* Functional Compartmentation of ATP and Creatine Phosphate in Heartmuscle. J. Mol. Cell. Cardiol. **1** 325–339 (1970).

5. *Keul, J., E. Doll, H. Stein, H. Homberger, H. Kern, H. Reindell:* Über den Stoffwechsel des Herzens bei Hochleistungssportlern. Z. Kreislaufforschg. **55** 190 (1965).
6. *Kübler, W., P. G. Spieckermann:* Regulation of Glycolysis in the Ischemic and the Anoxic Myocardium, J. Mol. Cell. Cardiol. **1** 351–377 (1970).
7. *Neely, J. R., H. E. Morgan:* Relation between Carbohydrate and Lipid Metabolism and the Energy Balance of the Heart, Ann. Rev. Physiol. **36**, 413–459 (1974).
8. *Oliver, M. F., V. A. Kurien, T. W. Greenwood:* Relation between Serum Free Fatty Acid and Arrhythmias and Death after Acute Infarction, Lancet **1968/I,** 710.
9. *Schraven, E.:* Influence of Carbocromene on Free Fatty Acid Metabolism of the Heart. Rec. Advanc. in Cardiac Struct. and Metabol. **11**, 363–367 (1978).
10. *Seifart, H. J., U. Delabar, M. Siess:* The Influence of Various Precursors on the Concentration of Energy-Rich Phosphates and Pyridine Nucleotides in Cardiac Tissue and its Possible Meaning for Anoxic Survival. Basic Res. Cardiol. **75,** 57–61 (1980).
11. *Siess, M.:* Influences on the Efficiency of Cardiac Work. Basic Res. Cardiol. **72,** 299–305 (1977).
12. *Siess, M., H. J. Keller, E. Schare, J. Geissler, G. Müller:* The Continuous and Simultaneous Measurement of O_2 Consumption, Rate of Decarboxylation of ^{14}C-Substrates and the Performance of Spontaneously Beating Isolated Heart Atria of Guinea Pigs. J. Mol. Cell. Cardiol. **1**, 261 (1970).
13. *Siess, M., H. J. Seifart:* Anoxic Energy Production and Contractile Activity in Mammalian Cardiac Muscle: Advances in Myocardiology (1979), Vol. 2. Baltimore, Ed. *Tajuddin, M., B. Bhatia, H.H. Siddiqui, G. Rona (1979, in press).*
14. *Süsskand, K., J. R. Sauter, M. Siess:* Effects of Carbocromene on Substrate Oxidation and Performance of Isolated Atria; Basic Res. Cardiol. **75,** 62–65 (1980).
15. *Wollenberger, A., E. G. Krause:* Metabolic Control Characteristics of the Acutely Ischemic Myocardium, Amer. J. Cardiol. **22**, 349–359 (1968).

Authors' address:
Prof. Dr. med. *M. Siess,* Pharmakologisches Institut der Universität Tübingen, Wilhelmstr. 56, 7400 Tübingen, F.R.G.

Basic Res. Cardiol. **75**, 57–61 (1980)
© 1980 Dr. Dietrich Steinkopff Verlag, Darmstadt
ISSN 0300–8428

Paper, presented at the Erwin Riesch Symposium, Tübingen, April 3–7, 1979

Pharmakologisches Institut der Universität Tübingen

The influence of various precursors on the concentration of energy-rich phosphates and pyridine nucleotides in cardiac tissue and its possible meaning for anoxic survival

Der Einfluß verschiedener Prekursoren auf die Konzentration von Pyridinnukleotiden und energiereichen Phosphaten im Herzmuskel und seine mögliche Bedeutung für das Überleben in Anoxie

H. I. Seifart, U. Delabar, and *M. Siess*

With 1 figure and 1 table

Summary

A special "anoxia test" was developed with isolated guinea pig atria to test influences on the anoxic energy balance. Adenine, ribose, nicotinic acid or nicotinamide added as precursors to nutrition solutions inhibit the loss of cardiac adenine and pyridine nucleotides during anoxia and improve the energy balance under aerobic and anaerobic conditions in the myocardium.

Anaerobic glycolysis is the only source of energy supply during anoxia. Using the "Pasteur effect" a special "anoxia test" was developed with electrically driven left atria of guinea pigs (2, 3).

This test can be used to investigate influences on
1) force and duration of a strongly reduced anoxic contractile activity (= anoxic tolerance as mechanical energy consumption);
2) the rate of anaerobic glycolysis (anoxic energy production);
3) concentration of energy-rich phosphates (anoxic energy storage) and
4) concentration of pyridine nucleotides (NAD/NADH) as main restraint of anaerobic glycolysis (1).

A short report follows on the influence of the precursors adenine and ribose on the adenine nucleotide pool as well as the influence of the precursors nicotinamide (N_{am}) and nicotinic acid (N_a) on the NAD pool during the above mentioned anoxia test as well as under normoxic conditions.

Methods

The auxotonic contractile work per beat (c.w.b.) of electrically driven (0.5 Hz; 0.5 msec; 0.4–0.6 mA) left atria of guinea pigs, incubated in Krebs-Henseleit solution (+ 15 mM glucose) was measured under aerobic (1 hour) and following anaerobic conditions (2 hours) at 35 °C. In this "anoxia test" precursors have been added after the first hour of anoxia. The concentrations of energy-rich phosphates and NAD were determined after the second hour of anoxia. Influences of the mentioned precursors on spontaneously beating unloaded floating atria were also tested during a 24-hour period under normoxic and anoxic conditions at 30 °C.

Results

1. Anoxia test: According to the force-frequency relationship, the aerobic contractile work/beat at 0.5 Hz amounts to 35% of the maximal contractile activity reached at 1.5–2.0 Hz. The total contractile work could be determined to only 5% of the maximum at 4 Hz. At this strongly reduced *aerobic* contractile work, the O_2 consumption was therefore raised only by 10% above the resting O_2 consumption.

After 1 hour normoxia (95% O_2/5% CO_2), anoxia was started (95 N_2/5% CO_2). Anoxic glucose consumption measured as lactate production increased ~6 fold related to the aerobic glucose uptake (Pasteur-effect). The c.w.b. decreased during the first 30 minutes of anoxia to ~20% of the initial aerobic value and was improved in correlation to the increasing lactate production rate to 50–80%, reaching a steady state level after ~1 hour anoxia which lasted at least until the end of the second hour of anoxia.

At this point ATP was decreased by 30% and CP by 90%. Electrolyte concentrations were only slightly, but not significantly, shifted to a decrease of K^+ and Ca^{++} and an increase of Na^+ (3).

2. Addition of 0.1 mM adenine after the first hour of anoxia was followed by a positive inotropic action. This effect could be enhanced by

Tab. 1. Concentrations of ATP, ADP and AMP in isolated atria of guinea pigs at the end of the anoxia test (1 hour normoxia, 2 hours anoxia). Precursors were added after 1 hour of anoxia.

	ATP		ADP		AMP	
	nMol/mg protein	Δ%	nMol/mg protein	Δ%	nMol/mg protein	Δ%
O_2 control (15 mM glucose)	16.40 ± 1.25		4.51 ± 0.76		1.06 ± 0.23	
N_2 control (15 mM glucose)	11.57 ± 0.65		3.80 ± 0.32		1.37 ± 0.41	
N_2 adenine (0.1 mM)	19.89 ± 3.22	+71.91*	6.51 ± 0.80	+71.32**	1.54 ± 0.30	+12.41
N_2 adenine (0.1 mM) + ribose (15 mM)	16.78 ± 0.38	+45.03*	5.99 ± 1.92	+57.63	1.63 ± 0.41	+18.98

  * $P < 0.05$
  ** $P < 0.01$

addition of 15 mM ribose. During this one-hour period of anoxia, the anoxic lowered concentrations of the total adenine nucleotides (AN) as well as ATP and ADP increased significantly to the values under O_2. The anoxic loss of CP, however, could not be avoided (table). No significant increase of the lactate production rate could be observed during this second hour of anoxia. The NAD concentration was not determined in these experiments. Under aerobic control conditions with adenine and ribose similar effects could be observed on contractile force and adenine nucleotide concentrations.

3. Addition of 10 mM nicotinamide (N_{am}) during the second hour of anoxia increased the anoxic contractile activity considerably ($\Delta + \sim$ 100%). The NAD level was at the end of the one hour lasting period of anoxia with N_{am} significantly ($P < 0.05$) higher (2.98 ± 0.17 nMol/mg prot.) than the anoxic lowered control value (2.41 ± 0.13 nMol/mg prot.). The same higher level of NAD (3.2 ± 0.13 nMol/mg prot.) could be observed in the anoxia test if N_{am} (10 mM) was added to the K.H.-solution before preparation procedure. The *aerobic* control value showed after 3 hours a NAD level of 3.56 ± 0.22 nMol/mg prot.; however, if N_{am} was added

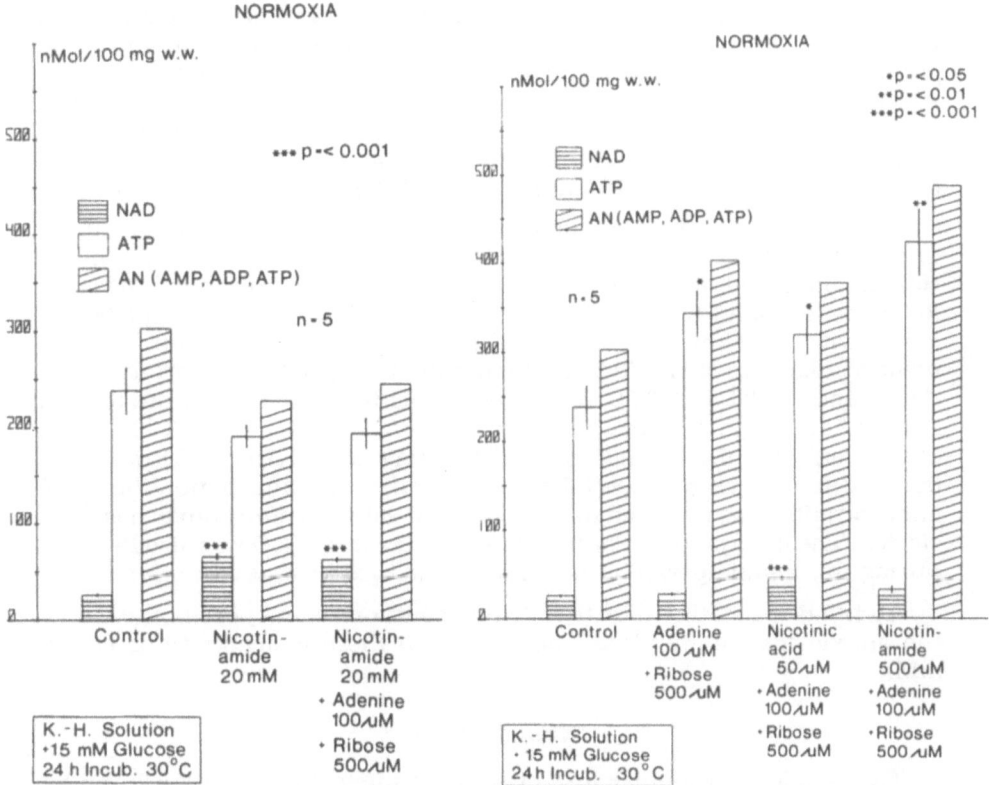

Fig. 1 (a and b). Concentrations of NAD, ATP and AN in spontaneously beating atria of guinea pigs after a 24 hours incubation period under normoxic conditions with various precursors of pyridine and adenine nucleotides.

already into the nutrition solution before preparation we found a NAD level of 4.73 ± 0.18 nMol/mg prot. ($\Delta = + 32.8\%$).

The ratio of anoxic NAD level/normoxic NAD level at the end of each experiment was calculated to 0.67 with or without addition of 10 mM N_{am} after 3 hours incubation time. The decline of the NAD level is presumably closely connected with a shift towards the NADH level which, however, could not be measured simultaneously. Thus there is evidence that N_{am} can preserve the NAD level during anoxia leading to an improved anoxic contractile activity.

4. Spontaneously beating atria showed under *normoxic conditions at 30 °C* after an incubation period of 24 hours with 20 mM nicotinamide an increase of the NAD concentration by 150% (fig. 1a). Simultaneously, ^{14}C-nicotinamide is incorporated as ^{14}C-NAD at a very high degree (1). The average NAD control value of 33 nMol/100 mg w.w. (range: $31.09 \pm 0.87 \leftrightarrow 36.12 \pm 3.02$ nMol) remained unchanged during an incubation period of 24 hours. Addition of 100 μM adenine + 500 μM ribose to the nutrition solution containing nicotinamide did not change this value, but the adenine nucleotide pool (AN) was not elevated as expected.

Nutrition solutions containing precursors in various concentrations were tested. Best results could be obtained with 50 μM nicotinic acid + 100 μM adenine + 500 μM ribose with a significant increase of ATP (+ 34%) and AN pool (+ 24%) as well as the NAD concentration (+ 72%) (fig. 1b). Addition of 500 μM nicotinamide instead of nicotinic acid leads to an increase of ATP by 77% and the total AN by 60% but the NAD concentration remained with $\Delta + 23\%$ in the range of the control value.

5. To test the behaviour of an *increased* NAD concentration under *anoxic conditions* atria were preincubated at 30 °C for 8 hours in a nutrition medium containing 20 mM nicotinamide. During this period the NAD level was elevated from 34.23 ± 0.03 nMol to 57.67 ± 4.89 nMol/100 mg w.w. with a simultaneous increase of the incorporation of ^{14}C-nicotinamide into NAD. At this 8-hour point the NADH concentration was determined to $20.79 + 3.36$ nMol, the NADH/NAD ratio therefore to 0.36. After 3 hours of anoxia the NAD concentration decreased to 26.89 ± 3.28, NADH only to 16.48 ± 1.36 nMol. Therefore the NADH/NAD ratio was doubled to 0.61. During the following 3 hours of reoxygenation the NAD concentration was reversed to the increased values before anoxia has been started. The incorporation of ^{14}C-nicotinamide into NAD was also lowered during this anoxic period and increased again after reoxygenation.

Addition of nicotinamide to nutrition solutions could possibly preserve the anoxic loss of pyridine nucleotides in these concentrations (10–20 mM).

Conclusions

The anoxic intracellular loss of adenine nucleotides and NAD can be avoided by addition of the precursors adenine, ribose, nicotinic acid or nicotinamide into nutrition solutions, combined with an improvement of the anoxic contractile activity in the "anoxia test".

Zusammenfassung

Ein besonderer „Anoxie-Test" wurde mit isolierten Meerschweinchen-Herzvorhöfen entwickelt, um Einflüsse auf das anoxische Energiegleichgewicht zu prüfen. Adenin, Ribose, Nikotinsäure oder Nikotinamid – als Prekursoren der Nährlösung zugegeben – verhindern den Verlust der kardialen Adenin- und Pyridinnukleotide während Anoxie und verbessern das Energiegleichgewicht im Herzmuskel unter aeroben und anaeroben Bedingungen.

References

1. *Delabar, U., M. Siess:* Synthesis and degradation of NAD in guinea pig cardiac muscle. I. Basic Res. Cardiol. **74**, p. 528–544 (1979), II. Basic Res. Cardiol. **74**, p. 571–593 (1979).
2. *Seifart, H. I.:* Funktionelle und biochemische Untersuchungen zur Anoxietoleranz des Herzmuskels und ihrer pharmakologischen Beeinflußbarkeit. Naturwissenschaftl. Diss. Tübingen 1978.
3. *Siess, M., H. I. Seifart:* Anoxic energy production and contractile activity in mammalian cardiac muscle: Advances in Myocardiology (1979), Vol. 2. (Baltimore) Ed. *Tajudin, M., B. Bhatia, H. H. Siddiqui, G. Rona* (1979, in press).

Authors' address:

Dr. *H. I. Seifart,* and Prof. Dr. med. *M. Siess,* Department of Pharmacology, University of Tuebingen, Wilhelmstr. 56, D-7400 Tuebingen, F.R.G.

Basic Res. Cardiol. **75**, 62–65 (1980)
© 1980 Dr. Dietrich Steinkopff Verlag, Darmstadt
ISSN 0300–8428

Paper, presented at the Erwin Riesch Symposium, Tübingen, April 3–7, 1979

Pharmakologisches Institut der Universität Tübingen

Effects of carbocromene on performance and oxidation of FFA and glucose in isolated atria

Wirkungen von Carbocromen auf Funktion und Oxidation von FFA und Glukose in isolierten Herzvorhöfen

K. Süsskand, J.R. Sauter, and *M. Siess*

With 1 figure

[14]C-FFA and ^{14}C-carbohydrate are oxidized by isolated atria with increasing concentrations according to an apparent Michaelis Menten kinetics. K_m-values and V_{max} of the substrates are different, which can be explained by variations of diffusion through the cell membrane, the mitochondrial membrane, and variations of the enzyme activities in the different pathways to the Krebs-cycle. In experiments with *combined substrates* the mutual competition and the participation of substrates in biological oxidation depends on the K_m- and V_{max}-values as well as the concentrations of the substrates (5, 4). Drugs can interfere here by activation or inhibition of key enzymes in the different pathways to the biological oxidation or by interaction in the penetration of substrates through the membranes.

Free fatty acids, which are not sufficiently oxidized or esterified to triglycerides in the heart muscle cell under extreme situations (hypoxia, ischemia), may interfere with Ca^{++}-fluxes during the contraction cycle and may be hazardous to the cardiac function together with other factors, i.e. catecholamines (1).

It would be therefore of interest if drugs could inhibit the penetration of FFA into the myocardial cell. *Schraven, E.* (2, 3) observed a decreased ^{14}C-palmitate uptake as well as a decreased [14]CO_2 production in ventricle strips of mice after addition of carbocromene to the incubation medium, whereas an enhanced [14]CO_2 production from labelled glucose occurred. He postulated from these findings a protective effect on the heart muscle cell. We have studied in electrically driven left atria of guinea pigs the effect of carbocromene on performance and oxidation rate of ^{14}C-labelled long and short-chain FFA and ^{14}C-glucose at combined incubation with 2 cross-labelled substrates.

Methods

Electrically driven left atria of guinea pigs (1.5 Hz) were incubated in Krebs-Henseleit solution (95 % O_2/5 % CO_2 and 30 °C) with ^{14}C-substrates and simultane-

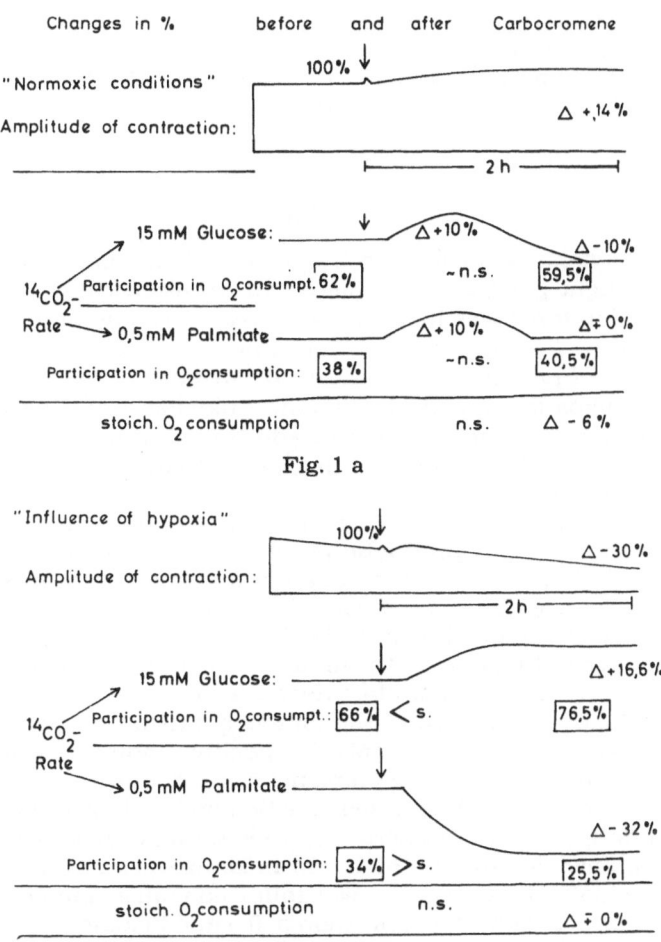

Fig. 1 a

Fig. 1 b

Fig. 1 a and b. Scheme of the effect of carbocromene (5×10^{-5} g/ml) on electrically driven (1.5 Hz) left guinea pig atria (Krebs-Henseleit solution 30 °C, 95 % O_2 + 5 % CO_2). After steady-state of contractile activity and of $^{14}CO_2$ rate of the cross-labelled substrate combination of 0.5 mM palmitate (n = 5) and glucose (n = 5), which was measured continuously, carbocromene (C.) was added. Total O_2 consumption with participation of each substrate was calculated stoichiometrically from the mean values of $^{14}CO_2$ rate.

a) The positive inotropic action of C. in atria, which has been incubated under normoxic conditions from the beginning, was followed by an transient increase of the oxidation rate ($^{14}CO_2$) of each substrate. No significant shift in the shares on total O_2 consumption could be observed.

b) Atria pretreated with hypoxia for 30 minutes showed at following normoxic conditions after addition of C. only a short and strongly reduced positive inotropic action. The contractile activity faded then continuously during 2 hours presumably due to a damage by the hypoxic pretreatment. Here the $^{14}CO_2$ rate of palmitate was significantly depressed by C. (− 32 %), whereas simultaneously glucose oxidation increased (+ 17 %). Therefore the share of palmitate on the total O_2 consumption decreased from 34 % to 25.5 % and that of glucose increased from 66 % to 76.5 %.

ously and continuously was registrated contraction force, frequency, and $^{14}CO_2$ production rate (5, 6). Experiments were carried out with cross-labelled combinations of 1) 0.5 mM palmitate bound to 0.5 % albumin + 15 mM glucose, or 2) 0.5 mM palmitate/0.5 % albumin + 2.0 or 0.5 mM hexanoate and 3) 0.5 or 2.0 mM hexanoate + 15 mM glucose. After steady state of $^{14}CO_2$ production rate, carbocromene $5 \cdot 10^{-5}$ g/ml = $1.4 \cdot 10^{-4}$ M was added.

Results

1. Carbocromene decreases the frequency of spontaneously beating atria with a slight positive inotropic effect. In electrically driven left atria, contraction force was increased by 15–20 % as maximum.
2. Correlating with the positive inotropic action a transient increase of oxidation of palmitate and glucose occurred (fig. 1a).
3. The participation of palmitate on the stoichiometrically calculated total O_2 consumption amounted before addition of carbocromene to 38 % and afterwards to 40.5 % and that of glucose to 62 % and to 59.5 % respectively (fig. 1a).
4. After preincubation of atria in *hypoxic* solutions for 30 minutes and steady state of $^{14}CO_2$ production under *normoxic* conditions, the palmitate oxydation-rate decreased at addition of carbocromene by 32 % and glucose increased by 17 % (fig. 1b), whereas the contractile activity faded due to the detrimental effects of the hypoxic pretreatment. The participation of glucose in the total O_2 consumption increases from 66 % to 76.5 % and that of palmitate decreases from 34 % to 25.5 % (fig. 1b).
5. At combined incubation of the long-chain palmitate (0.5 mM) with the short-chain hexanoate (2 mM) the positive inotropic effect of C. was followed by an increase of hexanoate oxidation (Δ + 14 %) whereas palmitate oxidation decreased. Participation of palmitate on total O_2 consumption was found here only to 8 % that of hexanoate to 92 %.
6. At combined incubation of 2 mM hexanoate and 15 mM glucose the positive inotropic effect of C. was followed with an increased hexanoate oxidation, at a lower concentration of 0.5 mM hexanoate, however, by an increase of glucose oxidation.

Conclusions

Carbocromene inhibits only in *hypoxic* injured atria the palmitate oxidation (− 32 %), whereas glucose oxidation-rate (+ 17 %) increased at the incubation with the combination of these 2 substrates. In the *normoxic controls*, however, the competition of substrates in the biological oxidation after the positive inotropic effect of C. was dependent on the V_{max}- and K_m-values of the oxidation-rate of each substrate as well as its concentration.

If carbocromene inhibits the palmitate oxidation in the stage of its penetration through the cell membrane or in the mitochondrial membrane or by other interference in the hypoxic injured atria cannot be decided yet.

Schlußfolgerungen

Carbocromen hemmt nur in *hypoxisch* geschädigten Vorhöfen die Palmitat-Oxidation (–32 %), während die Glucose-Oxidationsrate bei gleichzeitiger Inkubation mit beiden Substraten ansteigt (+17 %). Bei den *normoxischen* Kontrollen dagegen war der Anteil der beiden Substrate an der biologischen Oxidation nach dem positiv inotropen Effekt von Carbocromen abhängig von den V_{max}- und K_m-Werten der Oxidationsrate der jeweiligen Substrate und deren Konzentrationen.

Ob Carbocromen die Palmitat-Oxidation auf der Stufe der Penetration durch die Zellmembran, in der Mitochondrienmembran oder durch einen anderen Interferenzmechanismus im hypoxisch geschädigten Herzvorhof hemmt, kann noch nicht entschieden werden.

References

1. *Oliver, M.F., V.A. Kurien, T.W. Greenwood:* Relation between Serum Free Fatty Acid and Arrhythmias and Death after Acute Infarction, Lancet **1968/T** 710.
2. *Schraven, E.:* Regulation des Fett- und Kohlenhydratstoffwechsels des Herzens durch Carbocromen. Drug Res. **26**, 197–200 (1976).
3. *Schraven, E.:* Influence of Carbocromene on Free Fatty Acid Metabolism of the Heart. Adv. Cardiac Stru. and Metab. **11**, 363–367 (1978).
4. *Siess, M.:* Influence on the Efficiency of Cardiac Work. Basic Res. Cardiol. **72**, 299–305 (1977).
5. *Siess, M., H.J. Keller, E. Schare, J. Geissler, G. Müller:* The Continuous and Simultaneous Measurement of O_2 Consumption, Rate of Decarboxylation of ^{14}C-Substrates and the Performance of Spontaneously Beating Isolated Heart Atria of Guinea Pigs. J. Mol. Cell. Cardiol. **1**, 261 (1970).
6. *Süsskand, K.:* Stoffwechsel und Funktion des Herzmuskels unter langkettigen Fettsäuren. Naturwiss. Dissertation (Tübingen 1976).

Authors' address:

Dr. *K. Süsskand* and Prof. Dr. med. *M. Siess,* Pharmakologisches Institut der Univ. Tübingen, Wilhelmstr. 56, 7400 Tübingen, F.R.G.

Basic Res. Cardiol. **75**, 66–72 (1980)
© 1980 Dr. Dietrich Steinkopff Verlag, Darmstadt
ISSN 0300–8428

Paper, presented at the Erwin Riesch Symposium, Tübingen, April 3–7,1979

*Physiologisches Institut II, Institut für Submikroskopische Pathologie[1]),
Universität Tübingen*

Prospects of X-ray microanalysis in the study of pathophysiology of myocardial contraction*)

Perspektiven der Röntgenmikroanalyse für Untersuchungen über die Pathophysiologie der myokardialen Kontraktion

*M. F. Wendt-Gallitelli, H. Wolburg[1]), W. Schlote[1]),
M. Schwegler, C. Holubarsch,* and *R. Jacob*

With 3 figures and 2 tables

Summary

X-ray microanalysis was used to compare chemically untreated cryosections of quick-frozen myocardial tissue in "caffeine contracture" with cryosections of normal muscle. Our goal was to find out if it is possible by means of this method to detect changes in the calcium compartmentalization of the myocardial cell occurring by changes in its functional state. While it is possible to quantitate calcium in the cisternae of sarcoplasmic reticulum of the control muscle preparation, calcium could never be detected in these compartments of caffeine-contracted muscles.

In active microsomal fraction of ventricular myocardium it is possible to quantitate calcium and also to distinguish two components on account of their different ability to accumulate this element. The calcium content is different in the two components of the fraction.

Measurements of elemental composition in myocardial cell components in situ in various physiological and pathological conditions can aid understanding of the processes involving the regulation of Calcium transport within, into, and through heart muscle cells.

The combination of rapid freezing, cryoultramicrotomy, and X-ray microanalysis permits analysis of elemental composition of small cell compartments under simultaneous morphological observation, which is unique in biology. Nevertheless, serious preparative problems are still the limiting factors to date in the applicability of these techniques in the study of physiological processes (5).

The goal of our experiments was, firstly, to test the reliability of cryotechniques and electron probe microanalysis in a biochemically well-known material, such as fragmented myocardial sarcoplasmic reticulum. Secondly, we wished to determine whether the state of development of these methods already permits collection of detailed information about changes in calcium compartmentalization in the heart muscle cell under

---

*) Supported by the Deutsche Forschungsgemeinschaft

different pathophysiological conditions. Our intention was to reveal the feasibility of X-ray microanalysis in the planned study of some aspects of heart hypertrophy.

Material and methods

Rat papillary muscles were incubated in Tyrode solution (6) or in "caffeine-contracture" solution and stimulated as described by (3). Length-tension relations were recorded up to a few seconds before rapid freezing.

The muscle strips were rapidly frozen in liquid propane (-185 °C) or pressed, under vacuum, onto metal plates cooled to 4 °K. No prefixans or cryoprotectants were used. Ultrathin sections of the tissue were taken in a modified LKB cryo-ultramicrotome at temperatures between -120 and -140 °C. Translucent sections with interference colours were compressed in the cryochamber and freeze-dried at 10^{-5} Torr in a heavy brass box which warms up from -196 °C to room temperature during the night in the presence of a molecular sieve.

Some strips were freeze-substituted in acetone and embedded in araldite in order to test the morphology of the tissue after the freezing procedure (2).

The ultrathin freeze-dried muscle sections were carbon-coated and analysed in a Siemens Elmiskop 102 equipped with a Kevex energy dispersive detector (20 mm detector-probe distance) and a Siemens scanning transmission device. Our analysis conditions were: 4 μA beam current; about 20 nm spot diameter; 100 sec analysis time.

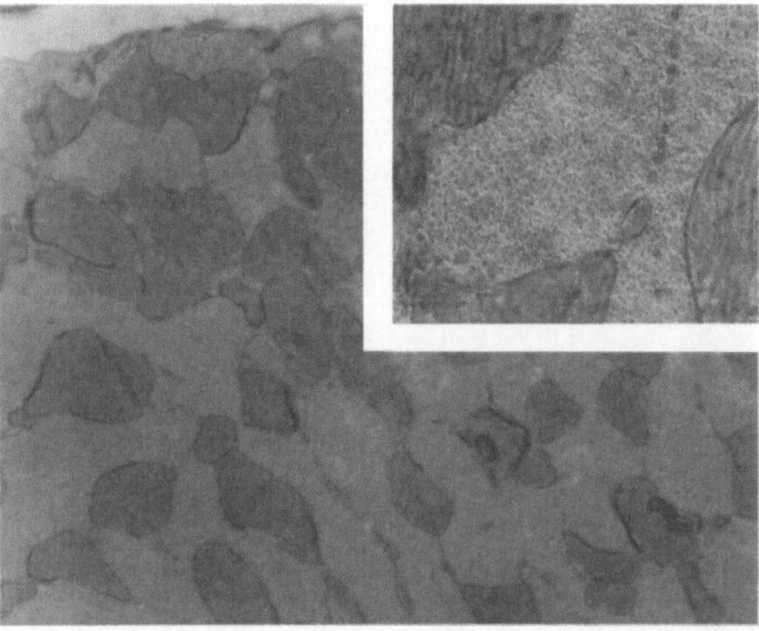

Fig. 1. Transversal section of contracted papillary muscle quickly frozen on metal plate at liquid He temp., freeze-substituted at – 80 °C with acetone. Mitochondria, myofibrils and SR elements have normal distribution. No important damages from growing ice crystals are present. Magnification × 16,000 (inset × 49,000).

We analysed adjacent compartments in myocardial cells of muscle strips which worked in normal Tyrode solution, and of such which worked in Tyrode solution under addition of caffeine (3).

For the quantitation of elements according to *Shuman* et al. (8), we used standards obtained from mixtures of phosvitin (containing chemically measured P content) and albumin. Binary crystals of elements in known stoichiometry were used to calculate the proportionality constants of Ca, K, Cl, Na, Mg, and S. The ventricular microsomal fractions were isolated as described in (11), quick-frozen and treated in the same way as the tissue.

Results and discussion

Preservation of the tissue after freezing

One important prerequisite for the availability of X-ray microanalysis of biological tissue is that no diffusion of elements takes place during treatment of the tissue. Because the muscle tissue in our papillary muscle strips is enveloped in endocardium many microns thick (10), this pre-requisites can be satisfied at least for superficial regions of the tissue by quick-freezing the material under vacuum on metal plates cooled to liquid Helium temperature. The preservation of the cardiac tissue at the subcel-lular level after quick freezing can be controlled by freeze-substituting the muscle strips. Such control experiments show that the morphology of the

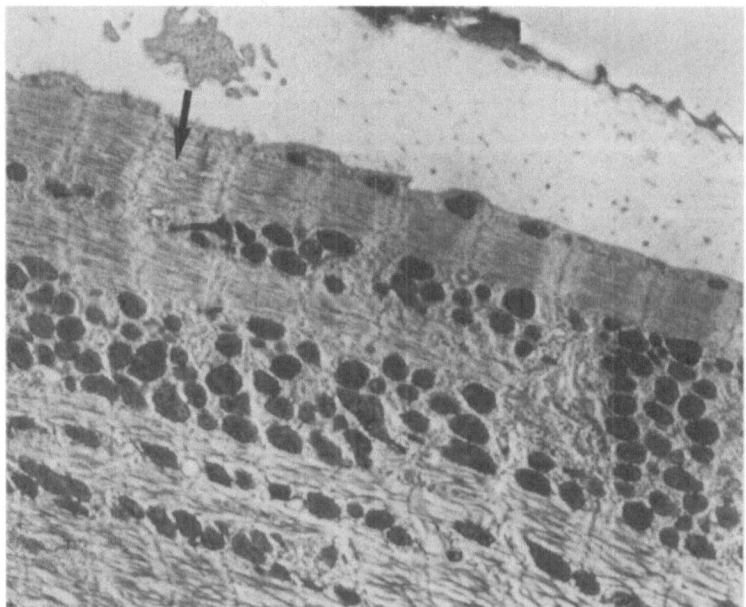

Fig. 2. Longitudinal section of papillary muscle frozen at –164 °C in liquid Freon$_{22}$ and freeze-substituted. Because of the thick endocardial layer (upper part of the picture), also in the superficial sarcomere layer), the arrangement of filament shows damages from growing ice crystals (arrow) during the freezing process. (Magnification × 8,900).

superficial muscle cells quick-frozen on a metal plate corresponds to that known from conventionally fixed and embedded muscles (fig. 1a). Actin and myosin filaments are not compressed by growing ice crystals (fig. 1b), as was the case in strips frozen in undercooled liquid $Freon_{22}$ (fig. 2). Also the sarcoplasmic reticulum and transversal-tubuli system have a normal morphology. Nevertheless, the morphological identification of subcellular structures in well-frozen, ultrathin and unstained cryosections is rendered difficult by the fact that, the better the freezing process and preservation of cellular structures, the poorer is the contrast of the unstained cryosections on the electron microscope (fig. 3).

Electron probe microanalysis

The analysis of microsomal fractions of cat myocardium shows that two populations of vesicles are present in the isolated active fraction which can be distinguished by their elemental composition and their ability to accumulate calcium (11). At a calcium concentration in the incubation medium of 60 nMol/mg fraction protein, "phosphate-vesicles" (probably corresponding to elements of longitudinal tubuli) show a calcium mass fraction of 432 mMol/kg dry weight ($\triangleq$ 160 mMol/l fraction protein) (Type a, table 2), while "oxalate-accumulating" vesicles (Type b, table 2, probably corresponding to cisternae of sarcoplasmic reticulum) show a calcium mass fraction of 666 mMol/kg dry weight.

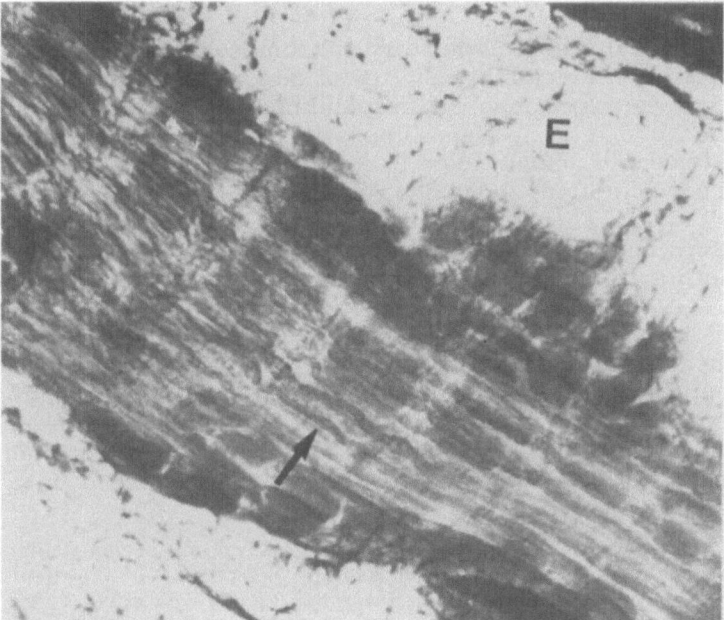

Fig. 3. Longitudinal section of chemically untreated papillary muscle quickly frozen in liquid propane, cryocut, and analysed. The poorer the contrast, the smaller the ice crystals (arrow = longitudinal system, E = endocardium. Magnification × 7,700).

Table 1. Elemental mass fractions in control and caffeine-calcium contracture muscle strips. Concentrations are expressed in mMol/kg dry weight, because the cryosections were freeze-dried. The continuum values (Wh) are given in counts/ 100 sec. Our continuum band is 5.5–6.0 keV. (Cyto. = cytoplasm; SR = cisternae of sarcoplasmic reticulum; Mito. = mitochondria). Data are means ± SD.

		No. of Analyses	P	Cl	K	Ca	Wh
Control	Cyto. + Mito.	20	224 ± 60	152 ± 49	697 ± 75	–	210 ± 40
	SR	20	209 ± 58	141 ± 52	575 ± 69	27 ±15	190 ± 49
Contracture	Cyto. + SR	20	194 ± 49	220 ± 47	530 ± 62	–	478 ± 80
	Mito.	20	204 ± 52	249 ± 42	583 ± 56	29,92 ±17	550 ± 75

The different concentration not only of calcium, but also of P, Cl, and K in the two types of vesicles show that X-ray microanalysis reveals heterogeneity in preparations which are considered biochemically homogeneous.

In normal working muscle strips calcium is unequivocally detectable in sites corresponding to the cisternae of sarcoplasmic reticulum (table 1). In adjacent regions, probably corresponding to longitudinal tubuli as well as in the sarcomeres it seems impossible to unequivocally quantitate calcium under our actually experimental conditions. The cytoplasmic low calcium concentrations show high standard deviation and high variability from cell to cell. Thus, data obtained to date from measurements in the cytoplasm must be interpreted with care (earlier data obtained from muscle strips frozen in Freon$_{22}$ show higher calcium (11) content in the cisternae).

In pilot experiments on caffeine-contracted papillary muscle which were otherwise treated in the same way as the control muscle, calcium was never found at the sites of the cisternae of sarcoplasmic reticulum, as was the case in the control experiment (table 1). Calcium was present in very low concentration in the cytoplasm both under control and contracture conditions. These last data must be considered with care.

Table 2. Mass fraction of elements in microsomal fraction of ventricular myocardium at calcium concentration of 60 nMol/mg SR protein in the medium. (The values are expressed in mMol/kg dry weight.)

	P	Cl	K	Ca
Vesicles type a	297 ± 30	294 ± 42	287 ± 67	432 ± 52
Vesicles type b	126 ± 28	512 ± 67	534 ± 40	666 ± 56

In contracture strip calcium is unequivocally detected in several mitochondria: The possibility that this moderate calcium accumulation in mitochondria could be the effect of preparative artifacts (formation of calcium granula (7, 9)) due to poor freezing procedure or melting during cryotomy can be excluded, firstly, because of the good preservation (poor contrast) of the tissue, and secondly, because the calcium concentration in such granula (9) is a manyfold of that found in our "contracture-muscles".

Moreover, in such muscles with artificially high calcium concentrations, the intracellular K content is generally low: This fact indicates that some cell damage has taken place during the treatment of the tissue, with consequent K diffusion and abnormal reduction in K intracellular concentration. In our successful muscle preparation, on the contrary, intracellular K concentrations are high (table 1) (150–200 mM) and correspond to the expected values.

The fact that calcium has often been detected in the "contracture experiment" in mitochondria, but never in the cisternae of sarcoplasmic reticulum, as was the case in the control experiment, possibly indicated that caffeine leads to increased calcium release from sarcoplasmic reticulum. This finding is consistent with biochemical results obtained on isolated fragmented sarcoplasmic reticulum (4). Under these contracture conditions at least part of the myocardial mitochondria can accumulate calcium and possibly play a role in the regulation of calcium transport (1).

We can conclude that changes in calcium compartmentalization occurring under different pathophysiological conditions can be revealed using the tested methods. Nevertheless our actual experimental and analytical conditions not yet permit unequivocal quantitation of the cytoplasmic calcium concentration.

Acknowledgements

We are particularly grateful to Dr. *P. Stöhr,* Physikalisches Institut, Universität Tübingen, for the design of the freezing-device.
The investigation was supported by the Deutsche Forschungsgemeinschaft.

Zusammenfassung

Ultradünne Kryoschnitte von chemisch unbehandeltem, schnell gefrorenem Myokardgewebe in Koffein-Kontraktur wurden verglichen mit Kontrollpräparaten mit der Methode der Röntgenmikroanalyse. Während in den Kontrollpräparaten Calcium in den Regionen nachweisbar ist, die den terminalen Zysternen des sarkoplasmatischen Retikulums entsprechen, ist dieses Element in den Kontrakturexperimenten nie in diesen Regionen nachweisbar. Häufig dagegen tritt dieses Element in den Mitochondrien auf.

In aktiven mikrosomalen Fraktionen aus dem Ventrikelmyokard ist es auch möglich, Calcium zu quantifizieren. Zwei Komponenten können in der Fraktion unterschieden werden, die sich auf Grund ihrer Fähigkeit, Calcium zu akkumulieren, unterscheiden. Der Calciumgehalt in den Komponenten kann bestimmt werden.

References

1. *Carafoli, E., M. Crompton:* In: Calcium transport and cell function. New York Acad. of Science, 269–285 (1978).

2. *Gonzales-Serratos, H., A. V. Somlyo, G. McClennan, H. Shuman, L. Borrero, A. P. Somlyo:* Composition of vacuoles and sarcoplasmic reticulum in fatigued muscle: Electron probe analysis. Proc. Natl. Acad. Sci. USA **75**, No. 3, 1329–1333 (1978).

3. *Holubarsch, Ch., R. Jacob:* Evaluation of elastic properties of myocardium. Experimental models of fibrosis and contracture in heart muscle strips. Z. Kardiol. **68**, 123–127 (1979).

4. *Katz, A. M., D. I. Repke, W. Hasselbach:* Dependence on Ionophore- and caffeine-induced calcium release from sarcoplasmic reticulum vesicles on external and internal calcium ion concentrations. J. Biol. Chemistry **252**, No. 6, 1938–1949 (1977).

5. *Lechene, P.:* Electron probe micro analysis, its present – its future. Am. J. Physiol. **232** (5), F 391–397 (1977).

6. *Jacob, R., G. Ebrecht, A. Kämmereit, I. Medugorac, M. F. Wendt-Gallitelli:* Myocardial function in different models of cardiac hypertrophy. An attempt at correlating mechanical, biochemical and morphological parameters. Basic Res. Cardiol. **72**, 160–167 (1977).

7. *Seveus, L., D. Brdiczka, T. Barnard:* On the occurrence and composition of dense particles in mitochondria in ultrathin frozen dry sections. Cell. Biol. Int. Rep. **2**, 155–162 (1978).

8. *Shuman, H., A. V. Somlyo, A. P. Somlyo:* Quantitative electron probe microanalysis of biological thin sections: methods and validity. Ultramicroscopy **1**, 317–339 (1976).

9. *Somlyo, A. V., J. Silcox, A. P. Somlyo:* Electron probe analysis and cryo-ultramicrotomy of cardiac muscle: mitochondrial granula. Proc. EMSA Meeting 532–533 (1975).

10. *Wendt-Gallitelli, M. F., H. Wolburg, W. Schlote:* Problems in the quantitation of diffusible ions in unstained heart muscle cryosections by X-ray microanalysis. 17. Dortmunder Gespräche: Crytotechniques for Microanalysis of Biological Objects. Arzneim.-Forsch./Drug Res. **29** (II), 11, 1814–1815 (1979).

11. *Wendt-Gallitelli, M. F., H. Wolburg, M. Schwegler, W. Schlote:* Electron probe X-ray microanalysis and cryoultramicrotomy of unstained myocardial fragmented and in situ sarcoplasmic reticulum. Experientia **35** (12), 1591–1593 (1979).

Authors' address:

Physiologisches Institut II, Institut für Submikroskopische Pathologie der Universität, 7400 Tübingen

Basic Res. Cardiol. **75**, 73–80 (1980)
© 1980 Dr. Dietrich Steinkopff Verlag, Darmstadt
ISSN 0300–8428

Paper, presented at the Erwin Riesch Symposium, Tübingen, April 3–7, 1979

Physiologisches Institut II, Universität Tübingen

Alterations in excitation of mammalian myocardium as a function of chronic loading and their implications in the mechanical events*)

Änderungen der Erregungsprozesse des Warmblütermyokards als Funktion chronischer Mehrbelastung und ihre Konsequenzen für das Kontraktionsgeschehen

R. W. Gülch

With 3 figures

Summary

It is shown that hypertrophied rat myocardium exhibits marked prolongation of its action potential during non-essential changes both in the resting potential, as well as in the amplitude of the action potential, and during a moderate but non-significant reduction in the maximum upstroke velocity.

When examining action potentials of various myocardial regions of the same heart, it can be demonstrated that high chronic loading involves broad action potentials both in rat and cat hearts.

After depression of the fast inward current either by TTX or by partial depolarization under high extracellular K^+ concentration, the prolongation of the Ca^{2+} mediated action potentials of myocardial cells under high chronic loading is still manifest.

The broadening of the action potential is certainly responsible to some extent for the prolonged activity of the corresponding myocardial cells, which is expressed in the significant increase in the isometric peak time and in the augmentation of isometric force.

In comparison to the nonhypertrophied mammalian myocardial cell, the hypertrophied cell reveals distinct alterations in transmembrane electrogenic properties. With nonsignificant alterations in the resting potential and amplitude, the action potentials of hypertrophied right ventricular cat myocardium are prolonged by approximately 20% as shown by *Tritthart* (1975).

However, in a recently published paper (*Gülch*, 1979) we reported up to a threefold prolongation of the action potential in hypertrophied left ventricular myocardium of *Goldblatt* rats. In 24-week-old spontaneously hypertensive rats we even found a 4.2-fold prolongation in comparison to

---
*) This work has been supported by grants from the Deutsche Forschungsgemeinschaft.

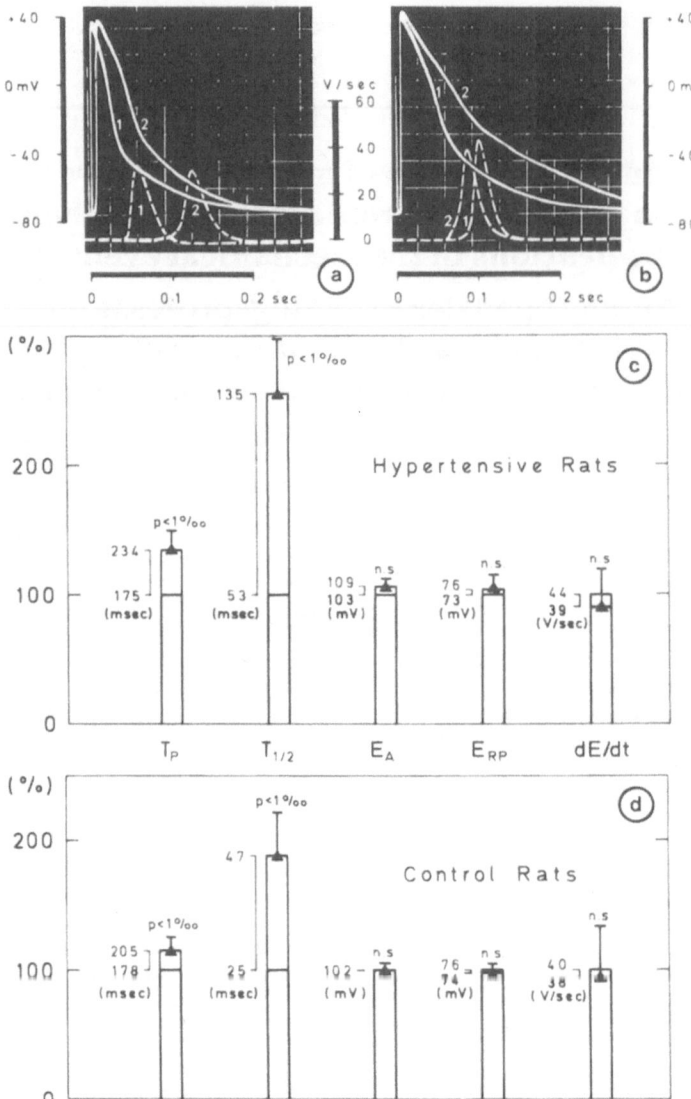

Fig. 1a and b. Oscilloscope recordings of representative action potentials of rat myocardium in the case of control (a) and hypertrophy (b). Signal 1 is obtained from a right ventricular, signal 2 from a left ventricular cardiac cell. The dashed traces show the corresponding first-time derivatives at tenfold sweep.

Fig. 1c and d. Statistical analysis of left and right ventricular action potentials of both groups. The left ventricular data are normalized with respect to the right ventricular values which have been set equal to 100%. The absolute values are indicated beside each column. Each vertical bar expresses the standard error (n = 19, 7–10 impalements). Note the highly significant increase in T_P and $T_{1/2}$ (p < 1‰) between left and right ventricular myocardium. $T_{1/2}$ represents the halfwidth, E_A the action potential amplitude, E_{RP} the resting potential, dE/dt the maximum upstroke velocity and T_P the isometric peak time.

the normotensive animals of the same age. A very important conclusion drawn from these investigations is that the prolongation of the action potentials is more marked, the more severe the degree of hypertrophy.

If these alterations can be interpreted as characteristic of hypertrophy then they pose the unavoidable question of whether they represent a general phenomenon equally affecting all myocardial cells of the hypertrophied heart, or whether single cells react in this manner but with varying degrees of prolongation depending on the extent of chronic loading.

The present study was designed to investigate the question of whether and to what extent the form of the action potential depends on the location and hence the chronic loading of the cells under consideration. That the time-course of the action potentials may be a function of the position of impalement within the heart can already be gathered from the studies of *Schaefer* (1943) or e.g. *Cohen* (1976).

Furthermore, the question of whether differences in myocardial performance could be explained by possible differences in the time-course of action potentials has been clarified.

Methods

All experiments were performed on isolated muscle preparations of hypertrophied hearts of *Goldblatt* rats and nonhypertrophied rat and cat hearts. The experimental conditions were the same as described in a recent paper (*Gülch*, 1979) with one exception: the measurements were performed simultaneously on two muscle strips from different regions of the same heart. The strips were mounted parallel to each other on two independent force transducers in the same muscle bath. By means of glass microelectrodes action potentials were alternatively recorded from each electrically stimulated muscle strip. This procedure permitted the use of Student's paired t-test for statistical analysis.

Results

In figure 1a and b original recordings of left and right ventricular action potentials of a hypertrophied and nonhypertrophied rat heart are shown. The selected examples are representative of the average behaviour of the respective groups. In both examples a clear prolongation of the left ventricular action potential is manifest in comparison to the right ventricular one.

A statistical analysis of both action potential types is demonstrated in figure 1c and d. The most important action potential parameters have been plotted by normalizing the left ventricular data with respect to the right ventricular values which have been set equal to 100%. Both diagrams reveal the uniform tendency of a highly significant increase in the duration of the action potential, the action potential being characterized by the halfwidth $T_{1/2}$. The slight alterations in amplitude E_A, resting potential E_{RP}, and even in the maximum upstroke velocity dE/dt are proved by statistics to be nonsignificant.

It is notable that the right ventricular action potentials of the *Goldblatt* rats (fig. 1c) are prolonged in comparison to corresponding controls (fig.

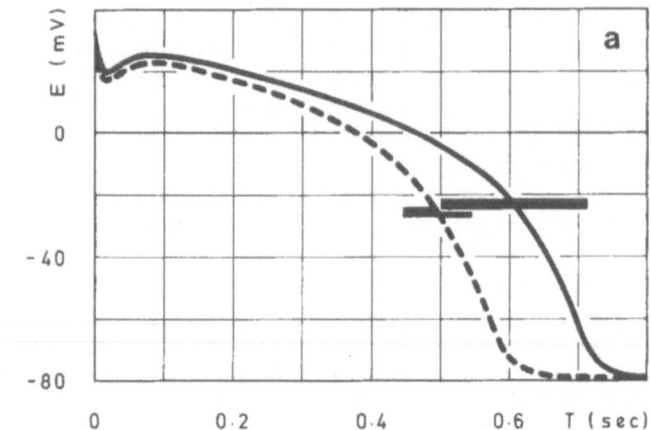

Fig. 2a. Mean action potentials constructed with data of all recorded action potentials of right ventricular (– – –) and left ventricular (——) cat myocardium. The horizontal bars indicate the (±) standard deviation (n = 13). The stimulation frequency was 0.2 Hz, the bath temperature 25 °C.

1d). This is in agreement with the slight degree of right ventricular hypertrophy of the *Goldblatt* rats which must be postulated on the basis of the approximately 20% increase in the weight of their right ventricles.

The isometric peak time T_P is also included in the diagrams. The left ventricular values are highly significantly augmented in hypertensive and normotensive rats.

That these phenomena do not turn out to be rat specific can be verified by the mean action potentials of 13 nonhypertrophied cat hearts shown in figure 2a. They were constructed using the statistical mean values of discrete points from all recorded action potentials of a group. The recordings were obtained simultaneously on a papillary muscle of the left and

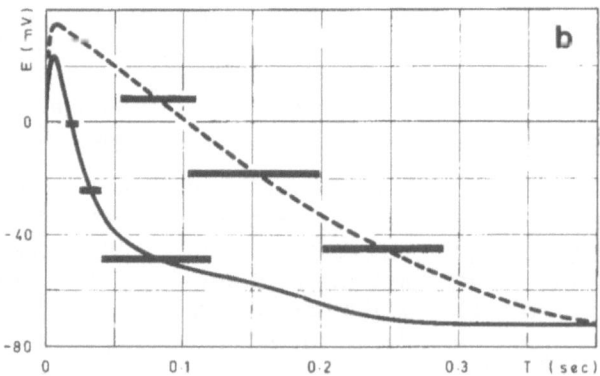

Fig. 2b. Mean action potentials of subendocardial (– – –) and subepicardial (——) left ventricular myocardium of hypertrophied rat heart. The horizontal bars indicate the (±) standard deviation (n = 7). The stimulation frequency was 0.2 Hz, the bath temperature 25 °C.

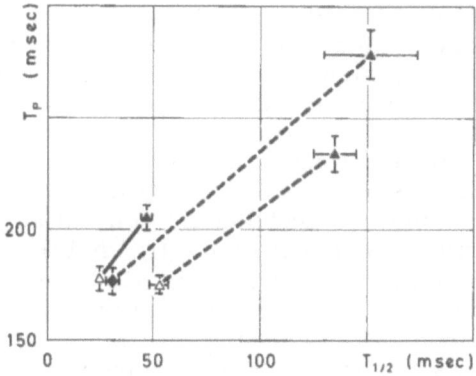

Fig. 3. Relationship between isometric peak time T_P and action potential halfwidth $T_{1/2}$ of rat myocardium. The single points represent statistical means of the following groups: ($\triangle$) right ventricular, ($\blacktriangle$) left ventricular subendocardial, ($\blacklozenge$) left ventricular subepicardial myocardium. The straight line connects data from control animals, the dashed lines data from *Goldblatt* rats. The horizontal and vertical bars indicate the corresponding ($\pm$) standard errors.

right ventricle of the same heart. The 23% prolongation based again on the halfwidth does not at first appear to be as spectacular as in the rat. Absolutely speaking, however, the increase of 110 msec which is verified as highly significant ($p < 0.1\%$) is very similar to the findings in the rat. Qualitatively similar, although less remarkable, results were obtained on guinea-pig hearts.

If one assumes that the differences in left and right ventricular action potentials can be attributed to the differing mechanical loading of the corresponding myocardial cells, then one must likewise propose differences in action potentials of subepicardial and subendocardial cells. For it is known that the wall layers located in the endocardial region are subjected to higher wall stress under the same inner pressure (*Hepp*, 1974).

In figure 2b simultaneous recordings on a subepicardial and subendocardial muscle strip from the same heart are shown, once again in the form of mean action potentials. Here again the tremendous 480% prolongation of the action potential of the cells under high chronic loading stands out. In contrast, the other action potential parameters are altered only slightly and nonsignificantly.

In figure 3 it is attempted to correlate the isometric peak time T_P with the action potential halfwidth $T_{1/2}$. The single points represent statistical means of the respective groups, whereby each pair which is connected by a straight line stems from the same experimental series. Although a uniform relation is not obvious, at least a tendency for a longer lasting mechanical activation to accompany a prolonged action potential can be recognized.

Discussion

As already described for the hypertrophied myocardium of *Goldblatt* rats (*Gülch*, 1979) and cats (*Tritthart*, 1975), the cardiac cell under high chronic loading exhibits the following alterations in the transmembrane electrogenic properties: the action potential duration is markedly prolonged whereas the amplitude E_A and the resting potential are only changed slightly but nonsignificantly. The alterations are very probably primarily the result of a delayed inactivation of the slow transmembrane influx. For the Ca^{2+} mediated action potentials, which can be recorded after inhibition of the fast inward current by tetrodotoxin or by partial depolarization under high extracellular K^+ concentration, also reveal a similar slow repolarization in hypertrophy (*Gülch*, 1979).

Additional reduction in the extracellular Ca^{2+} concentration in partially depolarized muscles leaves the shape of the Ca^{2+} mediated action potentials nearly unchanged with the exception of a reduction in amplitude. These facts can be interpreted as an indication of Ca^{2+} participation in the slow inward current.

The degree of the myocardial action potential alterations induced by cardiac hypertrophy is not found to be uniform in all cells of the same heart. The action potential duration is rather dependent on the position of the cell within the heart: a prolonged action potential is characteristic for cells which are exposed to high wall stress. This is the case for cardiac cells of subendocardial layers because of geometrical reasons, or for cells of left, in comparison to right ventricular papillary muscles because of the high left ventricular pressure. These phenomena which are already found in nonhypertrophied hearts are more pronounced in the case of cardiac hypertrophy.

The alteration in the action potentials described so far must naturally be of some consequence to cardiac performance. From the studies of *Antoni* (1969) it is known that an action potential broadening leads to a prolonged mechanical activity, which on its part might cause an increased peak force and a prolonged peak time. As demonstrated in figure 3, there is an unequivocal tendency toward longer peak time: a prolonged contraction accompanies a broader action potential.

Surprisingly, the increase in isometric force in hypertrophy (*Jacob*, 1977) or when comparing left and right ventricular contractions remains much below the expectations justified by the enormous action potential broadening. One reason for this may certainly lie in the external Ca^{2+} concentration of 2.2–2.5 mM which is commonly used for in vitro experiments on mammalian myocardium. The dose-response relation of rat myocardium for developed force seems to indicate that the region of saturation is nearly at this range of concentration (*Forester*, 1974). Thus an increased Ca^{2+} influx which must be postulated for a prolonged excitation can only minimally contribute to a further augmentation of force.

Yet delimitation of the effect of the changed excitation processes with respect to other alterations in electromechanical coupling is made difficult by the complexity of hypertrophy-induced alterations in cellular ultrastructure, such as the tubular system or myofibrillar content (*Wendt-Gallitelli*, 1977) and transport activity of the sarcoplasmic reticulum (*Ito*, 1974).

The precise etiology of the alterations in the excitation processes is at the moment beyond our knowledge. It is known, however, that many alterations at the sarcolemmal level accompany cardiac hypertrophy

(*Dhalla*, 1978). Thus it would seem straightforward to assume that those membrane structures which can be conceived of as channels are also involved. Changes in cell geometry could possibly play a role as well, since it is accepted that cell volume is increased in hypertrophy (*Hatt*, 1980).

Zusammenfassung

Es wird gezeigt, daß das hypertrophierte Rattenmyokard eine ausgeprägte Verlängerung seines Aktionspotentials aufweist bei unwesentlichen Veränderungen sowohl im Ruhepotential als auch in der Aktionspotentialamplitude und bei mäßiger, aber nichtsignifikanter Abnahme der maximalen Aufstrichgeschwindigkeit.

Vergleicht man Aktionspotentiale verschiedener Myokardbezirke desselben Herzens, so zeigt sich, daß eine erhöhte chronische Belastung mit breiteren Aktionspotentialen einhergeht. Dies ist an Ratten- wie auch an Katzenherzen nachweisbar.

Nach Blockade des schnellen Einwärtsstroms durch TTX oder durch partielle Vordepolarisation unter hoher extrazellulärer K^+-Konzentration erhält man im Falle chronischer Mehrbelastung sog. Ca^{2+}-Aktionspotentiale mit unvermindert langer Dauer.

Die Aktionspotentialverbreiterung ist sicher bis zu einem gewissen Grad für eine verlängerte Aktivierung der entsprechenden Herzmuskelzellen verantwortlich, die sich in einer signifikanten Zunahme der isometrischen Gipfelzeit und -kraft niederschlägt.

References

1. *Antoni, H., R. Jacob, R. Kaufmann:* Mechanische Reaktionen des Frosch- und Säugetiermyokards bei Veränderung der Aktionspotential-Dauer durch konstante Gleichstromimpulse. Pflügers Arch. **306**, 33–57 (1969).
2. *Cohen, I., W. Giles, D. Noble:* Cellular basis for the T-wave of the electrocardiogram. Nature **262**, 657–661 (1976).
3. *Dhalla, N. S., P. K. Das, G. P. Sharma:* Subcellular basis of cardiac contractile failure. J. Molec. Cell. Cardiol. **10**, 363–385 (1978).
4. *Forester, G. V., G. W. Mainwood:* Interval dependent inotropic effects in the rat myocardium and the effect of calcium. Pflügers Arch. **352**, 189–196 (1974).
5. *Gülch, R. W., R. Baumann, R. Jacob:* Analysis of myocardial action potential in left ventricular hypertrophy of Goldblatt rats. Basic Res. Cardiol. **74**, 69–82 (1979).
6. *Hatt, P. Y., K. Rakusan, P. Gastineau, M. Laplace, F. Cluzeaud:* Aorto-caval fistula in the rat. An experimental model of heart volume overloading. Basic Res. Cardiol. **75**, 105–108 (1980).
7. *Hepp, A., M. Hansis, R. Gülch, R. Jacob:* Left ventricular isovolumetric pressure-volume relations, "diastolic tone", and contractility in the rat heart after physical training. Basic Res. Cardiol. **69**, 516–532 (1974).
8. *Ito, Y., J. Suko, C. A. Chidsey:* Intracellular calcium and myocardial contractility. V. Calcium uptake of sarcoplasmic reticulum fractions in hypertrophied and failing rabbit hearts. J. Molec. Cell. Cardiol. **6**, 237–247 (1974).
9. *Jacob, R., G. Ebrecht, A. Kämmereit, I. Medugorac, M. F. Wendt-Gallitelli:* Myocardial function in different models of cardiac hypertrophy. An attempt at correlating mechanical, biochemical, and morphological parameters. Basic Res. Cardiol. **72**, 160–167 (1977).
10. *Schaefer, H., A. Pena, P. Schölmerich:* Der monophasische Aktionsstrom von Spitze und Basis des Warmblüterherzens und die Theorie der T-Welle des Ekg. Pflügers Arch. **246**, 728–745 (1943).

11. *Tritthart, H., H. Luedcke, R. Bayer, H. Stierle, R. Kaufmann:* Right ventricular hypertrophy in the cat – an electrophysiological and anatomical study. J. Molec. Cell. Cardiol. **7,** 163–174 (1975).
12. *Wendt-Gallitelli, M. F., G. Ebrecht, R. Jacob:* Morphological alterations and their functional interpretation in the hypertrophied myocardium of Goldblatt hypertensive rats. J. Molec. Cell. Cardiol. **11,** 275–287 (1979).

Author's address:

Dr. *R. W. Gülch,* Physiologisches Institut II der Universität Tübingen, Gmelin-straße 5, D-7400 Tübingen

Basic Res. Cardiol. **75**, 81–91 (1980)
© 1980 Dr. Dietrich Steinkopff Verlag, Darmstadt
ISSN 0300–8428

Paper, presented at the Erwin Riesch Symposium, Tübingen, April 3–7, 1979

*Division of Experimental Cardiology, Department of Physiology, Faculty of
Medicine, University of Manitoba, Winnipeg, Canada*

Subcellular changes during cardiac hypertrophy and heart failure due to bacterial endocarditis*)

Subzelluläre Änderungen des hypertrophierten und insuffizienten Herzens bei bakterieller Endokarditis

*N. S. Dhalla, A. Ziegelhoffer**), P. K. Singal, V. Panagia*, and
K. S. Dhillon

With 1 figure and 3 tables

Summary

Rabbits were catheterized and injected with saline (uninfected) or *Streptococcus viridans* (infected) to study the time course of changes in heart function, ultrastructure, membrane systems, myofibrils, and myocardial cations, cyclic AMP, norepinephrine and high energy phosphate contents. Myocardial hypertrophy in both infected and uninfected animals was found to follow increased activity of sympathetic nervous system as indicated by increased heart rate as well as norepinephrine and cyclic AMP contents. The decrease in sarcolemmal Na^+-K^+ ATPase activity was associated with contractile failure and preceded the observed decrease in myocardial K^+ and increase in Na^+ contents. The decrease in sarcolemmal Ca^{2+} binding activity may contribute in decreasing calcium entry and explain decreased myocardial Ca^{2+} contents and contractile activity; these changes were also accompanied by decreased microsomal calcium binding as well as depressed mitochondrial RCI. Depression in mitochondrial oxidative phosphorylation activity was found to result in declining high energy phosphate stores. Decreases in sarcolemmal, mitochondrial and myofibrillar ATPase activities as well as sarcolemmal adenylate cyclase activity were observed in late stages of bacterial endocarditis, at which time extensive myocardial cell damage was also apparent. These observations suggest that myocardial hypertrophy due to bacterial endocarditis may be a consequence of elevated levels of cyclic AMP whereas subsequent heart failure and cell damage in this disease may be due to defects in different membrane systems accompanied by a myocardial calcium deficiency.

Bacterial endocarditis can be easily produced by the insertion of a polyethylene catheter into the interior of the heart and subsequent injection of bacteria into the blood stream. Since the description of this procedure in rabbits (10), several investigators (2, 6, 7, 11, 12, 16, 19, 20) have successfully

---

*) Supported by the Manitoba Heart Foundation.
**) Visiting Professor supported by the Canadian Heart Foundation. Present
address: Department of Biochemistry, Institute of Experimental Surgery, Slovak
Academy of Sciences, Bratislava, Czechoslovakia.

employed this experimental model for studying the pathophysiology of this disease process. Earlier studies from our laboratory (19, 20) have revealed the occurrence of myocardial hypertrophy followed by heart failure in 100% of the catheterized rabbits upon injecting *Streptococcus viridans* within 6 days whereas only myocardial hypertrophy is seen in uninfected animals in which a catheter is inserted through the carotid artery and placed in the left ventricle. Although changes in heart function, myocardial untrastructure, different membrane systems, myofibrils and electrolyte distribution have been shown to occur at 3 and 6 days of bacterial infection (19–22), the information concerning the cause-effect relationship of these alterations during the development of endocarditis in these animals is not available in the literature. Furthermore, nothing is known about changes in the heart high energy phosphates, cyclic AMP and norepinephrine levels in the infected animals. It is therefore the purpose of this study to investigate the time-course of alterations in subcellular mechanisms during the development of myocardial hypertrophy and failure in rabbits with bacterial infection.

Materials and methods

Left heart endocarditis was induced in a New Zealand strain of male rabbits by implanting a catheter into the left ventricle through the right carotid artery and by injecting 10^7 organisms/kg of *Streptococcus viridans* intravenously 24 hr later. This method of producing bacterial endocarditis is similar to that described earlier (19, 20). Since it was found essential to keep the catheter in the left ventricle for producing cardiac hypertrophy and failure in 100% of the animals due to bacterial endocarditis, catheterized rabbits without bacterial infection (uninfected controls) were also used for the purpose of comparison. Healthy normal rabbits were employed for obtaining base-line values. After different time intervals of saline or bacterial injections, the animals were sacrificed by a blow on the head, their hearts removed and left ventricles employed for this investigation. The procedures for measuring left ventricle pressure (dP/dt) in the intact animals, morphological examination of the ventricles, isolation as well as determination of biochemical activities of mitochondria, fragments of the sarcoplasmic reticulum (microsomes), sarcolemma and myofibrils were the same as those described previously (19, 20, 22). Myocardial cation contents, heart norepinephrine, cyclic AMP as well as high energy phosphate compounds such as creatine phosphate (CrP) and ATP were measured by using procedures reported elsewhere (3, 8, 21). The results were analyzed statistically by using the Student's "t" test.

Results

From the data given in table 1, it can be seen that the rectal temperature of catheterized rabbits was significantly increased within one day after the bacterial injection whereas no change in the rectal temperature was noted in catheterized animals receiving the saline injection (control). A significant increase in the left ventricle wt/body wt ratio indicating hypertrophy of the left heart was evident at 2 days of infection or at 3 days in the uninfected catheterized control animals. The heart rates were significantly increased at 1, 2 and 3 days but decreased at 6 days of infection (table 1).

Table 1. Heart function, norepinephrine contents and myocardial electrolytes in rabbits at different times of bacterial infection. Each value is a mean ± S.E. of 4 to 6 animals.

	Rectal temp. (C°)	Left heart wt/ body wt.×10³	Heart rate beats/min	dP/dt mm Hg/sec	Norepinephrine contents (µg/g heart)	Cation contents µmol/g heart dry wt		
						Na⁺	K⁺	Ca²⁺
Normal	38.6 ± 0.11	1.34 ± 0.04	259 ± 7.2	460 ± 22	1.12 ± 0.16	118 ± 8.4	336 ± 12.1	7.4 ± 0.25
1 day control	38.6 ± 0.07	1.38 ± 0.07	268 ± 6.1	464 ± 24	1.15 ± 0.14	120 ± 7.9	340 ± 11.8	7.1 ± 0.26
1 day infected	39.2 ± 0.10*	1.45 ± 0.09	283 ± 6.4*	446 ± 22	1.57 ± 0.12*	129 ± 9.6	338 ± 14.2	6.8 ± 0.24
2 Day control	38.6 ± 0.04	1.45 ± 0.10	275 ± 6.6*	472 ± 24	1.30 ± 0.07	124 ± 8.6	332 ± 12.4	6.9 ± 0.32
2 day infected	39.7 ± 0.13*	1.68 ± 0.08*	309 ± 7.5*	380 ± 24*	1.92 ± 0.09*	148 ± 8.8	302 ± 10.5	5.4 ± 0.20*
3 day control	38.6 ± 0.07	1.61 ± 0.12*	286 ± 4.5*	448 ± 20	1.91 ± 0.09*	129 ± 10.5	318 ± 13.6	6.4 ± 0.28*
3 day infected	41.1 ± 0.14*	1.82 ± 0.09*	292 ± 6.1*	252 ± 23*	1.26 ± 0.08	166 ± 10.9*	282 ± 14.2*	4.2 ± 0.33*
6 day control	38.6 ± 0.06	2.06 ± 0.08*	302 ± 5.6*	394 ± 18*	1.81 ± 0.05*	214 ± 12.1*	262 ± 13.0*	5.5 ± 0.28*
6 day infected	40.8 ± 0.13	2.65 ± 0.11*	203 ± 5.9*	176 ± 16*	0.53 ± 0.07*	246 ± 13.2*	248 + 14.6*	5.6 ± 0.26*

*) Significantly different (P < 0.05) from normal values.

On the other hand, a progressive significant increase in heart rate was seen
in uninfected catheterized rabbits at 2 to 6 days. Significant depression in
the left ventricular dP/dt was apparent after 2 days of infection as well as
at 6 days of uninfected animals. The results in table 1 also indicate that
heart norepinephrine levels were significantly increased at 1 and 2 days
but decreased at 6 days of infection. Myocardial Na^+ was increased and K^+
was decreased significantly at 3 and 6 day of infected and 6 day uninfected
hearts whereas myocardial Ca^{2+} contents were decreased in 2, 3 and 6 day
infected and 3 and 6 day uninfected hearts (table 1).

The cyclic AMP levels in the heart were increased significantly at 1 and
2 days and decreased at 6 days of infection (table 2). The uninfected hearts
at 2 and 3 days also showed elevated levels of cyclic AMP. A significant
decrease in CrP levels was apparent at 3 and 6 days of infection, whereas
ATP levels were decreased only in 6 day infected hearts (table 2). Although
CrP levels were decreased in 6 day uninfected hearts, no change in ATP
contents was seen in these animals. The myofibrillar Ca^{2+} stimulated Mg^{2+}
dependent ATPase activity was depressed in 3 and 6 day infected and 6
day uninfected hearts. The mitochondrial respiratory control index (RCI)
was depressed at 2, 3 and 6 days of infection whereas mitochondrial
phosphorylation rate and ATPase activity was decreased at 3 and 6 days of
infection (table 2). Although there was a tendency of increase in
mitochondrial ATP-dependent calcium binding activity in infected and
uninfected hearts, significant difference was seen at 3 and 6 days of
infection.

The microsomal and sarcolemmal activities were also examined in
infected and uninfected hearts and the results are shown in table 3. The
microsomal ATP-dependent calcium binding, but not Ca^{2+}-stimulated
Mg^{2+} dependent ATPase activity, was decreased at 2, 3 and 6 day infected
and 6 day uninfected hearts. The sarcolemmal ATP-independent calcium
binding and Na^+-K^+ ATPase activities were decreased at 2, 3 and 6 day
infected and 6 day uninfected hearts. The sarcolemmal Mg^{2+} ATPase
activity was decreased significantly at 3 and 6 day infected and 6 day
uninfected hearts whereas sarcolemmal Ca^{2+} ATPase activity was depressed only at 6 days of infection. Although sarcolemmal adenylate
cyclase activities in the absence (basal) or presence of 100 μM epinephrine
were decreased in 3 and 6 day infected and 6 day uninfected hearts, the
stimulation of the enzyme activity due to epinephrine in these hearts was
not depressed in comparison to the normal preparations.

The sections of the left ventricles from infected and uninfected rabbits
were examined under the electron microscope. The ultrastructure of the
myocardium from 1, 2 and 3 day uninfected catheterized animals was not
different from the normal. However, in 6 day uninfected hearts the
changes observed were sporadic myofibrillar contracture, mild sarcotubular as well as mitochondrial swelling and slight degree of separation of the
intercalated disc in some sections. In contrast the damage to the structure
of infected hearts was quite pronounced and was related to the duration of
infection (fig. 1). Two day infected hearts showed mild but generalized
contracture of the myofibrils, swelling of the sarcotubular system,
intracellular edema throughout the cytoplasm as well as in the subsar-
colemmal regions (fig. 1A). No such changes were apparent in 1 day

Table 2. Cyclic AMP and high energy phosphate contents, myofibrillar Ca²⁺ ATPase, and mitochondrial oxidative phosphorylation, ATPase and calcium binding activities in rabbit hearts at different times of bacterial infection. Each value is a mean ± S.E. of 4 animals.

	Cyclic AMP (pmol/g heart)	CrP (μmol/g heart)	ATP (μmol/g heart)	Myofib. ATPase (μmol Pi/mg/min)	Mitochondria			
					Phosphory-lation rate (n atom Pi/mg/min)	RCI	ATPase (μmol Pi/mg/min)	Ca²⁺ binding nmol/mg/5 min
Normal	680 ± 41	11.2 ± 1.4	6.3 ± 0.5	0.25 ± 0.03	252 ± 18	7.2 ± 0.3	0.63 ± 0.05	60.5 ± 5.4
1 day control	675 ± 39	10.9 ± 1.1	6.1 ± 0.4	0.26 ± 0.04	248 ± 21	7.4 ± 0.4	0.67 ± 0.04	56.7 ± 5.4
1 day infected	1518 ± 72*	10.8 ± 1.2	6.2 ± 0.3	0.23 ± 0.03	264 ± 24	6.8 ± 0.4	0.59 ± 0.05	63.6 ± 4.3
2 day control	1276 ± 58*	9.3 ± 1.3	6.5 ± 0.6	0.21 ± 0.04	276 ± 15	7.2 ± 0.3	0.64 ± 0.06	61.8 ± 4.4
2 day infected	1134 ± 51*	9.7 ± 0.9	5.9 ± 0.4	0.18 ± 0.03	284 ± 17	6.0 ± 0.2*	0.52 ± 0.05	76.7 ± 6.2
3 day control	945 ± 44*	9.9 ± 1.2	6.0 ± 0.3	0.19 ± 0.04	281 ± 20	6.9 ± 0.5	0.62 ± 0.04	68.7 ± 4.1
3 day infected	724 ± 32	7.2 ± 0.6*	5.0 ± 0.4	0.14 ± 0.02*	198 ± 10*	5.0 ± 0.2*	0.46 ± 0.04*	89.1 ± 5.3*
6 day control	700 ± 40	8.1 ± 0.8*	5.8 ± 0.4	0.14 ± 0.02*	272 ± 16	6.6 ± 0.4	0.64 ± 0.05	74.2 ± 5.6
6 day infected	366 ± 28*	5.4 ± 0.4*	4.2 ± 0.2*	0.12 ± 0.01*	174 ± 9*	4.1 ± 0.2*	0.40 ± 0.03*	40.6 ± 3.4*

*) Significantly different (P < 0.05) from normal values.

Table 3. Microsomal and sarcolemmal ATPase and calcium binding and sarcolemmal adenylate cyclase activities in rabbit hearts at different times of bacterial infection. Each value is a mean ± S.E. of 4 animals.

| | Microsome | | Sarcolemma | | | | Adenylate cyclase (p mol cyclic AMP/mg/min) | |
| | Ca²⁺ATPase (μmol/mg/min) | Ca²⁺ binding (n mol mg/ 5 min) | ATPase (μmol Pi/mg/hr) | | | Ca²⁺ binding (nmol/ mg/5 min) | | |
			Mg²⁺ ATPase	Na⁺-K⁺ ATPase	Ca²⁺ ATPase		Basal	Epinephrine-stimulated
Normal	0.31 ± 0.04	42 ± 33	19.4 ± 1.3	7.6 ± 0.4	18.6 ± 1.0	45 ± 3.4	150 ± 9	224 ± 14
1 day control	0.32 ± 0.05	44 ± 41	19.1 ± 1.4	6.9 ± 0.5	18.1 ± 1.3	43 ± 3.8	146 ± 12	218 ± 12
1 day infected	0.32 ± 0.04	36 ± 36	19.0 ± 1.4	6.5 ± 0.4	18.0 ± 1.2	41 ± 4.1	154 ± 11	220 ± 14
2 day control	0.31 ± 0.04	38 ± 40	19.8 ± 1.5	7.1 ± 0.5	18.8 ± 0.9	38 ± 4.0	142 ± 10	217 ± 11
2 day infected	0.29 ± 0.03	$29 \pm 2.2^*$	17.6 ± 1.2	$5.8 \pm 0.3^*$	17.2 ± 0.8	$34 \pm 2.3^*$	135 ± 10	209 ± 13
3 day control	0.27 ± 0.04	35 ± 37	18.1 ± 0.9	6.4 ± 0.4	17.6 ± 0.9	37 ± 3.5	147 ± 12	206 ± 13
3 day infected	0.29 ± 0.05	$22 \pm 2.5^*$	$16.0 \pm 0.7^*$	$4.2 \pm 0.3^*$	16.6 ± 0.8	$32 \pm 2.9^*$	$109 \pm 8^*$	$170 \pm 8^*$
6 day control	0.28 ± 0.06	$28 \pm 2.9^*$	$15.9 \pm 0.6^*$	$5.5 \pm 0.4^*$	17.4 ± 1.0	$33 \pm 2.1^*$	$113 \pm 7^*$	$181 \pm 7^*$
6 day infected	0.27 ± 0.04	$19 \pm 2.1^*$	$13.8 \pm 0.8^*$	$3.4 \pm 0.3^*$	$15.0 \pm 0.6^*$	$22 \pm 2.0^*$	$92 \pm 6^*$	$152 \pm 9^*$

*) Significantly different ($P < 0.05$) from normal values.

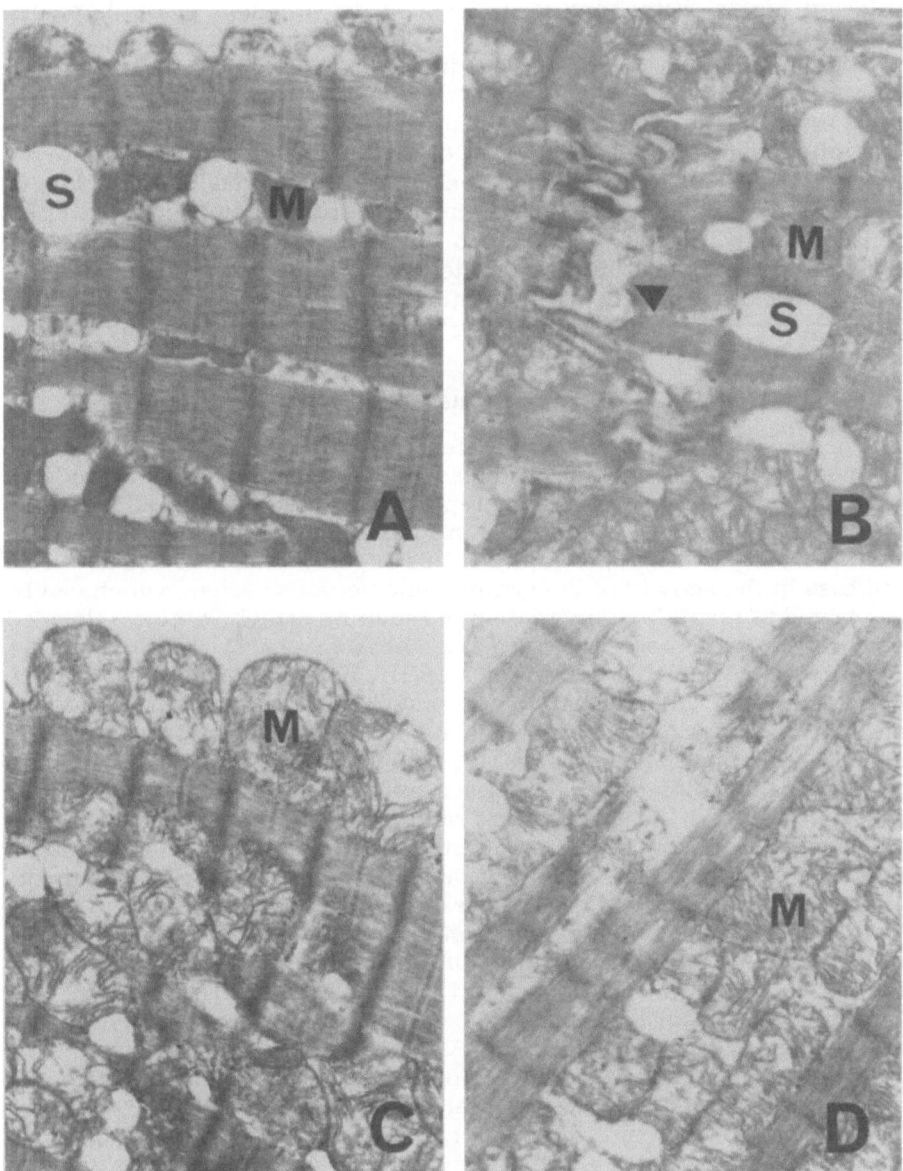

Fig. 1. Electron micrographs showing a portion of the left ventricle from rabbit hearts infected with *S. viridans* for 2 days (A), 3 days (B) and 6 days (C and D). Contracture of myofibrils and swelling of the sarcotubular system is apparent at all stages of infection. Separation of the intercalated disc (arrow) is quite evident in 3 day infected heart. Mitochondria in 2 day infected heart are normal but progressive damage to this organelle from 3 to 6 days of infection was noted. Damage to the microfilaments can be seen in 6 day infected heart. M, mitochondria; S, sarcotubules; Magnification × 16,500.

infected hearts. Mitochondria in 1 and 2 day infected hearts appeared normal and had electron dense interior as well as a normal arrangement of cristae; intercellular contacts in the intercalated disc of these hearts were also intact. In 3 day infected hearts the above mentioned changes had progressed further and also involved mitochondria (fig. 1B). Swelling of the mitochondria, some disruption of cristae and loss of electron dense material from the matrix were consistently observed in these hearts. Separation of the intercalated discs and interstitial edema were also apparent in 3 day infected hearts. In 6 day infected hearts, the structural damage to the myocardium was extensive (fig. 1C and D). Separation as well as loss of myofilaments in addition to marked changes in mitochondrial and sarcotubular membrane systems were observed in 6 day infected hearts.

Discussion

We have shown that bacterial infection, as reflected by an increase in body temperature of rabbits, produced an increase in left heart wt/body wt ratio in 2 days whereas cardiac norepinephrine and cyclic AMP contents as well as heart rate increased within 1 day of infection. It is possible that the observed cardiac hypertrophy in this experimental model is due to an increase in the activity of the sympathetic nervous system, which can be conceived to result in an increase in circulating catecholamines, elevated levels of cardiac norepinephrine and cyclic AMP as well as high heart rate. Catecholamines have been implicated in the manifestation of cardiac hypertrophy (15, 23). Myocardial norepinephrine and cyclic AMP contents have also been shown to increase before heart hypertrophy becomes evident in myopathetic hamsters (13, 17). Furthermore, myocardial hypertrophy in the uninfected catheterized animals was also preceded by or associated with an increase in heart rate as well as cardiac norepinephrine and cyclic AMP contents. On the other hand, cyclic AMP and norepinephrine contents of the heart have also been reported to decrease in late stages of hypertrophy (14, 18). This is exactly what we have seen in hearts from animals after 6 days of infection. However, this situation most probably reflects decreased sympathetic activity as well as cardiac contractile failure and cell damage. It should also be pointed out that catecholamine-induced myocardial cell damage has been associated with elevated levels of myocardial cyclic AMP (1). Thus it appears likely that an increase in sympathetic activity would release catecholamines in the circulation and increase myocardial cyclic AMP, which may produce cardiac hypertrophy and subsequent contractile failure and cell damage. Although initial increase in cyclic AMP content was not associated with an increase in the sarcolemmal adenylate cyclase activity, the late decline in cyclic AMP content may be a consequence of decreased adenylate cyclase activity.

In this study myocardial K^+ decreased whereas Na^+ content increased in 3 and 6 day infected and 6 day uninfected hearts. These changes may be due to decreased sarcolemmal Na^+-K^+ ATPase activity. On the other hand, myocardial Ca^{2+} contents were decreased in 2 to 6 day infected and 3 to 6 day uninfected hearts and this may possibly be due to a decreased entry of calcium in the myocardium. Although sarcolemmal calcium binding also decreased in 2 to 6 day infected hearts, a significant decrease in sarcolemmal calcium binding was noted only in 6 day uninfected hearts. Furthermore, sarcolemmal Ca^{2+} ATPase, which has been implicated in the entry of calcium into the myocardium (5), was decreased only in 6 day infected hearts. In addition, increased sympathetic activity in both infected and uninfected animals should favour increased entry of calcium into the myocardium (9). Thus the exact reason for the observed decrease in myocardial Ca^{2+} contents in the uninfected hypertrophied heart is not clear at present whereas in the infected hearts decreased sarcolemmal Ca^{2+} binding and Ca^{2+} ATPase activities may partly explain the decreased entry of calcium into the myocardium and subsequent decrease in myocardial Ca^{2+} contents. Such a calcium deficiency in the myocardium may also contribute to the development of contractile failure and loss of structural integrity. Intracellular calcium deficiency has already been implicated in the pathogenesis of cardiac contractile failure and cell damage (4).

Alterations observed in microsomal, sarcolemmal, mitochondrial and myofibrillar activities in 3 and 6 day infected as well as in 6 day uninfected hearts confirm our earlier findings (21, 22). In addition, it was found that microsomal calcium binding, sarcolemmal calcium binding and Na^+-K^+ ATPase activities were decreased at 2 days of infection and these changes were associated with a decline in ventricular performance. Decreased calcium binding by sarcolemmal and microsomal membranes can be conceived to decrease calcium stores and thus less calcium will be released upon excitation of the myocardium (4, 5); this may partly explain the observed decrease in ventricular dP/dt in the infected hearts. Although mitochondrial RCI was significantly decreased indicating a loose coupling of the oxidative phosphorylation activities at 2 days of infection, mitochondrial phosphorylation as well as Ca^{2+} binding and ATPase activities were not altered significantly at this time. While increased calcium binding activity of mitochondria at 3 days of infection may represent an adaptive mechanism, decreased mitochondrial calcium binding in 6 day infected heart may contribute in the pathogenesis of contractile failure at this stage of endocarditis. At any rate, decreased mitochondrial oxidative phosphorylation activity at 3 and 6 days of infection can be taken to reflect a defect in the process for energy production. This view is consistent with our observations that the high energy phosphate stores were decreased at this late stage. Whether depressed myofibrillar ATPase activity as well as mitochondrial and sarcolemmal ATPase activities at 3 and 6 days of infection represent adaptive mechanism for conserving energy or reflect defects in the process of energy utilization cannot be stated with certainty. Decreased sarcolemmal adenylate cyclase activity as well as myocardial cyclic AMP levels may also contribute for the observed contractile failure in late stages of infection. From the observations reported in this study it is evident that changes in different membrane systems and myofibrillar ATPase at late stages of bacterial endocarditis are associated with ultrastructural damage and contractile failure and it is likely that these generalized defects may in fact be responsible for severe congestive heart failure and subsequent death of individuals with infective endocarditis.

Zusammenfassung

Bei katheterisierten Kaninchen wurde Streptococcus viridans bzw. Kochsalzlö-
sung (bei Kontrolltieren) injiziert und der Zeitverlauf der Veränderungen in der
Herzaktion der myokardialen Ultrastruktur (Membransysteme, Myofibrillen) sowie
dem Gehalt an Kationen, zyklischem AMP, Noradrenalin und energiereichem
Phosphat verfolgt. Sowohl bei in infizierten als auch bei den nichtinfizierten Tieren
ergab sich, daß die Myokardhypertrophie einer verstärkten Aktivität des sympathi-
schen Nervensystems folgt, wie aus der Steigerung der Herzfrequenz sowie des
Gehaltes an Noradrenalin- und zyklischem AMP hervorging. Der Rückgang in der
Aktivität der sarkolemmalen Na^+-Ka^+-ATPase-Aktivität war von kontraktilem Ver-
sagen begleitet und ging einem Abfall des myokardialen K^+-Gehalts und einem
Anstieg des Na^+-Gehalts voraus. Die Minderung der sarkolemmalen Ca^{2+}-Bin-
dungsaktivität könnte zu einem Rückgang der Ca^{2+}-Aufnahme beitragen und die
Minderung des myokardialen Ca^{2+}-Gehaltes und der kontraktilen Aktivität erklären. Diese Veränderungen waren auch von einer reduzierten mikrosomalen Ca^{2+}-
Bindung und von einer verminderten mitochondrialen RCI begleitet. Eine redu-
zierte Aktivität der oxidativen Phosphorylierung in den Mitochondrien bewirkte
einen Rückgang der Vorräte an energiereichem Phosphat. Ein Abfall der sarkolemmalen, mitochondrialen und myofibrillären ATPase-Aktivität und der sarkolemmalen Adenylatcyclase wurde in späteren Stadien der bakteriellen Endokarditis beobachtet, in denen auch ausgedehnte Zellschädigungen vorlagen. Diese Beobachtungen lassen vermuten, daß die myokardiale Hypertrophie bei bakterieller Endokarditis Folge eines erhöhten Spiegels an zyklischem AMP ist, während das nachfol-
gende Herzversagen und die Zellschädigung bei dieser Erkrankung auf Defekte
verschiedener Membransysteme – begleitet von myokardialem Ca^{2+}-Defizit – bezogen werden kann.

References

1. *Bhagat, B., J. M. Sullivan, V. W. Fischer, E. M. Nadel, N. S. Dhalla:* cAMP
   activity and isoproterenol-induced myocardial injury in rats. Recent Advances
   in Studies on Cardiac Structure and Metabolism. **12,** 465–470 (1978).
2. *Carrizosa, J., K. Kaye, W. Kobasa:* Experimental Streptococcal endocarditis.
   Arch. Pathol. Lab. Med. **102,** 518–521 (1978).
3. *Dhalla, N. S., B. D. Bhagat, P. V. Sulakhe, R. E. Olson:* Catecholamine stores in
   the isolated heart perfused with substrate-free medium. J. Pharmacol. Exptl.
   Therap. **177,** 96–101 (1971).
4. *Dhalla, N. S., P. K. Das, G. P. Sharma:* Subcellular basis of cardiac contractile
   failure. J. Mol. Cell. Cardiol. **10,** 363–385 (1978).
5. *Dhalla, N. S., A. Ziegelhoffer, J. A. C. Harrow:* Regulatory role of membrane
   systems in heart function. Can. J. Physiol. Pharmacol. **55,** 1211–1234 (1977).
6. *Durack, D. T.:* Experimental bacterial endocarditis. IV. Structure and evolution
   of very early lesions. J. Pathol. **115,** 81–89 (1975).
7. *Durack, D. T., P. B. Beeson:* Experimental bacterial endocarditis. I. Coloniza-
   tion of a sterile vegetation. Brit. J. Exp. Path. **53,** 44–49 (1972).
8. *Fedelesova, M., N. S. Dhalla:* High energy phosphate stores in the hearts of
   genetically dystrophic hamsters. J. Mol. Cell. Cardiol. **3,** 93–102 (1971).
9. *Fleckenstein, A., J. Janke, H. J. Doring, O. Leder:* Myocardial fiber necrosis due
   to intracellular Ca overload – a new principle in cardiac pathophysiology.
   Recent Advances in Studies on Cardiac Structure and Metabolism. **4,** 563–580
   (1974).
10. *Garrison, P. K., L. R. Freedman:* Experimental endocarditis. I. Staphylococcal
    endocarditis in rabbits resulting from placement of a polyethylene catheter in
    the right side of the heart. Yale J. Biol. Med. **42,** 394–410 (1970).

11. *Gutschik, E., N. Chritensen:* Experimental endocarditis in rabbits. I. Technique and spontaneous course of non-bacterial thrombic endocarditis. Acta path. microbiol. scand. Sect. B. **86,** 215–221 (1978).
12. *Gutschik, E., N. Chritensen:* Experimental endocarditis in rabbits. 2. Course of untreated Streptococcus faecalis infection. Acta path. microbiol. scand. Sect. B. **86,** 223–228 (1978).
13. *Harrow, J. A. C., J. N. Singh, G. Jasmin, N. S. Dhalla:* Studies on adenylate cyclase-cyclic AMP system of the myopathic hamster (UM–X7.1) skeletal and cardiac muscles. Can. J. Biochem. **53,** 1122–1127 (1975).
14. *Kramer, R. S., D. T. Mason, E. Braunwald:* Augmented sympathetic neurotransmitter activity in the peripheral vascular bed of patients with congestive heart failure and cardiac norepinephrine depletion. Circulation **38,** 629–634 (1968).
15. *Laks, M. M., F. Morady:* Norepinephrine – The myocardial hypertrophy hormone. Amer. Heart J. **91,** 674–675 (1976).
16. *Lowy, F., N. H. Steigbigel:* Infective endocarditis. Part III. Prevention of bacterial endocarditis. Amer. Heart J. **96,** 689–695 (1978).
17. *Sole, M. J., C. M. Lo, C. W. Laird, E. H. Sonnenblick, R. J. Wurtman:* Norepinephrine turnover in the heart and spleen of the cardiomyopathic Syrian hamster. Circulat. Res. **37,** 857–862 (1975).
18. *Stewart, D., D. T. Mason, J. Wikman-Coffelt:* Changes in cAMP concentrations during chronic cardiac hypertrophy. Basic Res. Cardiol. **73,** 648–658 (1978).
19. *Tomlinson, C. W., N. S. Dhalla:* Myocardial cell damage during experimental infective endocarditis. Lab. Invest. **33,** 316–323 (1975).
20. *Tomlinson, C. W., N. S. Dhalla:* Alterations in myocardial function during bacterial infective cardiomyopathy. Amer. J. Cardiol. **37,** 373–381 (1976).
21. *Tomlinson, C. W., N. S. Dhalla:* Alterations in calcium metabolism in cardiac hypertrophy and failure caused by bacterial infection. Recent Advances in Studies in Cardiac Structure and Metabolism. Vol. **12,** 191–198 (1978).
22. *Tomlinson, C. W., S. L. Lee, N. S. Dhalla:* Abnormalities in heart membranes and myofibrils during bacterial infective cardiomyopathy in the rabbit. Circulat. Res. **39,** 82–92 (1976).
23. *Womble, J. R., M. K. Haddox, D. H. Russell:* Epinephrine elevation in plasma parallels canine cardiac hypertrophy. Life Sci. **23,** 1951–1958 (1978).

Authors' address:

Dr. *Naranjan S. Dhalla*, Professor of Physiology, Faculty of Medicine, University of Manitoba, Winnipeg, Canada R3E OW3

Basic Res. Cardiol. **75,** 92–96 (1980)
© 1980 Dr. Dietrich Steinkopff Verlag, Darmstadt
ISSN 0300-8428

Paper, presented at the Erwin Riesch Symposium, Tübingen, April 3–7, 1979

Universität Konstanz, Fakultät für Biologie

Characterization of cardiac microsomes from spontaneously hypertonic rats*)

Charakterisierung der Mikrosomenfraktion von Herzen spontan hypertonischer Ratten

C. Heilmann, T. Lindl, W. Müller, and *D. Pette**)*

With 2 figures and 1 table

Summary

Capacity of Ca^{2+} sequestration was found to be significantly lowered in microsomal preparations of hearts from spontaneously hypertonic rats. A decrease to 40% of the control level was found for basal and extra ATPase. A similar reduction existed in initial and total Ca^{2+} uptake. These findings are correlated with a lower concentration of the Ca^{2+} transport ATPase in SDS gel electrophoresis, a lower density of the 7–9 nm intramembraneous particles and higher half-lives of phosphoprotein. Altered contractility of hypertrophied myocardium may thus be partially explained by the dysfunction of the Ca^{2+} sequestering system.

Decreased contractility and failing of hypertrophied myocardium (1) has been mainly related to a deranged homeostasis of intracellular $[Ca^{2+}]$ (2). Attempts have been made to explain the latter in terms of dysfunctions of membrane systems regulating intracellular $[Ca^{2+}]$ such as mitochondria, sarcolemma and sarcoplasmic reticulum (for review see 2). In the present study spontaneously hypertensive rats (SHR) which develop severe hypertrophy of the myocardium were chosen as a model for studying function and ultrastructure of sarcoplasmic reticulum (SR) in the hypertrophied heart. The data from SHR are compared to those from normotensive Wistar rats (NR).

Methods

SR was prepared from left ventricles of SHR and NR by differential centrifugation using 0.3 M sucrose and 5 mM Hepes (pH 7.5) as isolation medium. All measurements were performed on freshly prepared SR. Methods for determining ATPase activities, Ca^{2+} uptake, SDS gel electrophoresis and phosphoprotein formation have been described (3, 4). For ultrastructural analyses, negative staining with phosphotungstic acid and freeze-fracturing were performed.

---

*) This study was supported by the Deutsche Forschungsgemeinschaft, Sonderforschungsbereich 138 "Biologische Grenzflächen und Spezifität".
**) To whom requests for reprints should be addressed.

Results and discussion

Systolic blood pressure was 195 mm Hg in SHR and 120 mm Hg in NR. Weight of left ventricles relative to body weight (mg/g) was 1.9 in NR and 3.3 in SHR. Microsomal preparations were obtained at similar yields both from NR and SHR. Measurements of ATPase inhibition by ouabain and of mitochondrial marker enzymes indicated a contamination with 10% sarcolemmal membranes and about 30% mitochondrial fragments.

Table 1 summarizes results obtained for ATPase activities, Ca^{2+} uptake characteristics and phosphoprotein formation in SR preparations of NR and SHR. Both Mg^{2+}- and Ca^{2+}-dependent ATPase activities were markedly reduced in SHR. Ca^{2+} dependence of extra ATPase was unaltered as shown by identical values for Ca^{2+} concentration for half maximal rate. Corresponding changes existed in initial and total Ca^{2+} uptake which both were reduced to about 40% as compared to SR of NR (table 1). On the other hand, Ca^{2+} dependence as well as efficiency of Ca^{2+} transport proved to be not significantly changed in SHR (table 1). The changes in Ca^{2+} uptake of SHR were much smaller if measurements were performed in the absence of oxalate. The reason for this is so far unclear. Measurements of Ca^{2+} release from ^{45}Ca-oxalate preloaded SR vesicles provided no evidence for changes in SHR. This argues against a defective vesicular membrane in the sense of leakiness as was suggested by *Aoki* et al. (5).

Electrophoretic peptide patterns of SR from NR and SHR are compared in figure 1. It is seen that no qualitative differences exist. However, a distinct reduction of the 115.000-Mr Ca^{2+} pumping protein is obvious in figure 1 and was found in all SHR preparations studied. The identity of

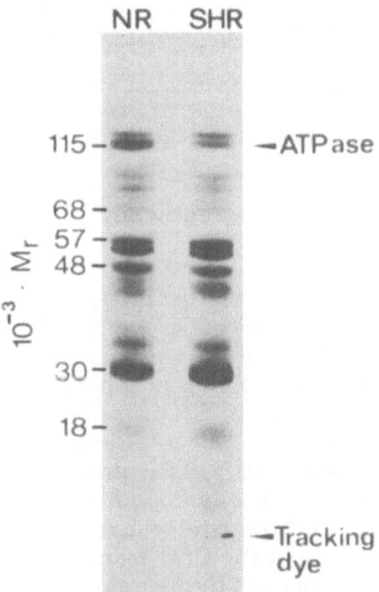

Fig. 1. Sodium dodecylsulfate polyacrylamide gel electrophoreses of cardiac microsomes from NR and SHR.

Table 1. Comparison of some functional and kinetic properties of SR from left heart ventricles of NR and SHR. Measurements of ATPase activities, Ca^{2+} uptake and ^{32}P incorporation were performed as previously described (3, 4).

Cardiac microsomes	NR	SHR	NR/SHR
Yield of microsomes (mg protein/g wet weight)	2.0	2.0	1.0
Mg^{2+}-dependent (basal) ATPase (U/mg)	2.4	1.04	2.3
Ca^{2+}-dependent (extra) ATPase (U/mg)	0.05	0.022	2.27
Extra ATPase/total ATPase	0.02	0.02	1.0
K_m (μM Ca^{2+})	1.4	1.4	
Initial Ca^{2+} uptake (nmol/mg × min)	66.2	27.5	2.4
Capacity of Ca^{2+} uptake (nmol/mg × 40 min)	525	187	2.8
K_m (μM Ca^{2+})*	1.66	1.34	
Efficiency of Ca^{2+} transport (mol Ca^{2+}/mol ATP)	1.3	1.22	
Initial Ca^{2+} uptake in the absence of oxalate (nmol/mg × min)	6.4	5.2	1.23
Maximal Ca^{2+} uptake in the absence of oxalate (nmol/mg × 8 min)	12.1	11.1	1.1
^{32}P incorporation (pmoles ^{32}P/mg) in the presence of:**			
Mg^{2+} + EGTA	22.4	26.9	0.83
Ca^{2+}	158.5	147.3	1.08
Ca^{2+} + Mg^{2+}	234.4	170.0	1.38
Half-lives (sec) of total phosphoprotein formed in the presence of:***			
Mg^{2+} + EGTA	24.6	27.9	0.88
Ca^{2+}	48.6	133.2	0.36
Ca^{2+} + Mg^{2+}	18.6	33.3	0.56

   * Half-maximal activation of Ca^{2+} uptake was determined in the presence of 0.5 mM oxalate.
  ** Data for maximal phosphoprotein formation were obtained by extrapolation to zero time from the initial linear portion of a semilogarithmic plot.
*** Half-lives of total phosphoprotein were calculated from a semilogarithmic plot.

this peptide was proved radioautographically by the Ca^{2+}-dependent ^{32}P-phosphoprotein intermediate.

Phosphoprotein formation in microsomal preparations from SHR was lower by about 30% in the presence of Ca^{2+} and Mg^{2+}. The differences were much smaller when phosphorylation was performed in the presence of either Mg^{2+} or Ca^{2+} alone (table 1). Remarkable differences were found in the dephosphorylating activities in SR from NR and SHR. This is indicated by data for phosphoprotein half-lives in table 1. Half-lives for phosphoprotein formed by SR from SHR in the presence of Ca^{2+} and Mg^{2+} and with Ca^{2+} alone were higher by a factor of 1.8 and 2.7, respectively, as compared to NR. These findings suggest a delayed hydrolysis of the phosphoprotein intermediate of the Ca^{2+} transport ATPase in cardiac SR from SHR. Lower activities of Ca^{2+}-dependent ATPase and Ca^{2+} transport in SHR may be partially explained by the delayed dephosphorylation of the phosphoprotein intermediate since the latter is the rate limiting step during Ca^{2+} uptake by the SR (6).

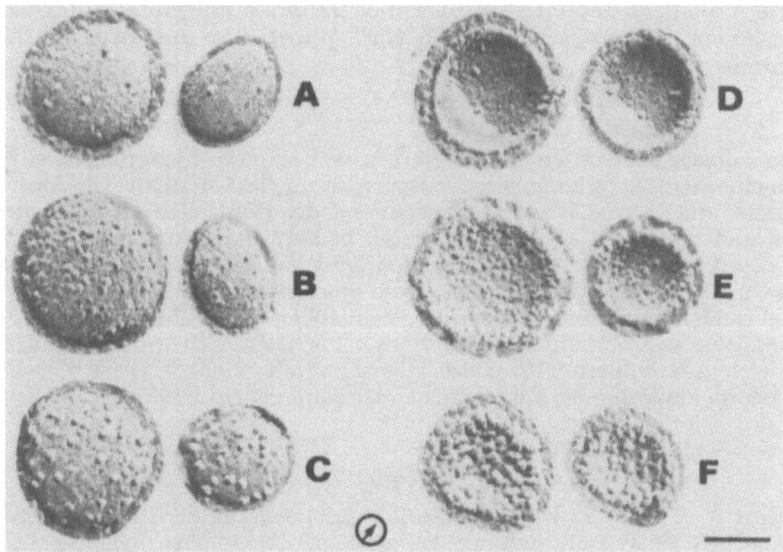

Fig. 2. Freeze-fracturing faces of microsomes from rat cardiac muscle. Typical examples of convex (A, B, C) and concave (D, E, F) vesicle faces are shown. For each class of faces two images are presented and oriented according to the direction of platinum shadowing (encircled arrow). Magnification: × 110.000; bar = 0.1 μm.

Ultrastructural studies by negative staining revealed a considerable heterogeneity of the vesicle preparation of both NR and SHR. No significant differences existed with regard to the vesicle types in NR and SHR. Freeze-fracturing of the vesicles made it possible to distinguish six different fracture faces (fig. 2, A–F) derived from various vesicle types. Intramembranous particles (IMP) were classified according to size and density per unit membrane area. Among these, IMP of 7–9 nm found in concave fracture faces (fig. 2, E) were interpreted as being morphological correlates of the Ca^{2+} pumping ATPase or an oligomer of it, in analogy to the findings on SR vesicles from rabbit skeletal muscle (7, 8). The density of these IMP was about half that seen in SR vesicles of fast-twitch skeletal muscle.

2000–3000 7–9 nm IMP per μm^2 were counted on concave faces E (fig. 2) of cardiac SR from NR, while 4000–6000 7–9 nm IMP per μm^2 were counted on the respective faces of SR from rabbit skeletal muscle. This indicates a lower density of Ca^{2+} transport ATPase per unit area of the membrane in rat cardiac SR. Fracture faces E (fig. 2) represented about one half of the concave faces of our preparations. Comparing density of these IMP between NR and SHR revealed a decrease by about 30% in the latter.

It may be concluded that Ca^{2+} homeostasis in hypertrophied left heart ventricles from SHR is disturbed in consequence of a decreased rate and capacity of Ca^{2+} sequestration by the SR. The molecular basis of the observed malfunction of the Ca^{2+} sequestering system may be explained by both a delayed dephosphorylation of the phosphorylated intermediate and a lower concentration of the Ca^{2+} pump per unit area of the SR membrane.

Zusammenfassung

Mikrosomale Präparationen aus Herzen von spontan hypertonischen Ratten zeigten eine signifikant herabgesetzte Kapazität zur Ca-Aufnahme. Die Aktivitäten von basaler und Extra-ATPase waren gegenüber den Kontrollen auf 40% erniedrigt. Initiale und gesamte Ca-Aufnahme waren in ähnlichem Ausmaß herabgesetzt. Diese Befunde lassen sich mit einer erniedrigten Konzentration der Ca-Transport-ATPase in SDS-Gelelektrophoresen sowie einer niedrigeren Dichte der 7–9-nm-Partikel in Membrangefrierbrüchen und schließlich den erhöhten Werten der für Phosphoproteine ermittelten Halbwertszeiten korrelieren. Die veränderte Kontraktilität des hypertrophierten Myokards läßt sich somit möglicherweise teilweise auf eine gestörte Funktion der mikrosomalen Membranen zurückführen.

References

1. *Alpert, N. R., M. S. Gordon:* Myofibrillar Adenosine Triphosphatase Activity in Congestive Heart Failure. Amer. J. Physiol. **202,** 940 (1962).
2. *Dhalla, N. S., D. K. Prasun, S. P. Gyan:* Subcellular Basis of Cardiac Contractile Failure. J. Mol. Cell. Cardiol. **10,** 363 (1978).
3. *Heilmann, C., D. Brdiczka, E. Nickel, D. Pette:* ATPase Activities, Ca^{2+} Transport and Phosphoprotein Formation in Sarcoplasmic Reticulum Subfractions of Fast and Slow Rabbit Muscles. Eur. J. Biochem. **81,** 211 (1977).
4. *Heilmann, C., D. Pette:* Molecular Transformations in Sarcoplasmic Reticulum of Fast-Twitch Muscle by Electro-Stimulation. Eur. J. Biochem. **93,** 437 (1979).
5. *Aoki, K., N. Ikeda, K. Yamashita, K. Hotta:* ATPase Activity and Ca^{2+} Interaction of Myofibrils and Sarcoplasmic Reticulum Isolated from the Hearts of Spontaneously Hypertensive Rats. Jap. Heart J. **15,** 475 (1974).
6. *Hasselbach, W.:* The Reversibility of the Sarcoplasmic Calcium Pump. Biochim. Biophys. Acta **515,** 23 (1978).
7. *Baskin, R. J., D. W. Deamer:* Comparative Ultrastructure and Calcium Transport in Heart and Skeletal Muscle Microsomes. J. Cell. Biol. **43,** 610 (1969).
8. *MacLennan, D. H., Ph. Seeman, G. H. Iles, C. C. Yip:* Membrane Formation by the Adenosine Triphosphatase of Sarcoplasmic Reticulum. J. Biol. Chem. **246,** 2702 (1971).

Authors' address:

Dr. *Claus Heilmann,* Medizinische Universitätsklinik, Hugstetter Str. 55, D-7800 Freiburg i. Br.
Dr. *Toni Lindl,* Hormon-Chemie München, Freisinger Landstr. 74, D-8000 München 45
Dr. *Werner Müller,* Zahnärztliches Institut der Universität Zürich, Abteilung für orale Strukturbiologie, Plattenstr. 11, CH-8028 Zürich
Prof. Dr. *Dirk Pette,* Universität Konstanz, Fachbereich Biologie, Postfach 55 60, D-7750 Konstanz 1

Basic Res. Cardiol. **75**, 97–104 (1980)
© 1980 Dr. Dietrich Steinkopff Verlag, Darmstadt
ISSN 0300–8428

Paper, presented at the Erwin Riesch Symposium, Tübingen, April 3–7, 1979

Institute of Physiology I, University of Goettingen

Functional alterations of cardiac subcellular structures during energy deficiency in relation to the metabolic state of the heart muscle cell*)

Funktionelles Verhalten subzellulärer Strukturen des Myokards während Sauerstoffmangel in Relation zum Metabolitstatus der Herzmuskelzelle

P. G. Spieckermann, M. M. Gebhard, G. G. Göring, H. Kahles, V. A. Mezger, C. J. Preuße, and *M. Stellwaag*

With 3 figures

Summary

The functional behaviour of membrane systems of the cardiac cell during oxygen deficiency was analyzed and the alterations were related to the metabolic state of the tissue as an index of injury.
1. The retention function of the cell membrane for proteins. With increasing energy deficiency the cardiac sarcolemma loses its ability to retain macromolecules (myoglobin, enzymes) within the cell. Close correlations exist between protein release and oxygen supply as well as ATP content of the tissue.
2. Function of isolated mitochondria after ischemia. In parallel with a strong impairment of oxidative phosphorylation (decrease of Q_{O_2}, RCI values, phosphorylation rates) the Ca^{++}-transporting activity of mitochondria is continuously depressed with decreasing myocardial ATP.
3. Function of isolated sarcoplasmic reticulum after ischemia. With breakdown of high energy phosphates during ischemia rate and extent of Ca^{++} binding both decrease markedly.

The balance of energy in the myocardium can be equalized only under aerobic conditions. During an oxygen deficïency, anaerobic glycolysis can secure only a part of the myocardial energy demand. This automatically causes a deficiency in energy that manifests itself in the disturbance of all energy-consuming processes and can finally lead to irreversible damage of the tissue. The functional, structural and biochemical changes during ischemia or anoxia have been extensively analysed, but surprisingly, little is known about the function of subcellular structures in relation to the metabolic state of the tissue.

The primary events of myocardial damage during an energetic disequilibrium must occur on a subcellular and molecular level. We have therefore examined the functional behaviour of myocardial membrane systems during oxygen deficiency and tried to relate the alterations to the metabolic state of the heart muscle.

*) Supported by the Deutsche Forschungsgemeinschaft, SFB 89 – Kardiologie Goettingen.

1. The retention function of the cell membrane for proteins

The organization of a cell is – thermodynamically seen – a very improbable state. Enzyme retention or the "prevention of enzyme leakiness" *(Zierler)* therefore seems to be – directly or indirectly – an energy-consuming process. We have examined in which way the retention function of the cell membrane for proteins changes during states of imbalance of myocardial energy metabolism.

Experiments were carried out on the Langendorff-perfused guinea pig heart. In a first group of experiments, myocardial enzyme release under reduced energy supply was examined. The hearts were subjected to a) total heart ischemia of different duration and b) hypoxic or anoxic perfusion.

During aerobic reperfusion after ischemic periods of 5, 10, 20 or 30 minutes, the shape of the enzyme release curve was always the same: After an initial maximum of enzyme release, in all cases preischemic control values were reached within 5–7 minutes of reperfusion period *(Sakai* et al. 1975). Plotting integral postischemic enzyme release during 5 minutes against duration of perfusion stop resulted in a direct correlation between these two determinants (fig. 1, left above). Because irreversible cell damage under our conditions is not to be expected after only 5 or 10 minutes of ischemia, myocardial enzyme release, therefore, occurs significantly prior to myocardial cytolysis *(Spieckermann* et al. 1973, *De Leiris* et al. 1969).

For examining protein release under different O_2-deficiency conditions, the perfusate was equilibrated with gas mixtures containing 0, 5, 10 or 25% O_2 in 5% CO_2 and N_2. During this stepwise reduction of oxygen supply the enzyme and myoglobin release was stepwise elevated. The correlation between O_2-supply and enzyme release follows an inverse power function (fig. 1, right above) *(Gebhard* et al. 1977).

After analysing the effects of reduced energy supply in a second group of experiments, the myocardial enzyme release during reduced energy demand of the heart was examined. The energy requirements were varied by reducing perfusion temperature, by β-blockade or reserpinisation.

The release of MDH, LDH, and CPK during anoxic perfusion at 15 °C in comparison with 25 or 35 °C was significantly lowered.

The correlation between perfusion temperature and enzyme release could be quantified in the Arrhenius plot (fig. 1, lower left). There resulted temperature coefficients of nearly 2–2.5 for release of these enzymes similar to those found for metabolic parameters such as anaerobic ATP breakdown, heart rate, or O_2 consumption in the myocardium. Q_{10} values for enzyme loss during aerobiosis between 1.2 and 1.5 may indicate that for physiological enzyme liberation mainly physicochemical factors are responsible *(Gebhard* et al. 1977). Myocardial β-blockade or reserpinisation resulted in a marked reduction of enzyme release (see also *De Leiris* et al. 1972) with a surprisingly strong effect of propranolol *(Sakai* and *Spieckermann* 1975).

These experimental results support the assumption that there is a strong relationship between energy metabolism and enzyme release. Reducing energy supply to the heart – as is done by total heart ischemia or

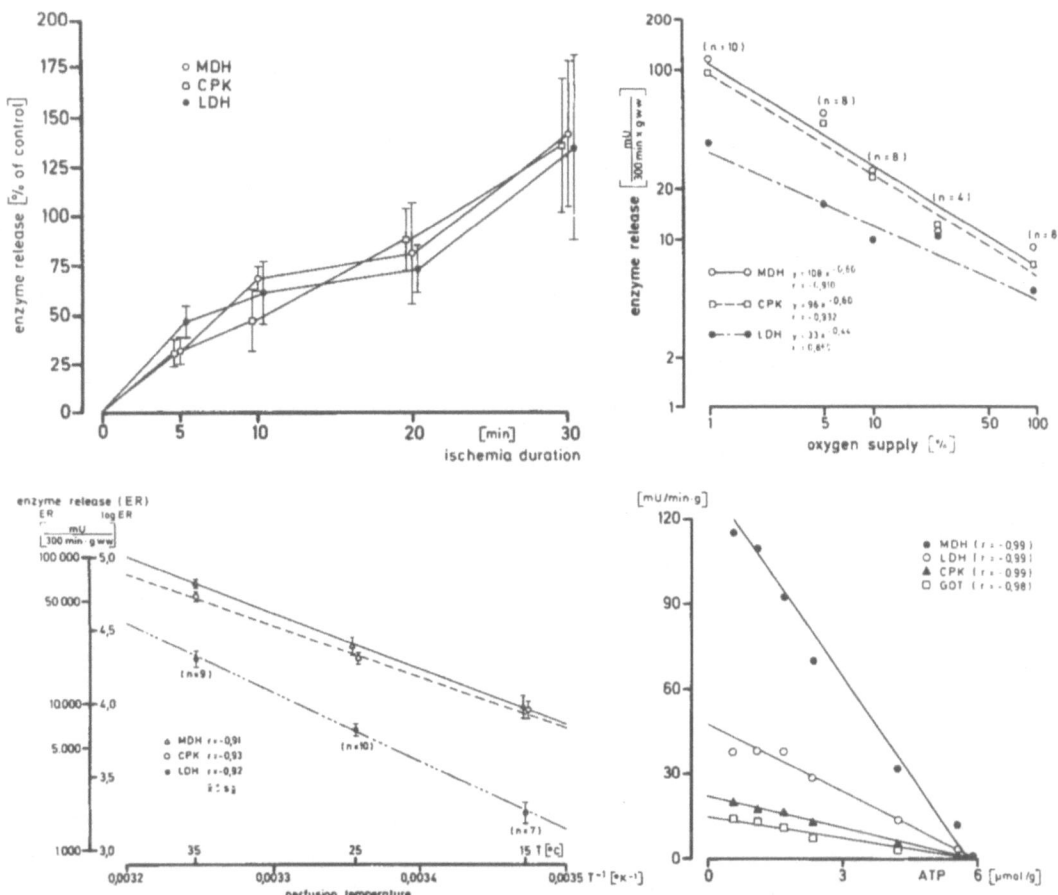

Fig. 1. Myocardial enzyme release and energy metabolism. Above: Relations between postischemic enzyme liberation and ischemia duration (left) and between enzyme release and oxygen supply (right). Below: Influence of temperature on integral enzyme release during 300 min anoxic perfusion (Arrhenius-plot) (left). Enzyme release rate in relation to the ATP-content (ww) of the left ventricle (right).

hypoxic perfusion – is followed by cellular enzyme release. Reducing energy demand during reduced energy supply situations – by β-blockade or reserpinisation or lowering temperature during anoxia – decreases enzyme release. Hence, we may conclude that, for the membrane "permeability" and cell enzyme release, the relation between energy supply and energy demand is decisive. Myocardial cell plasma membranes become permeable for intracellular enzyme proteins if cells come into an energy deficient state. Moreover, the relationship between postischemic enzyme release and ischemia duration, the correlation between enzyme release and O_2 supply in hypoxia and also the temperature dependency of the anoxia caused enzyme release show that cellular enzyme loss increases with rising energy deficiency of the cell.

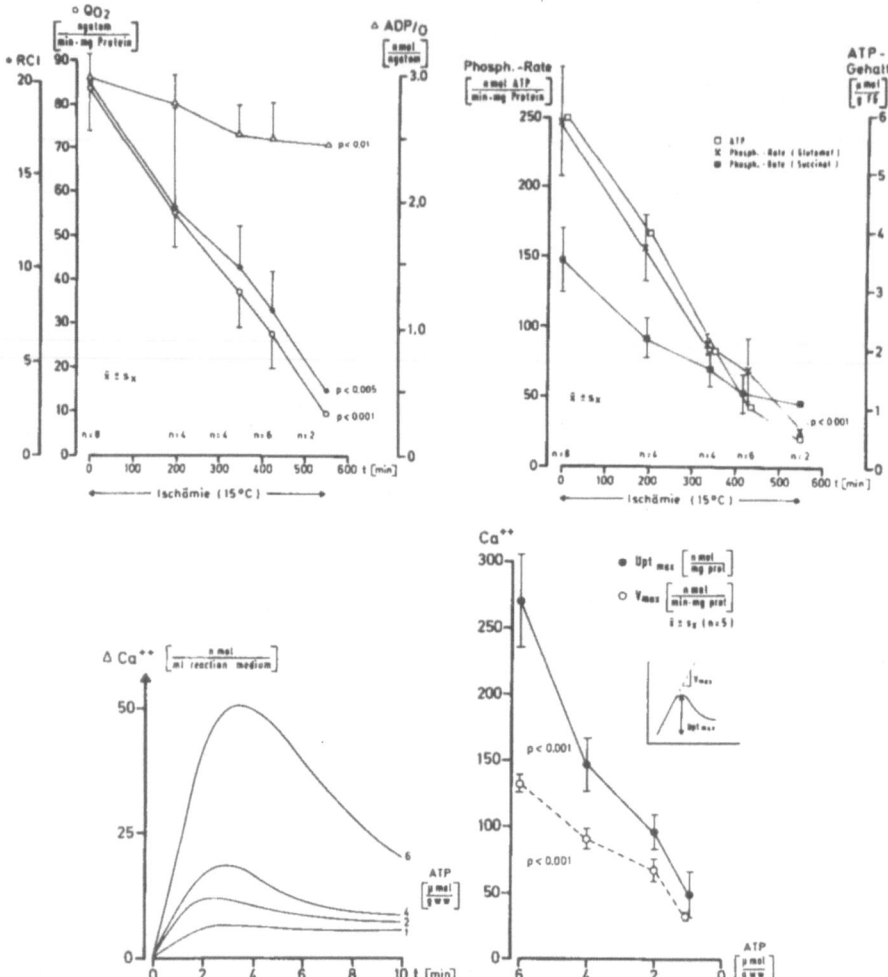

Fig. 2. Oxidative phosphorylation and Ca++-transport parameters of canine heart mitochondria isolated after different durations of ischemia (cardioplegia). Above: Oxygen consumption, ADP/$_0$-ratios and RCJ-values (left) as well as phosphorylation rates and myocardial ATP content (right) after different durations of ischemia. Below: Superimposed original records of mitochondrial Ca++-transport in relation to the metabolic state (ATP) of the myocardium (left). Mitochondrial Ca++-uptake (upt$_{max}$) and uptake rate (v$_{max}$) as a function of myocardial ATP content.

If these conclusions are correct, one may expect that there is a correlation between intramyocardial metabolic parameters and enzyme release (*Spieckermann* et al. 1975).

10 isolated dog hearts were subjected to a non-recirculatory anoxic perfusion at 25 °C with Tyrode-glucose-solution after an aerobic steady state period. In 5 experiments the appearance of enzymes in the sinus effluent, in the remaining experiments the left ventricular tissue contents of creatine phosphate, ATP and lactate were determined. This was done in order to eliminate effects of mechanical cell disruption during sampling

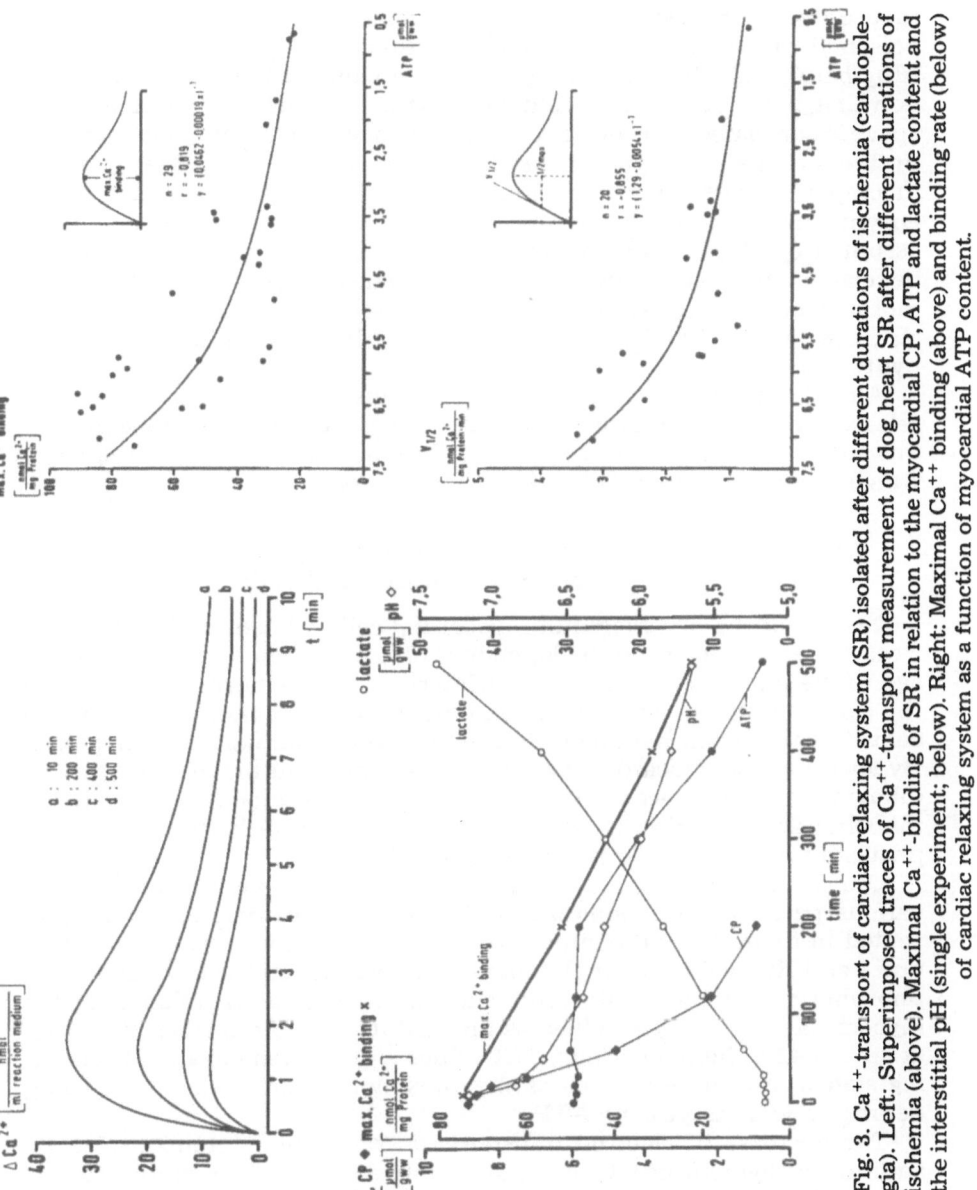

Fig. 3. Ca^{++}-transport of cardiac relaxing system (SR) isolated after different durations of ischemia (cardioplegia). Left: Superimposed traces of Ca^{++}-transport measurement of dog heart SR after different durations of ischemia (above). Maximal Ca^{++}-binding of SR in relation to the myocardial CP, ATP and lactate content and the interstitial pH (single experiment; below). Right: Maximal Ca^{+} binding (above) and binding rate (below) of cardiac relaxing system as a function of myocardial ATP content.

on enzyme activities. The experimental conditions were otherwise identical in both groups.

The rate of enzyme release was the higher the smaller the myocardial ATP content (fig. 1, right below). Similar results have been reported for mouse livers infected by virus hepatitis (*Mancini* et al. 1966) and also for poisoned or substrate free incubated human red cells and leucocytes (*Englhardt* et al. 1969). These findings are incompatible with the assumption that the occurrence of cellular enzyme proteins in the extracellular space is correlated to a certain critical state of cell structure as is supposed by the so-called cytolysis theory of cell enzyme release. They are also incompatible with the supposition that the extracellular occurrence of cell enzymes is correlated to a certain critical state of cell metabolism as assumed by *Hearse* and *Chain* (1973) for the isolated rat heart. They may be related, however, to new plasma membrane concepts such as the "fluid mosaic model" which suggest the plasma membrane to be a very dynamic structure, whose "fluidity", for example, clearly can be influenced by ATP hydrolysis.

Already in 1958 *Zierler*, on the basis of his studies in cellular enzyme release, postulated plasma membrane to be oscillating; permeability of this membrane he proposed to be a function of oscillation frequency which might be a metabolism-dependent factor.

2. Calcium transport and oxidative phosphorylation of isolated mitochondria after "in situ" ischemia

20–30% of the dry weight of myocardial cells related to mitochondria. Because the myocardium is dependent on aerobic energy delivery, damage to the mitochondria must be deleterious for the normal functions of the cell. Our studies were made on mitochondria isolated by differential centrifugation from hypothermic canine myocardium after cardioplegia. By lowering the myocardial energy requirements, this model permits us to follow the consequences of ischemia in a slow motion manner. Parallel to mitochondrial function analysis the tissue content of high energy phosphates during the course of ischemia was determined.

Oxidative phosphorylation parameters of mitochondria isolated after various periods of ischemia during hypothermic cardiac arrest are presented in figure 2: on the left above the ADP/O ratios, oxygen consumption – and RCI values with glutamate as substrate, on the right above the phosphorylation rates with glutamate and succinate in relation to the myocardial ATP content. Whereas the ADP/O ratio diminishes little even at advanced ischemic periods, RCI values and oxygen consumption during state-3 respiration as well as the phosphorylation rates are markedly depressed with decreasing ATP.

The decrease of electron transport can be partially compensated by addition of cytochrome C to isolated mitochondria. This stimulation is more effective in mitochondria isolated after advanced durations of myocardial ischemia (*Kahles* et al. 1977). In addition to the successive reduction of electron flow during ischemia the calcium transport of mitochondria is also impaired. Ca transport across mitochondrial membranes was analysed continuously with a Dual-wavelength spectrometer and murexide as a Ca-sensitive indicator. Mitochondria take up Ca and this Ca can be partially released if the Ca/mitochondrial protein ratio in the test exceeds a critical level ($\sim$ 400 nmol Ca/mg$_{Prot}$) (*Göring* et al. 1977). This can bee seen in analogy to the findings of *Katz*. As in SR, a Ca-induced Ca release must also be discussed for mitochondria.

Figure 2 lower left shows superimposed traces of original records. With decreasing moycardial ATP the Ca transport activity is depressed. The relationship between ATP and two parameters of Ca transport activity – the maximal uptake and the uptake velocity v_{max} – appears in the diagram right below. The decrement of both parameters with decreasing ATP is with $p < 0.001$ highly significant (*Göring* and *Spieckermann* 1978). These changes during ischemia may help to understand early processes in myocardial cell damage such as, for example, contracture phenomena.

3. Calcium transport of isolated sarcoplasmic reticulum

In parallel to these measurements we analysed in the same specimens the Ca transport properties of the cardiac relaxing system after isolation by differential centrifugation. Similar to the behaviour of mitochondria, the vesicles show Ca-binding and release phenomena (fig. 3 left above). With increasing duration of ischemia the curves were depressed. In the lower left portion of figure 3 the maximal Ca binding is related to metabolic parameters of the tissue as CP, ATP, lactate, and the intramyocardial pH.

This diagram gives the protocol of a single experiment, in the right two figures all measurements of binding (above) and binding velocity (below) are plotted against the myocardial ATP content. The points are best fitted by hyperbolic functions with correlation coefficients between 0.8 and 0.9. Similar correlations we found for lactate and the interstitial pH (*Stellwaag* et al. 1979).

These findings give a phenomenology of functional changes of subcellular structures during oxygen deficiency. Proceeding from these results we hope to find possibilities of restimulating mitochondria and the relaxing system and restoring the barrier function of the cell membrane.

Zusammenfassung

Das funktionelle Verhalten von Membransystemen der Herzmuskelzelle während Sauerstoffmangel wurde untersucht und die Veränderungen in Beziehung gesetzt zum Metabolitstatus des Gewebes als Index für die Zellschädigung.
1. Die Retentionsfunktion der Zellmembran für Proteine. Mit zunehmendem Energiedefizit verliert die Zellmembran die Fähigkeit, Makromoleküle (Myoglobin, Enzyme) innerhalb der Zelle zu retinieren. Zwischen Proteinfreisetzung und O_2-Versorgung bzw. Gewebs-ATP bestehen enge Korrelationen.
2. Funktion isolierter Mitochondrien nach Ischämie. Parallel zur Einschränkung der oxidativen Phosphorylierung (Abnahme von Q_{O_2}, RCI-Werten, Phosphorylierungsraten) nimmt die Ca^{++}-Transport-Aktivität der Mitochondrien mit Abfall des Gewebs-ATP kontinuierlich ab.
3. Funktion des isolierten sarkoplasmatischen Retikulums nach Ischämie. Mit dem Zerfall der energiereichen Phosphate während Ischämie werden Rate und Ausmaß der Ca^{++}-Bindung an das SR stark eingeschränkt.

References

1. *De Leiris, J., D. Breton, D. Feuvray, E. Coraboeuf:* Lactico-dehydrogenase release from perfused rat heart under the effect of abnormal media. Arch. Int. Physiol. Biochem. **77**, 749 (1969).
2. *De Leiris, J., D. Feuvray, C. Come:* Acetylcholine-induced release of lactate dehydrogenase from isolated perfused rat heart. J. Molec. Cell. Cardiol. **4**, 357 (1972).
3. *Englhardt, A., G. Schmidt-Sodingen, H. Lange:* Metabolitgehalt und Enzympermeabilität isolierter menschlicher Blutzellen bei Substratmangel und Zusatz von Stoffwechselgiften. Enzym. biol. clin. **10**, 258 (1969).
4. *Gebhard, M. M., H. Denkhaus, K. Sakai, P. G. Spieckermann:* Relations between energy metabolism and enzyme release. J. Molec. Med. **2**, 271 (1977).
5. *Göring, G. G., W. G. Nayler, P. G. Spieckermann:* The release of calcium from cardiac mitochondria: The importance of the Ca/protein ratio. Basic Res. Cardiol. **72**, 77 (1977).
6. *Göring, G. G., P. G. Spieckermann:* Ca^{2+} uptake and -release phenomena from cardiac mitochondria under normal and ischemic conditions. Basic Res. Cardiol. **73**, 126 (1978).
7. *Hearse, D. J., E. B. Chain:* Effect of glucose on enzyme release from, and recovery of the anoxic myocardium. In: *Dhalla, N. S.* (Ed.): Myocardial metabolism. Recent advances in studies on cardiac structure and metabolism, Vol. 3, p. i (Baltimore 1973).
8. *Kahles, H., G. Göring, H. Nordbeck, C. J. Preusse, P. G. Spieckermann:* Functional behaviour of isolated heart muscle mitochondria after in situ ischemia. Polarographic analysis of mitochondrial oxidative phosphorylation. Basic Res. Cardiol. **72**, 563 (1977).
9. *Katz, A. M.:* Regulatory effects adenosinetriphosphate on the cardiac contractile process. Basic Res. Cardiol. **75**, 103 (1980).
10. *Mancini, A., B. Galanti, G. Gnisti:* Veränderungen des ATP-Gehaltes im Lebergewebe der Maus bei experimenteller Virus-MHV-3-Hepatitis. Enzym. biol. clin. **6**, 279 (1966).
11. Sakai, K., P. G. Spieckermann: Effects of reserpine and propranolol on enzyme release resulting from anoxia in the isolated perfused guinea pig heart. Naunyn.-Schmiedebergs Arch. Pharmacol. **291**, 123 (1975).
12. *Sakai, K., M. Gebhard, P. G. Spieckermann, H. J. Bretschneider:* Enzyme release resulting from ischemia in the isolated perfused guinea pig heart. J. Molec. Cell. Cardiol. **7**, 827 (1975).
13. *Spieckermann, P. G., M. Gebhard, K. Kalbow, D. Knoll, F. Kohl, H. Nordbeck, K. Sakai, H. J. Bretschneider:* Freisetzung von Enzymen aus der Herzmuskelzelle während Sauerstoffmangel. Verh. dtsch. Ges. Kreisl.-Forschg. **39**, 193 (1973).
14. *Spieckermann, P. G., M. M. Gebhard, H. Nordbeck:* Role of energy metabolism in enzyme retention. A study on isolated perfused canine hearts. Experientia **31**, 1046 (1975).
15. *Stellwaag, M., M. M. Gebhard, G. G. Göring, H. Kahles, C. J. Preusse, P. G. Spieckermann:* Functional behaviour of isolated cardiac relaxing system after 'in situ' ischemia. Pflügers Arch. **379**, Suppl. R 59 (1979).
16. *Zierler, K. L.:* Increased muscle permeability to aldolase, produced by depolarisation and by metabolic inhibitors. Amer. J. Physiol. **193**, 534 (1958).

Authors' address:

Prof. Dr. med. *P. G. Spieckermann,* Institute of Physiology I, University of Goettingen, Humboldtallee 7, D-3400 Goettingen

Basic Res. Cardiol. **75**, 105–108 (1980)
© 1980 Dr. Dietrich Steinkopff Verlag, Darmstadt
ISSN 0300–8428

Paper, presented at the Erwin Riesch Symposium, Tübingen, April 3–7,1979

*Unité de Recherches de Pathologie Cardiovasculaire de l'I.N.S.E.R.M., Hôpital
Léon Bernard, 94450 Limeil-Brévannes (France)*

Aorto-caval fistula in the rat. An experimental model of heart volume overloading

Aorto-kavaler Kurzschluß bei der Ratte. Ein experimentelles Modell für das volumenbelastete Herz

P. Y. Hatt, K. Rakusan, P. Gastineau, M. Laplace,
and *F. Cluzeaud*

Summary

Abdominal aorto-caval fistula was experimentally induced in rats, and animals were sacrificed 5 days, 1 month, and 6 months later.

Cardiac weight almost doubled the normal weight during the first month. Cell length increased to the same extent as the cell width, indicating harmonious growth. Increase in cell volume, as well as the amount of degenerative changes, were more pronounced in subendocardium than in midwall and subepicardium.

Cytological features of active cellular growth was found not only in the early stages (5 days and 1 month) but also 6 months after the operation. This finding is consonant with proteosynthesis stimulation not only in the early period of constitution of hypertrophy but also in the later stages.

Most of the procedures experimentally utilized to reproduce human heart hypertrophy (and failure) induce either subacute heart failure or heart hypertrophy of only moderate degree. This may explain some differences between human and animal: heart can double or triple its normal weight in human, although it rarely exceeds more than 150% of the control weight in animal. Beyond a "critical weight" cell hypertrophy could be replaced by hyperplasia (2, 12) in man, that was never confirmed in animal. Polyploidy often found in nuclei from human cardiac myocytes (16) was very rarely detected in experimental conditions (10).

The purpose of the present study was to produce slowly developing heart hypertrophy by experimental aorto-caval fistula in the rat and to study the increase in heart weight, myocardial cells' dimensions and cytology at different stages of the load.

Female Wistar rats with an average body weight of 200 g were subjected to a 1.5 mm wide aorto-caval fistula, between abdominal aorta (below the origin of left renal artery) and vena cava.

Animals were sacrificed after 5 days, 1 month and 6 months respectively. Only animals with largely patent fistula (vena cava stretched, reddish and pulsatile) were retained. Heart was fixed in vivo by an intra-aortic perfusion of fixative and subsequently examined in light and electron microscope.

The permeability of the fistula was verified by serial sections.

Heart weight as well as heart-weight-to-body-weight ratio increased significantly after 1 and 6 months. This increase reached 182% within the first month and regained the normal rate of growth during the 5 further months.

Cell dimensions were estimated in subendocardial and midwall layers on longitudinal sections. Cell width was easy to estimate. But cell length was not, for a least two reasons: true longitudinal sections were rare, and distances between intercalated discs vary from one cell to the other and within the same cell (1, 9, 11, 15).

Therefore the length-to-width ratio was recorded in a great number of myocytes with well-defined boundaries and the results were pooled separately for control and operated animals. In both groups, the length-to-width ratio being similar, it was used for our estimates of cell volume from cell width and assuming a cylindrical model.

Cell width and volume were, in controls, similar in subendocardial and midwall regions while, in experimental animals, they increased moderately in the midwall region and considerably in the subendocardium.

A comparison between the relative increase in heart weight and cell volume showed rather complex features: within the first month, heart weight increased as much as subendocardial cell volume, and more than midwall cell volume. After 6 months, subendocardial cell volume continued to increase out of proportion with heart weight, while midwall cell volume regained a normal rate of growth. The relative increase in the average cell volume was rather parallel to the increase in heart weight.

It is difficult to interprete these data as we don't know the exact contribution of each layer to the total heart weight.

Nevertheless the rather parallel evolution of heart weight and average cell volume seems to indicate that most if not all cardiac growth was due to simple hypertrophy.

Something new is the predominance of cell hypertrophy in subendocardium, which was previously found in rats subjected to transitory abdominal aorta constriction (7). It let us suppose an unequal distribution of either the work performed or the blood supply throughout the ventricular wall, as formerly proposed by *Holtz* et al. (8).

Some cytological features may be related to active cellular growth. The size of the nucleolus and of its nucleolonema, the number of nucleoli per nucleus were significantly increased not only at 5 days but still after 1 and 6 months of overloading. Similar finding was quoted in human heart hypertrophy (3).

Rudimentary myofibrils taking place under the sarcolemma at the periphery of the cell could signify some process of centrifugal growth of the myocyte. Similar aspects were found formerly during the early stages of a two steps overloading in the rat (6).

Intercalated disc was rather disorganized as well as neighbouring myofibrils. These figures are very similar to other ones found in the early stages of aortic insufficiency in the rabbit (6). They are very similar to other pictures of sarcomerogenesis depicted in various types of embryonic muscle during growth.

Such features of active growth were encountered in the present experimentation not only at the end of the first month but even after 6 months in some animals. This observation is consonant with the persistence of cell growth and increased proteosynthesis not only in the period of stable compensatory hypertrophy but also in later stages. This is in contradiction to the usual opinion in that matter (13).

Mitochondria had a general tendency to proliferate, increase their number and decrease their size. Similar findings were encountered in a two steps overloading (6) where they were morphologically confirmed.

Cell lesions were few and present at 6 months in only one rat (out of 7). Some of these lesions displayed the characteristics of cell damage recently described under the name of "Shredding" (4). Some others looked like oldier, with isolated myocytes and interstitial histiocytosis.

Most often, myocytes looked like only hypertrophied, with an apparently active nucleus. In two rats this total absence of any lesions was coincident with evident heart failure: subcutaneous edema, liver and lung congestion.

This latter point confirms the old statement of *Aschoff*, recalled by *Linzbach* (12), according to whom heart failure was a matter for physiologists and not for morphologists.

In conclusion aorto-caval fistula is a convenient model of volume overloading easy to be performed. It induces chronically developing heart hypertrophy and eventually heart failure. The gain in ventricle weight attains about twice the control weight within the first month.

As other types of volume load, it induces an harmonious growth of the myocardial cells with preservation of length-to-width ratio.

Two peculiar findings evidenced in this experiment are that

1) cell hypertrophy is not homogeneous throughout the ventricular wall. It predominates in the subendocardial layers.

2) Cytological features of active cellular growth were found not only in the early stages but also in the later stages of overloading.

Zusammenfassung

Bei Ratten wurde eine aorto-kavale Fistel erzeugt. Die Tiere wurden 5 Tage, 1 Monat bzw. 6 Monate nach dem Eingriff getötet. Während des ersten Monats kam es annähernd zu einer Verdoppelung des Herzgewichts. Die Länge der Zelle nahm um dasselbe Ausmaß zu wie der Querdurchmesser, als Hinweis für harmonisches Wachstum. Sowohl die Zunahme des Zellvolumens als auch das Ausmaß degenerativer Veränderungen traten subendokardial stärker in Erscheinung als in Wandmitte oder subepikardial. Zytologische Charakteristika aktiven Zellwachstums wurden nicht nur in·den Frühstadien gefunden (nach 5 Tagen bzw. 1 Monat), sondern auch noch 6 Monate nach der Operation. Dieser Befund ist in Einklang mit einer Stimulierung der Proteinsynthese nicht nur im Anfangsstadium der Hypertrophiebildung, sondern auch in späteren Stadien.

References

1. *Angelakos, E. T., P. Bernardini, W. C. Barrett:* Myocardial fiber size and capillary-fiber ratio in the right and left ventricles of the rat. Anatomical Record **149**, 671–676 (1964).

2. *Astorri, E., R. Bonognesi, B. Colla, A. Chizzola, O. Visioli:* Left ventricular hypertrophy: A cytometric study on 42 human hearts. Journal of Molecular and Cellular Cardiology **9**, 763–775 (1977).
3. *Bloom, S., D. Egli:* Variation of myocardial nucleolar abundance with heart weight. Proceedings of the Society for Experimental Biology and Medicine **130**, 1019–1021 (1969).
4. *Cuenoud, H. F., I. Joris, G. Majno:* Ultrastructure of myocardium after pulmonary embolism. A study in the rat. American Journal of Pathology **92**, 421–458 (1978).
5. *Edington, D. W., A. C. Cosmas:* Effects of maturation and training on mitochondrial size distributions in rat heart. Journal of Applied Physiology **33**, 715–718 (1972).
6. *Hatt, P. Y.:* Cellular changes in mechanically overloaded heart. Basic Research in Cardiology **72**, 198–202 (1977).
7. *Hatt, P. Y., P. Jouannot, J. Moravec, J. Perennec, M. Laplace:* Development and reversal of pressure-induced cardiac hypertrophy. Light and electron microscopic study in the rat under temporary aortic constriction. Basic Research in Cardiology **73**, 405–421 (1978).
8. *Holtz, J., W. von Restorff, P. Bard, E. Bassenge:* Transmural distribution of myocardial blood flow and or coronary reserve in canine left ventricular hypertrophy. Basic Research in Cardiology **72**, 286–292 (1977).
9. *Korecky, B., K. Rakusan:* Normal and hypertrophic growth of the rat heart: changes in cell dimensions and number. American Journal of Physiology **243**, 123–128 (1978).
10. *Kuhn, H., P. Pfitzer, K. Stoepel:* DNA content and DNA synthesis in the myocardium of rats after induced renal hypertension. Cardiovascular Research **8**, 86–91 (1974).
11. *Laks, M. M., M. J. Nisenson, H. J. Swan:* Myocardial cells and sarcomere lengths in the normal dog heart. Circulation Research **21**, 671–678 (1967).
12. *Linzbach, A. J.:* Heart failure from the point of view of quantitative anatomy. American Journal of Cardiology **5**, 370–382 (1960).
13. *Meerson, F. Z.:* The myocardium in hyperfunction, hypertrophy and heart failure. Circulation Research **25** (n° 1 suppl. II), 1–163 (1969).
14. *Rakusan, K., O. Poupa:* Changes in the diffusion distance in the rat heart during development. Physiologia Bohemoslovica **12**, 220–227 (1963).
15. *Rakusan, K., S. Raman, R. Layberry, B. Korecky:* The influence of ageing and growth on the post natal development of cardiac muscle in the rats. Circulation Research **42**, 212–218 (1978).
16. *Sandritter, W., C. P. Adler:* Numerical hyperplasia in human heart hypertrophy. Experientia **27**, 1435–1437 (1971).
17. *Weibel, E. R., S. K. Gonzague, F. L. Walter:* Practical stereological methods for morphometric cytology. Journal of Cell Biology **30**, 23–38 (1966).

Authors' address:

Dr. *P. Y. Hatt*, Unité de Recherches de Pathologie Cardiovasculaire de l'I.N.-S.E.R.M., Hôpital Léon Bernard, 94450 Limeil-Brévannes (France)

Basic Res. Cardiol. **75**, 109–117 (1980)
© 1980 Dr. Dietrich Steinkopff Verlag, Darmstadt
ISSN 0300–8428

Paper, presented at the Erwin Riesch Symposium, Tübingen, April 3–7, 1979

Max-Planck-Institut für physiologische und klinische Forschung, W.-G.-Kerckhoff-Institut, 6350 Bad Nauheim, West Germany

Quantitative ultrastructure of the myocardium in chronic aortic valve disease

Quantitative ultrastrukturelle Befunde des Myokards bei Patienten mit chronischen Aortenklappenvitien

F. Schwarz, D. Kittstein, B. Winkler, and *J. Schaper*

With 3 figures and 2 tables

Summary

Light and electron microscopic morphometry was carried out in tissue samples which were obtained from the left ventricular free wall in 29 patients with chronic aortic valve disease during open-heart surgery. 6 patients had aortic stenosis, 9 had aortic insufficiency and 14 had a mixed aortic valve lesion. Hemodynamics were studied before operation. Patients with mixed aortic valve disease had a higher left ventricular mass, a lower ejection fraction and mean circumferential fiber shortening rate than patients with aortic stenosis. Peak systolic wall stress was comparable between groups. The intracellular content of contractile material was lower and the sarcoplasmic volume was higher in mixed aortic valve disease than in aortic stenosis. Mitochondrial volume and interstitial fibrosis were not different between groups. Patients with aortic insufficiency showed no significant difference of parameters as compared to both other groups. We conclude that an intracellular deficiency of myofibrils causes lack of contractility in advanced hypertrophy due to mixed aortic valve disease.

It is generally accepted that myocardial failure develops in advanced left ventricular hypertrophy due to work overload. It was suggested that an increased amount of fibrotic content of the myocardium may be the cause of myocardial failure (1). Recently ultrastructural degenerative changes of the myocardium have been detected and these changes were advocated as morphological correlates of depressed cardiac function in hypertrophied hearts (2). We were able to show in an earlier study that degenerative cell changes can be found in the myocardium of patients with pressure- or volume-overloaded left ventricles due to aortic valve disease. We also found that the degree of fibrotic content of the myocardium did not correlate with the degree of left ventricular dysfunction as estimated during heart catheterization and angiography (3). Furthermore, surgical correction of the diseased valve produced complete recovery of myocardial function even in cases with cardiac failure preoperatively. Therefore the significance of the ultrastructural findings in chronic aortic valve disease remains debatable.

This study quantitates
1. the intracellular content of contractile material, mitochondria and sarcoplasm (empty space) and
2. the interstitial myocardial fibrosis. It was then attempted to correlate ultrastructural changes and hemodynamic findings in these patients.

Methods

We studied 29 patients with isolated aortic valve disease between 2 and 6 weeks before aortic valve replacement. Predominant aortic stenosis was found in 6 patients, predominant aortic insufficiency in 9 patients and a mixed aortic valve lesion in 14 patients (aortic stenosis plus aortic insufficiency). Aortic stenosis was defined as a transvalve gradient without significant aortic regurgitation as estimated by aortic root angiography (4). Aortic insufficiency was defined as a significant aortic regurgitation without any transvalve gradient. All remaining cases were assembled as mixed aortic valve disease. Associated mitral valve disease was excluded in all patients. Obstructive coronary artery disease was not found in any patient of this series during selective coronary arteriography using the Judkins technique.

Patients were studied during heart catheterization. A no. 8.5 F Brockenbrough catheter was positioned in the left ventricle transseptally, and a no. 8 F pigtail catheter was inserted into the ascending aorta. Before injection of contrast material, right and left heart pressures were measured (P 23 Db Statham transducers). Single plane 35 mm cineangiograms of the left ventricle were filmed at a rate of 48 frames per second in the 30° right anterior oblique projection after injection of 50 ml Urografin 76. Simultaneously the aortic pressure was recorded with a paper speed of 100 mm per second. In all patients aortic root angiography was performed to estimate the degree of regurgitation.

From the cineangiograms, left ventricular end-diastolic and end-systolic volumes were calculated using the area length method (5). Left ventricular mass, ejection fraction, mean circumferential fiber shortening rate, and peak systolic wall stress were calculated according to standard formula (6, 7).

Tissues were obtained by biopsy from each patient at the time of open heart surgery. We used a Tru-cut biopsy needle (Travenol laboratories) to take a transmural biopsy specimen from the left ventricular anterior free wall. The specimen was taken before crossclamping of the aorta from the beating heart. Immediately after biopsy the tissues were fixed as previously described (3). Semithin sections of 1 to 2 μm thickness were prepared and stained with alkaline toluidine blue for light microscopy. Each block measured 1 to 4 mm² in area. Morphometry for fibrosis was carried out with the light microscope using a grid with 110 points. According to the basic principles of morphometry (8), counting of the number of points overlying a structure results in a quantitative determination of the volume of the structure in relation to the volume of the entire tissue under the grid. Longitudinal sections at a magnification of 250 × were evaluated and blood vessels and perivascular interstitial cells were excluded. For quantitative determination of intracellular structures photographs of ultrathin sections were made using a Philips electron microscope 300. Photographs were made in a random sampling manner using a magnification of 10.000 ×. Intracellular structures were determined by counting of at least 40 photographs in each patient. The average value for contractile material, mitochondria, and empty space in each patient was taken as the representative value. The fractional volume of these 3 structures was expressed as %.

Table 1. Mean values ± SD for hemodynamic, angiographic and morphometric data in patients with aortic stenosis (AS), insufficiency (AI), and patients with mixed aortic valve disease (AS & AI).

	AS (n = 6)	AI (n = 9)	AS + AI (n = 14)	AS vs AI	AI vs AS + AI	AS vs AS + AI
Hemodynamic data						
Heart rate (min^{-1})	72.8 ± 9.8	83.5 ± 15.1	81.7 ± 14.8	ns	ns	ns
Left ventricular systolic pressure (mm Hg)	198.7 ± 16.1	146.0 ± 14.5	200.1 ± 42.3	< 0.001	< 0.001	ns
Peak to peak systolic transvalvular gradient (mm Hg)	76.8 ± 25.7	0.0 ± 0.0	81.1 ± 46.0	< 0.001	< 0.001	ns
Left ventricular end-diastolic pressure (mm Hg)	21.8 ± 4.9	17.1 ± 9.6	26.7 ± 8.8	ns	< 0.05	ns
Mean left atrial pressure (mm Hg)	12.7 ± 5.7	11.3 ± 6.5	20.9 ± 7.8	ns	< 0.05	< 0.05
Right ventricular systolic pressure (mm Hg)	37.2 ± 6.5	33.1 ± 12.4	45.9 ± 14.1	ns	< 0.05	ns
Right ventricular end-diastolic pressure (mm Hg)	8.3 ± 2.7	8.0 ± 2.8	8.1 ± 3.6	ns	ns	ns
Angiographic data						
Aortic regurgitation (angiographic degree 1–5)	1.0 ± 0.9	4.2 ± 0.7	3.5 ± 0.7	< 0.001	< 0.05	< 0.001
End-diastolic volume (ml/m^2)	90.8 ± 18.3	184.4 ± 43.8	142.0 ± 46.4	< 0.01	< 0.05	< 0.01
Left ventricular mass (g/m^2)	155.3 ± 30.4	174.0 ± 56.1	195.7 ± 41.8	ns	ns	< 0.05
Ejection fraction (%)	63.0 ± 12.1	52.4 ± 11.5	48.1 ± 13.5	ns	ns	< 0.05
Mean circumferential fiber shortening rate (edcirc/sec)	1.08 ± 0.37	0.86 ± 0.25	0.74 ± 0.29	ns	ns	< 0.05
Peak systolic wall stress (dynes × 10^3/cm^2)	315.2 ± 64.3	380.4 ± 80.1	375.2 ± 69.5	ns	ns	ns
Morphometric data						
Contractile material (%)	49.7 ± 3.7	44.5 ± 6.0	41.7 ± 4.4	ns	ns	< 0.01
Empty space (%)	29.3 ± 4.1	32.9 ± 8.2	36.5 ± 4.7	ns	ns	< 0.01
Mitrochondria (%)	21.6 ± 2.2	22.8 ± 4.4	21.9 ± 3.6	ns	ns	ns
Fibrotic content of the myocardium (%)	17.1 ± 5.5	16.0 ± 4.6	15.0 ± 4.2	ns	ns	ns

Results

Table 1 compares hemodynamic, angiographic, and morphometric data in patients with aortic stenosis, aortic insufficiency and patients with mixed aortic valve disease. Heart rate was comparabel between groups. Left ventricular systolic pressure and peak transvalvular gradient were higher in aortic stenosis and mixed aortic valve disease as compared to aortic insufficiency. Left ventricular end-diastolic pressure and mean left atrial pressure were higher in mixed aortic valve disease than in aortic insufficiency. Mean left atrial pressure was also higher in mixed aortic valve disease than in aortic stenosis. Right ventricular systolic pressure and end-diastolic pressure were comparable between groups.

The degree of aortic regurgitation was higher in aortic insufficiency than in both other groups but was also higher in mixed aortic valve disease than in pure aortic stenosis. Left ventricular end-diastolic volume showed a parallel behaviour and was higher in aortic insufficiency than in both other groups and was again higher in mixed aortic valve disease than in aortic insufficiency (table 1). Left ventricular mass was higher, ejection fraction and mean circumferential fiber shortening rate were lower in mixed aortic valve disease as compared to aortic stenosis. These parameters were not different between both other groups (fig. 1). Peak systolic wall stress was not significantly different between groups (fig. 1).

The intracellular content of contractile material was reduced and the empty space was augmented in mixed aortic valve disease as compared to aortic stenosis (fig. 2). Mitochondrial volume and the fibrotic content of

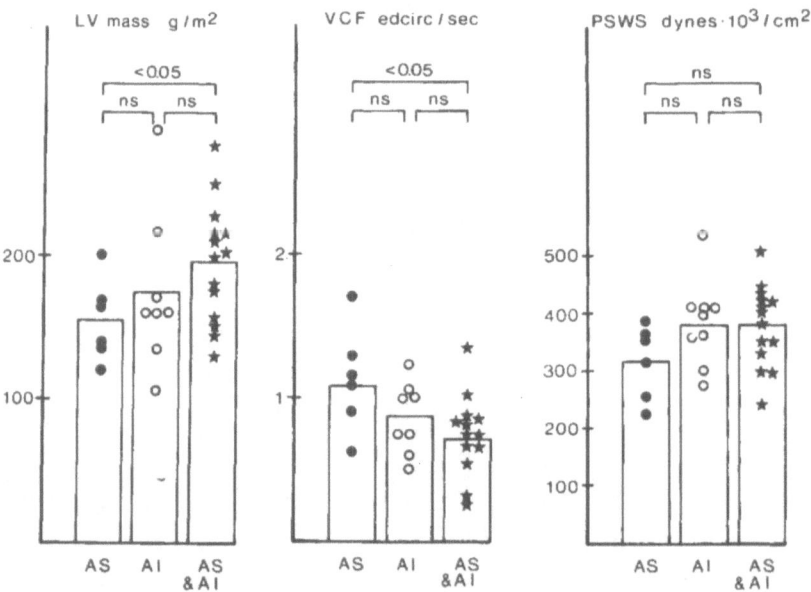

Fig. 1. Individual data and mean values for left ventricular mass, mean circumferential fiber shortening rate (VCF), and peak systolic wall stress (PSWS). AS = aortic stenosis, AI = aortic insufficiency, AS & AI = mixed aortic valve disease.

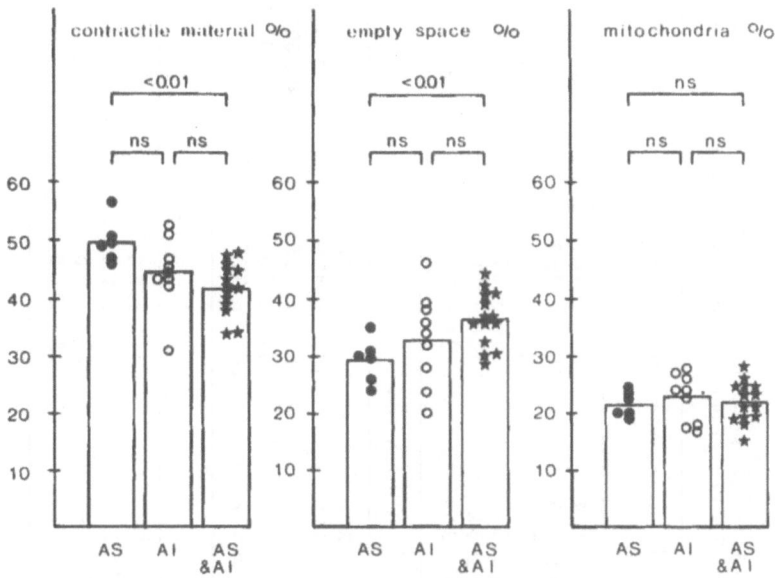

Fig. 2. Individual data and mean values of contractile material, empty space, and mitochondria.

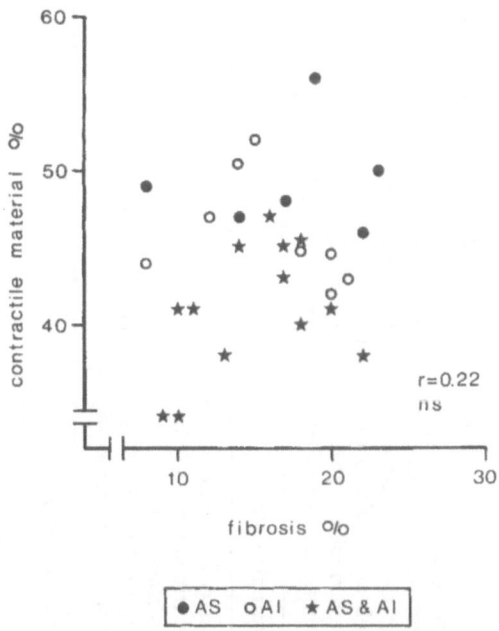

Fig. 3. Lack of correlation between percentage interstitial fibrosis and intracellular content of contractile material.

Table 2. Mean values ± SD for hemodynamic, angiographic and morphometric data in patients with aortic valve disease and control individuals. The morphometric control data were collected from 5 patients operated for atrial septal defect.

Hemodynamic data	Controls (n = 10)	Aortic valve disease (n = 29)	p value
Heart rate (min^{-1})	75.4 ± 11.4	80.3 ± 14.1	ns
Left ventricular systolic pressure (mm Hg)	123.2 ± 14.6	184.4 ± 39.7	< 0.001
Left ventricular end-diastolic pressure (mm Hg)	11.2 ± 3.7	22.9 ± 9.1	< 0.001
Mean left atrial pressure (mm Hg)	6.8 ± 2.1	16.6 ± 8.2	< 0.001
Right ventricular systolic pressure (mm Hg)	29.1 ± 3.2	40.6 ± 13.2	< 0.001
Right ventricular end-diastolic pressure (mm Hg)	6.9 ± 2.5	8.1 ± 3.1	ns
Angiographic data			
End-diastolic volume (ml/m^2)	76.7 ± 20.9	143.1 ± 52.0	< 0.001
Left ventricular mass (g/m^2)	72.6 ± 14.2	180.9 ± 45.8	< 0.001
Ejection fraction (%)	68.7 ± 6.9	52.5 ± 13.5	< 0.001
Mean circumferential fiber shortening rate (edcirc/sec)	1.31 ± 0.2	0.85 ± 0.3	< 0.001
Peak systolic wall stress (dynes × 10^3/cm^2)	292.8 ± 59.2	363.8 ± 73.7	< 0.01
Morphometric data			
Contractile material (%)	58.9 ± 5.4	44.2 ± 5.6	< 0.001
Empty space (%)	16.1 ± 5.7	33.9 ± 6.4	< 0.001
Mitochondria (%)	25.4 ± 4.4	22.1 ± 3.5	ns
Fibrotic content of the myocardium (%)	16.4 ± 4.8	15.8 ± 4.5	ns

the myocardium were not different between groups. No correlation was found between the degree of myocardial fibrosis and the intracellular content of contractile material (r = 0.22, n.s., fig. 3).

Data of all patients with aortic valve disease were pooled and compared to data obtained in 10 normal individuals. Control data for morphometry were obtained from 5 patients with atrial septal defect. As shown in table 2, left ventricular systolic pressure, left ventricular end-diastolic pressure, mean left atrial pressure and right ventricular systolic pressure were elevated in aortic valve disease as compared to controls. Right ventricular end-diastolic pressure was normal in aortic valve disease. Left ventricular end-diastolic volume, left ventricular mass, and peak systolic wall stress were higher in aortic valve disease than in controls, while ejection fraction and mean circumferential fiber shortening rate were significantly lower. The content of contractile material was considerably and significantly reduced in aortic valve disease as compared to controls while the empty space was augmented. Mitochondrial volume and percentage fibrosis were within normal limits.

Discussion

Mixed pressure- and volume-overloaded hearts revealed the highest degree of hypertrophy in this series when compared to pressure overload. This group also showed depressed left ventricular function and reduced amount of intracellular contractile material. The fibrotic content of the myocardium, however, was normal. These findings suggest that the intracellular content of myofibrils is more closely correlated to mechanical myocardial function than interstitial myocardial fibrosis. The group with mixed aortic valve disease revealed a combination of overloads (table 1). Left ventricular systolic pressure was significantly increased as in patients with pure pressure overload. In addition, a significant regurgitation was present in these cases and end-diastolic volume was considerably augmented as in aortic insufficiency. This combination of overloads may be the cause of the excessive degree of hypertrophy (196 g/m^2 versus 73 g/m^2 in controls). It is interesting to note that peak systolic wall stress was not different in mixed aortic valve disease when compared to both other groups. Peak systolic wall stress defines the relation between left ventricular load (pressure times radius of the chamber) and the degree of the compensatory hypertrophy (wall thickness). When peak wall stress was not elevated in mixed aortic valve disease as compared to pure aortic stenosis, this signifies that the compensatory mechanism was well functioning over a wide range of overload. An inadequate adaptation should be detectable by an increased peak systolic wall stress. Our patients with mixed aortic valve disease showed no significant increase of peak systolic wall stress but a reduction of shortening velocity and a reduction of intracellular myofibrils when compared to aortic stenosis. We therefore assume that not an inadequate degree of hypertrophy but an intracellular deficiency of myofibrils causes the lack of contractility in mixed aortic valve disease. Thus, in hypertrophied cells the production of sarcomeres seems to be significantly impaired. This is a new finding in human hearts. The sarcomerolysis obviously is not correlated to the development of interstitial myocardial fibrosis (fig. 3), and the mechanism of this phenomenon is unclear. *Hatt* et al. (9) produced an acute aortic constriction of the abdominal aorta in experimental animals and described a reduction of the fractional volume of myofibrils associated with an increase of the sarcoplasmic volume in the early phase after production of pressure overload. After correction of overload, normalization of these changes occurred. We have no ultrastructural data of patients after correction of overload. Our postoperative hemodynamic data, however, showed a significant reduction of hypertrophy after removal of overload and a normalization of contractile function. When cases with left ventricular hypertrophy were compared to controls, contractile function was clearly depressed in hypertrophied hearts, but the degree of fibrosis was normal. This finding is in contrast to some studies that gave evidence that fibrosis might be increased in some hypertrophied hearts (1, 10). It has to be noted that all our cases had normal coronary arteries. In this study, however, only data from an isolated sample could be analyzed, and we did not study papillary muscles which are known to be more vulnerable than other parts of the hypertrophied heart. On the other hand, the previous studies were postmortem studies of patients who died from their disease while we studied symptomatic patients who underwent corrective valve surgery.

Zusammenfassung

Licht- und elektronenoptische Morphometrie wurde an Gewebeproben des linken Ventrikels durchgeführt, die bei der Herzoperation entnommen wurden. 6 Patienten hatten eine Aortenstenose, 9 eine Aorteninsuffizienz und 14 ein kombiniertes Aortenvitium. Hämodynamische Messungen wurden vor der Operation durchgeführt. Patienten mit kombiniertem Aortenvitium hatten eine höhere linksventrikuläre Masse, eine niedrigere Ejektionsfraktion und Verkürzungsgeschwindigkeit als Patienten mit Aortenstenose. Der systolische „Wall Stress" war vergleichbar in den 3 Gruppen. Der intrazelluläre Gehalt an Myofibrillen war geringer, und der sarkoplasmatische Raum war höher bei kombinierten Aortenvitien als bei Aortenstenose. Das Mitochondrienvolumen und die interstitielle Fibrose waren nicht unterschiedlich in den Gruppen. Patienten mit Aorteninsuffizienz zeigten keinen signifikanten Unterschied zu den beiden anderen Gruppen. Wir schließen daraus, daß eine intrazelluläre Verarmung von kontraktilem Material die Ursache der eingeschränkten Myokardfunktion bei fortgeschrittener Hypertrophie infolge kombinierten Aortenvitiums ist.

References

1. *Linzbach, A. J.:* Heart failure from the point of view of quantitative anatomy. Amer. J. Cardiol. **14**, 370–382 (1960).
2. *Maron, B. J., V. J. Ferrans, W. C. Roberts:* Myocardial ultrastructure in patients with chronic aortic valve disease. Amer. J. Cardiol. **35**, 725–739 (1975).
3. *Schwarz, F., W. Flameng, J. Schaper, F. Langebartels, M. Sesto, F. Hehrlein, M. Schlepper:* Myocardial structure and function in patients with aortic valve disease and their relation to postoperative results. Amer. J. Cardiol. **41**, 661–669 (1978).
4. *Hunt, D., W. A. Baxley, J. W. Kennedy, T. P. Judge, J. E. Williams, H. T. Dodge:* Quantitative evaluation of cineaortography in the assessment of aortic regurgitation. Amer. J. Cardiol. **31**, 696–700 (1973).
5. *Kasser, I. S., J. W. Kennedy:* Measurement of left ventricular volumes in man by single-plane cineangiography. Invest. Radiol. **4**, 83–90 (1969).

6. *Trenouth, R. S., N. C. Phelps, W. A. Neill:* Determinants of left ventricular hypertrophy and oxygen supply in chronic aortic valve disease. Circulation **53**, 644–650 (1976).
7. *Schwarz, F., W. Flameng, J. Thormann, M. Sesto, F. Langebartels, F. Hehrlein, M. Schlepper:* Recovery from myocardial failure after aortic valve replacement. J. Thorac. Cardiovasc. Surg. **75**, 854–864 (1978).
8. *Weibel, E. R., S. K. Gonzagne, F. Walter:* Practical stereological methods for morphometric cytology. J. Cell. Biol. **30**, 23–38 (1966).
9. *Hatt, P. Y., P. Jouannot, J. Moravec, J. Perennec, M. Laplace:* Development and reversal of pressure induced cardiac hypertrophy. Light and electron microscopic study in the rat under temporary aortic constriction. Basic Res. Cardiol. **73**, 405–421 (1978).
10. *Wigle, E. D.:* Myocardial fibrosis and calcareous emboli in valvular heart disease. Brit. Heart J. **19**, 539–549 (1957).

Authors' address:

Priv.-Doz. Dr. *F. Schwarz,* Abteilung Innere Medizin III (Kardiologie) der Mediz. Universitätsklinik, Bergheimer Str. 58, 6900 Heidelberg, West Germany

Basic Res. Cardiol. **75**, 118–125 (1980)
© 1980 Dr. Dietrich Steinkopff Verlag, Darmstadt
ISSN 0300–8428

Paper, presented at the Erwin Riesch Symposium, Tübingen, April 3–7, 1979

Institute of Pathology, University of Düsseldorf (Head: Prof. Dr. W. Hort)

Differences between transmitter depletion in human heart hypertrophy and experimental cardiac hypertrophy in Goldblatt rats

Transmitterverarmung bei Herzhypertrophie des Menschen und bei experimenteller Herzhypertrophie der Goldblatt-Ratten

F. Borchard

With 3 figures

Summary

The transmitter depletion of the myocardium in hypertrophy and especially insufficiency has formerly been attributed to a decrease of certain enzymes that are involved in the neurotransmitter synthesis. However, we could show in human auricles recently that one main reason for the catecholamine depletion is the distension of the adrenergic ground plexus in the course of hypertrophy of the myocardial muscle cells. At the same time, electron microscope investigations revealed various changes of the axonal ultrastructure, especially in heart insufficiency. Additional experimental work in renal hypertension of rats should answer the question whether this process occurs also in other parts of the heart and whether it can be followed sequentially during the development of hypertension. In this preliminary report about these studies, attention is drawn to focal transmitter depletion in areas of severe vascular necrosis and inflammation, especially in the right ventricular wall. During the first three months after the beginning of the experiment, the total noradrenaline content decreased only slightly, whereas the concentration of this transmitter is lowered significantly by myocardial growth in both ventricles. It is concluded that there are essential differences between hypertrophy in experimental renal hypertension and human cardiac hypertrophy.

Many investigators have found a decrease of adrenergic transmitter concentration in human and experimental heart failure (7, further ref. see 1). The decrease of the rate limiting enzyme for the noradrenaline (NA) synthesis, tyrosine hydroxilase, was accused to be the main reason for the transmitter depletion in cardiac insufficiency (10). In the course of a multi-methodological approach to this problem, however, basic topographical and histochemical changes of the adrenergic ground plexus during hypertrophy development were considered to be more important (1). First of all, structural characteristics of the normal adrenergic ground plexus in different parts of the heart had to be demonstrated by morphometry; since such histochemical studies were not possible in post-mortem human hearts because of the autolysis, the rat myocardium was chosen as a model. In different parts of the rat heart, the catecholamine concentration significantly (p = 0.007) depends on the density of the adrenergic ground plexus (1). The pattern of adrenergic innervation in human cardiac auricles obtained during heart surgery was quite similar. During hypertrophy and insufficiency, changes of the distribution, transmitter content and fine structure of the adrenergic nerves occurred that have been reported already in detail (1). The main aspects of these alterations are summarized again in comparison with changes which were seen in cardiac hypertrophy in the course of experimental renal hypertension (coarctation of one renal artery with contralateral nephrectomy).

Hypertrophy in human hearts

In 43 human auricles the noradrenaline (NA) concentration and the adrenaline (A) concentrations were determined by column chromatography and fluorimetry. The medium fibre width of atriocytes and the connective tissue content were established by light microscopical morphometry. The distribution of adrenergic nerves was visualized according to their NA content by means of the Falck method, and their arrangement was studied by morphometry. Additional electron microscopical studies were performed related to the structure of adrenergic nerves and to the volume density of so-called 'specific' atrial granules, since it was suggested that these structures might contain catecholamines (5).

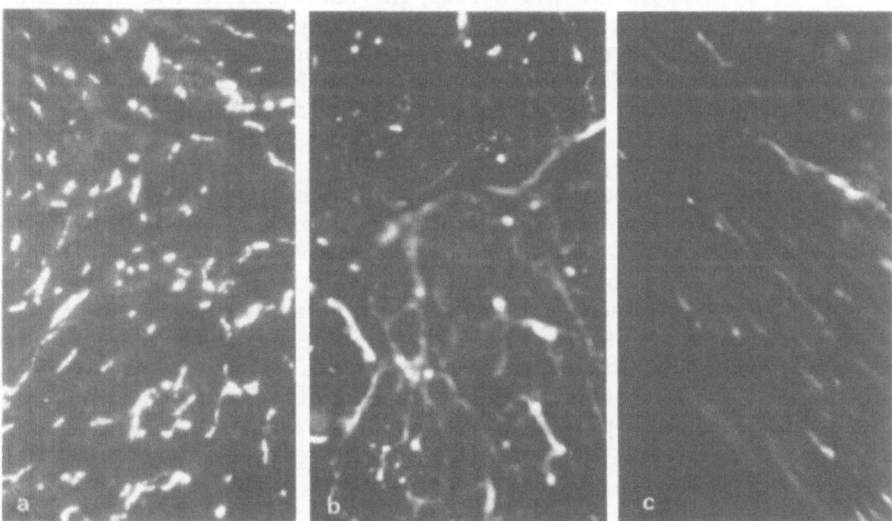

Fig. 1. Adrenergic nerves in the human cardiac auricle as visualized by the adrenergic transmitters (Falck-method, reflected light, 125 ×):
a) Dense adrenergic ground plexus in a child
b) Distended adrenergic ground plexus in an adult with slight myocardial hypertrophy
c) Few residual adrenergic fibres in severe hypertension and heart insufficiency

It was shown that in accordance with other authors (ref. 1) the main cardiac transmitter is NA (95%), whereas there is only a small amount of A (5%). Histochemically NA is nearly exclusively situated in the adrenergic nerves. No specific transmitter fluorescence could be traced in the atrial myocardial cells. Therefore the hypothesis that the atrial granules might contain catecholamines could neither be substantiated by these results nor by the correlation analysis of transmitter concentration with the volume density of the so-called specific atrial granules in different auricles. By morphometrical analysis of the histochemical results, we could demonstrate that the depletion of cardiac catecholamine stores is partly due to a distension of the adrenergic ground plexus, partly to focal transmitter fading (fig. 1). As one possible reason for these alterations of the transmitter fluorescence, a spectrum of regressive changes of autonomic cardiac nerves could be seen by electron microscopy.

As we were interested in the question whether such changes also occur in other regions of the heart and in other species, we performed additional experimental work in renal hypertension, for this was considered as an appropriate model.

Experimental renal hypertension

This extensive work was done together with Dr. *Völker* and Dr. *Stoepel* from the Bayer Pharma-Forschungszentrum in Wuppertal and is under publication in greater detail now (3). In this study, the transmitter content, the distribution of adrenergic nerves, the cardiac fibre width, and the ultrastructure of cardiac autonomic nerves were also studied systematically in 79 female Wistar rats by the same methods as mentioned above. These items were investigated mainly in the first 12 weeks, but morphological pilot studies were also performed in later periods of the experiment.

After one month hypertension with systolic values of more than 200 mm Hg is fully developed. During the first 12 weeks after the operations, there is an average increase of the total heart weight from about 0.65 g to 1.2 g compared to 0.75 g in the control group. This hypertrophy is mainly due to an enlargement of the left cardiac ventricular wall which grew from 0.43 to 0.95 g in experimental animals in comparison with 0.53 g in control rats. Only in experimental animals a further increase of weight of the right ventricular wall plus atria from 0.2 to 0.4 g was observed, partly due to edema, partly due to severe morphological changes described below, and partly due to hypertrophy: The average fibre diameter was measured across the entire wall in the median line of both ventricles. It averaged 12.1

Fig. 2. Morphological alterations of the myocardium in experimental renal hypertension.
a) Severe necrotic changes of small arteries in the right ventricular wall with reactive inflammation in the region of perivascular nerves (cf. fig. 3a; HE, 75 ×)
b) Necrosis of a myocardial cell 2 weeks after operation (electr. micr. 2000 ×)
c) Patchy scarring of the myocardium, 10 weeks after operation (El.-van Gieson, 75 ×)

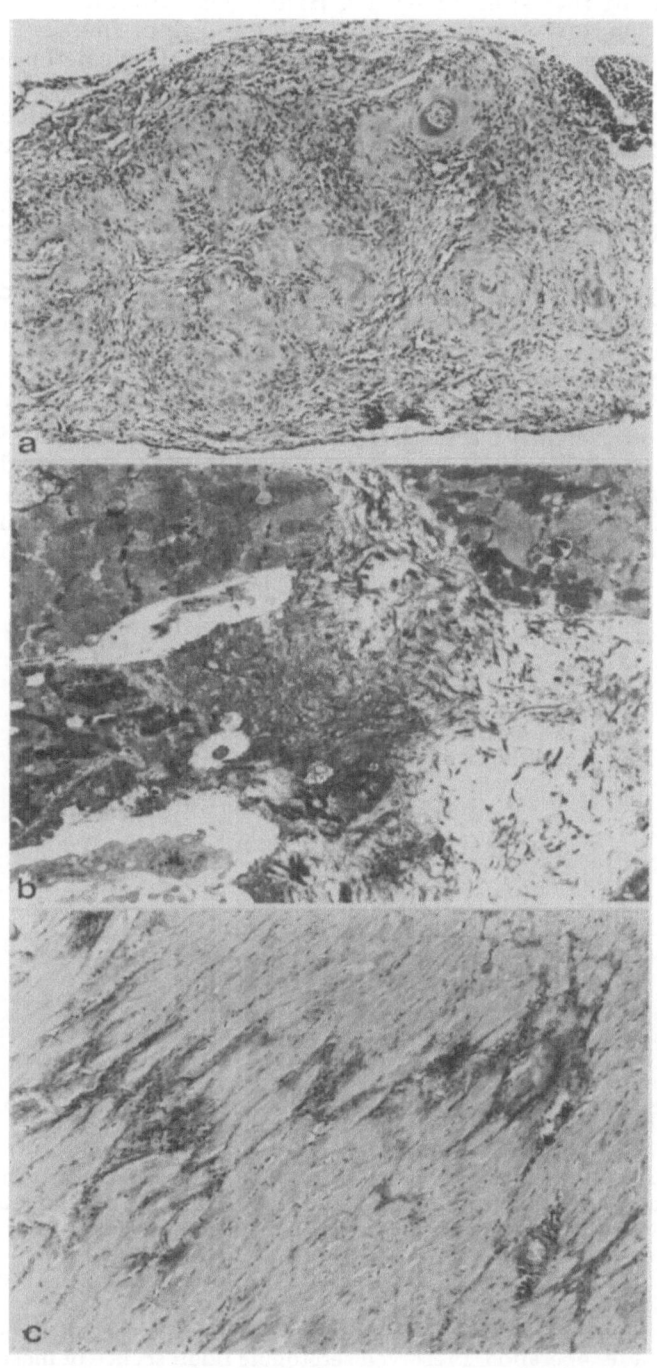

µm in both ventricles' walls in the control group irrespective of the duration of the experiment compared to 17.0 µm in the left ventricular wall in Goldblatt rats after 12 weeks. Histological investigations showed in some rats severe necrotic alterations of the wall of smaller arteries, especially in the region of the right ventricular wall. Near these alterations, there was a severe inflammatory reaction (fig. 2a, 3a), and sometimes also necroses could be shown in the myocardium by light and electron microscopy (fig. 2b). In later stages perivascular fibrosis and foci of intramyocardial scarring were seen (fig. 2c).

The transmitter determinations revealed only a very small loss of the total cardiac NA content of about 7.2% in the entire heart, of 3% in the left ventricular wall and of 15.4% in the right ventricular wall. However, referring to the same mass of tissue, the concentration of NA decreased by 32.6% in the left and even 36.6% in the right ventricular wall compared to control values.

The histochemical investigations showed that there are at least two sites of reduction of the specific transmitter fluorescence: in the first place, there is nearly a total decay of transmitter fluorescence in the region of severe perivascular inflammation (fig. 3a) and in the second place, there is a focal fading of the specific fluorescence between the myocardial muscle fibres (fig. 3b). In pilot studies of later stages of experimental renal hypertrophy, there was almost an entire loss of NA fluorescence in

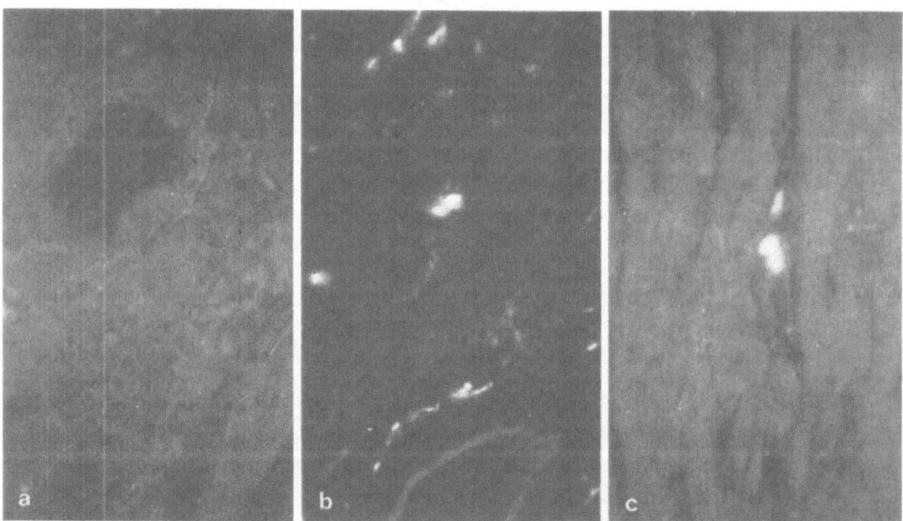

Fig. 3. Adrenergic nerves in experimental renal hypertension as visualized by the adrenergic transmitters (Falck-method, transmitted light, 125 ×):
a) Total loss of transmitter fluorescence in the region of perivascular inflammatory changes
b) Focal fading of adrenergic nerves in the intramural plexus, 6 weeks after operation
c) Nearly total loss of transmitter fluorescence in the adrenergic ground plexus 12 weeks after operation. Preserved serotonine fluorescence of mast cells.

adrenergic nerves, while the serotonine fluorescence of the mast cells was retained (fig. 3c). Additional electron microscopic investigations showed that in initial stages of the experiment, some findings point to a tendency of forming new adrenergic nerves, whereas in later stages there are partly severe degenerative changes in the autonomic nerves of the heart (3).

Discussion

The results show that several mechanisms may be involved in the depletion of transmitter stores in the development of cardiac hypertrophy and insufficiency. The main principle is the distension of the adrenergic nerves by growth of the myocardial fibres in the course of hypertrophy. This process does not obviously induce a decrease of transmitter in the single nerve fibre initially; however, in later stages of the disease this process also takes place as evidenced by our histochemical findings (1) and those of *Vogel* and co-workers (14). Beside these mechanisms in human auricles also the inhibitory role of scarring for transmitter liberation has been discussed (1). In the experimental Goldblatt hypertension very special conditions are given during the development of hypertrophy, e.g. the muscle cell necroses and the severe perivascular inflammation in the course of hypertensive arteriolar damage. As we could find a fading of adrenergic nerves in the region of such inflammatory changes and finally also an immuration of nerve processes in the perivascular scar tissue, these changes are obviously peculiarities of the renal hypertension which cannot be compared with conditions of hypertension development in man.

An important question is concerned with the consequences of transmitter depletion for the hypertrophied heart. In human auricles we have discussed the critical value to be 0.6 µg NA/g wet tissue below which overt heart failure could usually be found. We have also shown ultrastructural damage of the cardiac autonomic nerves in severe hypertrophy which was normally accompanied by heart insufficiency.

Cardiac transplantation, however, have shown that surgical neural ablation does not abolish the contractility, but only the adaptability of the heart to functional demands. So the transmitter loss in severe hypertrophy means the loss of adaptation by defect of one decisive mechanism for the increase of contractility (4, 1). One may ask for the significance of adrenergic nerves for the development of hypertension which is beyond the scope of this paper and has been delineated already earlier (1). It is quite clear that under certain conditions catecholamines and sympathomimetic drugs may induce hypertrophy. We do not know whether the renal hypertension belongs to this group. Since an increased turnover of catecholamines under these conditions has been reported by *Velly* et al. (13) one has to doubt if the lowered NA concentration that we found in our experiment reflects the functional role of the adrenergic system appropriately which might possibly induce myocardial growth. Certainly, the interaction between the renin-angiotensin-mechanism and the catecholamine metabolism is very complex and cannot be fully discussed here (ref. see: 9, 12, 8, 6, 11). Some experimental and clinical results, however, confirm the assumption that the adrenergic system plays its part in the fixation of renal hypertension.

Zusammenfassung

Die bekannte Transmitter-Verarmung des Myokards bei Herzhypertrophie und besonders bei Herzinsuffizienz wurde früher auf eine Verarmung des Myokards an bestimmten Enzymen der Katecholaminsynthese zurückgeführt. In eigenen Untersuchungen an menschlichen Herzohren wurde kürzlich nachgewiesen, daß die Ausweitung des adrenergen Grundplexus im Verlauf der Hypertrophie der Herzmuskelzellen eine wesentliche Ursache für die Katecholaminverarmung des Myokards darstellt. Elektronenmikroskopische Untersuchungen zeigten gleichzeitig unterschiedliche Schäden der axonalen Ultrastruktur.

Ergänzende Experimente bei renaler Hypertonie sollten die Fragen beantworten, ob dieser Prozeß auch in anderen Herzabschnitten auftritt und ob er schrittweise während der Entstehung der Hypertonie verfolgt werden kann. In diesem vorläufigen Bericht wird besonders auf die herdförmige Transmitterverarmung im Bereich von Gefäßwandnekrosen mit Begleitentzündung vorwiegend im Bereich der rechten Kammerwand hingewiesen. Während der ersten drei Monate nach Versuchsbeginn ist der gesamte Noradrenalingehalt beider Kammerwände nur geringfügig verändert, wohingegen die Transmitterkonzentration signifikant durch das Muskelwachstum sinkt. Das Experiment zeigt, daß wesentliche Unterschiede zwischen der experimentellen Hypertrophie beim Goldblatt-Versuch und der menschlichen Herzhypertrophie bestehen.

References

1. *Borchard, F.:* The adrenergic nerves of the normal and the hypertrophied heart, in: Normale und Pathologische Anatomie (Eds.: *W. Bargmann, W. Doerr)* Vol. 33 (Stuttgart 1978).
2. *Borchard, F., H. J. Völker* (a. G.); *K. Stoepel* (a. G.), *K. Karcenski* (a. G.): Katecholamingehalt und adrenerge Nerven des Rattenherzens bei experimenteller renaler Hypertonie. Verh. Dtsch. Ges. Path. **62**, 340 (1978).
3. *Borchard, F., H. J. Völker, K. Stoepel:* Adrenergic nerves and catecholamine content in experimental renal hypertension (in prep.)
4. *Braunwald, E.:* The autonomic nervous system in heart failure, in: The myocardium: Failure and Infarction (Ed.: *E. Braunwald,* p. 59–69 (New York 1974).
5. *Büchner, F., S. Onishi, A. Wada:* Cardiomyopathy associated with systemic myopathy. Genetic defect in actomyosin influencing muscular structure and function (Baltimore 1978).
6. *Bunaq, R. D.:* Circulatory effects of angiotensin, aus: Handbuch der experimentellen Pharmakologie, Bd. 37: Angiotensin (Berlin 1974).
7. *Chidsey, C. A., E. Braunwald, G. Morrow, D. T. Mason:* Myocardial norepinephrine concentration in man. Effects of reserpine and congestive heart failure. N. Engl. J. Med. **269**, 653–658 (1963).
8. *Dempsey, P. J., T. Cooper:* Pharmacology of the coronary circulation. Annu. Rev. Pharmacol. **12**, 99–110 (1972).
9. *Peach, M. J., F. M. Bumpus, Khairallah:* Inhibition of norepinephrine uptake in hearts by angiotension II and analogs. J. Pharmacol. Exp. Ther. **167**, 291–299 (1969).
10. *Pool, P. E., J. W. Covell, M. Levitt, J. Gibb, E. Braunwald:* Reduction of cardiac tyrosine hydroxylase activity in experimental congestive heart failure. Circulat. Res. **20**, 349–353 (1967).
11. *De Schaepdryver, A. F., E. J. Moerman:* Experimentele renale hypertensie en noradrenerge mechanismen. Verh. K. Akad. Geneeskd. Belg. **36** (1974).

12. *Starke, K., U. Werner, H. J. Schüman:* Wirkung von Angiotensin auf Funktion und Noradrenalinabgabe isolierter Kaninchenherzen in Ruhe und bei Sympathicusreizung. Arch. Pharm. **265,** 170–186 (1969).
13. *Velly, J., J. Karasz, J. L. Imbs, J. Schwartz:* Hypertensions artérielles rénovasculaire et neurogène du rat: Synthèse et turnover de la noradrénaline dans le cœur, l'aorte et l'artère rénale. Thérapie **28,** 1029–1042 (1973).
14. *Vogel, J. H., D. Jacobowitz, C. A. Chidsey:* Distribution of norepinephrine in the failing bovine heart. Correlation of chemical analysis and fluorescence microscopy. Circulat. Res. **24,** 71–84 (1969).

Author's address:

Prof. Dr. *F. Borchard,* Pathologisches Institut der Universität Düsseldorf, 4000 Düsseldorf, Moorenstr. 5 (W. Germany)

Basic Res. Cardiol. **75**, 126–138 (1980)
© 1980 Dr. Dietrich Steinkopff Verlag, Darmstadt
ISSN 0300–8428

Paper, presented at the Erwin Riesch Symposium, Tübingen, April 3–7, 1979

Institute of Pathology, Ludwig-Aschoff-House, University of Freiburg/Br.

Alterations of substances (DNA, myoglobin, myosin, protein) in experimentally induced cardiac hypertrophy and under the influence of drugs (isoproterenol, cytostatics, strophanthin)

Veränderungen von Substanzen (DNS, Myoglobin, Myosin, Protein) bei experimenteller Herzhypertrophie und unter dem Einfluß von Medikamenten (Isoproterenol, Zytostatika, Strophanthin)

C. P. Adler and *W. Sandritter*

With 5 figures

Summary

In growing human hearts the biochemically estimated *total amount of DNA* increases from 20 mg to 50–100 mg, and in hypertrophied hearts the increase may be threefold compared with normal hearts. Whereas most animal hearts have nearly only diploid muscle cells, in human hearts most muscle cell nuclei are polyploid. According to the grade of hypertrophy a pronounced *polyploidisation* of heart muscle cells occurs. The quantitative ratio of noncondensed chromatin/condensed chromatin remains constant 4:1 in all grades of hypertrophy. The *amount of myoglobin* in hearts above 500 g weight is more than 100% compared with normal hearts and is correlated with the width of the heart muscle fibres. In hypertrophied hearts an irregular and higher *double refraction of myosin* can be seen indicating an early stage of necrosis. In concentric cardiac hypertrophy the *dry weight* of the muscle fibres is more increased than in eccentric hypertrophy. The *protein concentration* within the muscle fibres increases with rising heart weight. Some *cytostatics* cause a decrease of the myocardial DNA content, a reduction of the ploidy level and a diminishing of the number of connective tissue cells. *Isoproterenol* effects, within the first 3 weeks after administration, a severe reduction of the cell number; after 2 months a pronounced polyploidisation of the heart muscle cells occurs and the cell number increases again above the normal level indicating the regeneration capabilities of the myocardium.

During normal growth, the weight of the heart increases from 20 g right after birth up to 350 g in adult life. A prolonged functional activity of the heart results in a further growth of the heart muscle which is called *hypertrophy*. This goes along with an increased volume of the heart muscle cells which become lengthened and enlarged (*Adler,* 1972). Quantitative histochemical investigations revealed that changes had occurred in certain parts of the heart muscle cells in growing or hypertrophied human and animal hearts.

A. Myocardial DNA

Biochemical DNA determinations of the *human myocardium*[1]) showed that the *total amount of DNA* increases from 20 mg in newborns to 50–100 mg in adults (*Adler,* 1971, 1976; fig. 1a). The increase of the amount of DNA up to fivefold results from an increase in volume of the myocardial fibres, an increase of the connective tissue cells and an increase of the DNA within the heart muscle cells. The amount of the DNA content of the heart muscle is correlated with the weight of the heart. In excessively hypertrophied hearts the total amount of the DNA may be increased as much as threefold in comparison with normal hearts.

In *animal hearts* varying greatly in size a direct correlation could be seen between the weight of the heart muscle and the DNA content of the myocardium: In hearts of mice showing a weight of the myocardium between 0.16 to 0.24 g, the DNA content ranges from 0.073 to 0.132 mg. In hearts of horses weighing between 1270 and 3475 g, the total amount of DNA varies from 191.3 mg to 445.5 mg.

B. Polyploidisation

By means of biochemical DNA determinations the total DNA content of the myocardium is obtained which originates from the connective tissue cells as well as from the heart muscle cells. On the basis of morphological (*Klinge,* 1970) and autoradiographic investigations (*Grove* et al., 1968), that did not reveal regular mitotic figures or labeling of DNA in the heart muscle nuclei, *Rumyantsev* (1965), *Fanburg* (1970) and others believe that the augmentation of DNA in growing hearts and in cardiac hypertro-

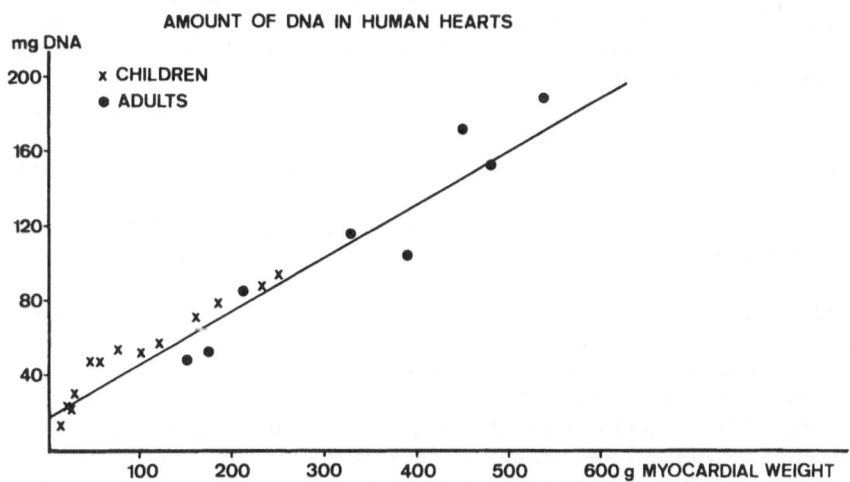

Fig. 1a. Biochemically estimated amount of total DNA in growing, normal and hypertrophied human hearts. The increase of the DNA amount is correlated with the weight of the myocardium.

---

[1]) diphenylamine reaction (*Dische,* 1930; *Burton,* 1956)

phy is exclusively due to a proliferation of the connective tissue elements of the heart muscle.

This view differs greatly, however, from our own investigations of the myocardial nuclei, since by means of cytophotometric measurements of Feulgen-stained heart muscle cells we were able to quantitatively determine the DNA content of the heart muscle nuclei. We have studied so far a total of nearly 500 hearts by carrying out measurements with a *Deeley* integrating microdensitometer (1955). From the diagram of the *distribution of the ploidy classes* expressed as percentage (fig. 1b) it is evident that polyploidisation of myocardial cells occurs in *human hearts.* This was first described in 1964 by *Sandritter* and *Scomazzoni* and was confirmed by later studies (*Adler,* 1971; *Pfitzer,* 1971). From birth to age 7, 80–90% of the nuclei are diploid with only 7–16% tetraploid nuclei. From age 7 to 12 a physiological polyploidisation of the myocardial nuclei occurs (*Adler,* 1976). In normal hearts of adults the number of tetraploid cells dominates with 60%, and 20% of the cells are octoploid. In cardiac hypertrophy under the influence of longstanding cardiac hyperfunction an additional, very pronounced polyploidisation of the myocardial cells is seen. In hearts weighing about 800 g, the diploid cells are entirely absent (10% 4c-, 55% 8c-, 30% 16c- and 5% 32c-nuclei), but there is an occurrence of 16-ploid and 32-ploid, occasionally even 64-ploid nuclei (*Adler,* 1971; *Pfitzer,* 1971). Our findings reveal that polyploidisation of the heart muscle cell nuclei depends on the degree and the duration of prolonged functional activity of the myocardium.

In accordance with others (*Pfitzer* and *Kuhn,* 1970) our investigations of *animal hearts* did not show a polyploidisation of the myocardial cells. The hearts of animals which we examined revealed as little as 0.33% to 4% tetraploid cells; nearly all cells were diploid. Our findings showed that also in experimentally induced cardiac hypertrophy the degree of polyploidisation of the myocardial cells is by far less pronounced than in man (*Grove* et al., 1968; *Meerson,* 1969).

Polyploidisation of the nuclei of the heart muscle which will result in hypertrophy of the heart is caused by cardiac hyperfunction which also produces morphological changes in the size and form of heart muscle nuclei and influences the distribution of *chromatin structures* (*Adler* et al., 1977). In 30 hypertrophied human hearts and in 70 hypertrophied hearts of rats we made an analysis of the nuclei by means of measurements obtained from an universal microspectrophotometer[2]) and from computer material. These measurements led to the following results: Although in hypertrophied human hearts the nuclear areas increase with a rising degree of hypertrophy, the quantitative ratio of non-condensed chromatin in comparison with condensed chromatin remains constant 4:1 inspite of the polyploidisation of the nuclei. The portion remaining of the condensed chromatin expressed as surface percentage of the whole nuclear area is approximately 20%. Only in extremely hypertrophied hearts could an increase in condensed chromatin of up to 38% be seen. But in any case, of the 80% non-condensed chromatin only 10% is genetically active. – In rats, in which cardiac hypertrophy had been produced as a result of a long-term

---

[2]) UMSP I, Zeiss Manufactures, Oberkochen/Württ.

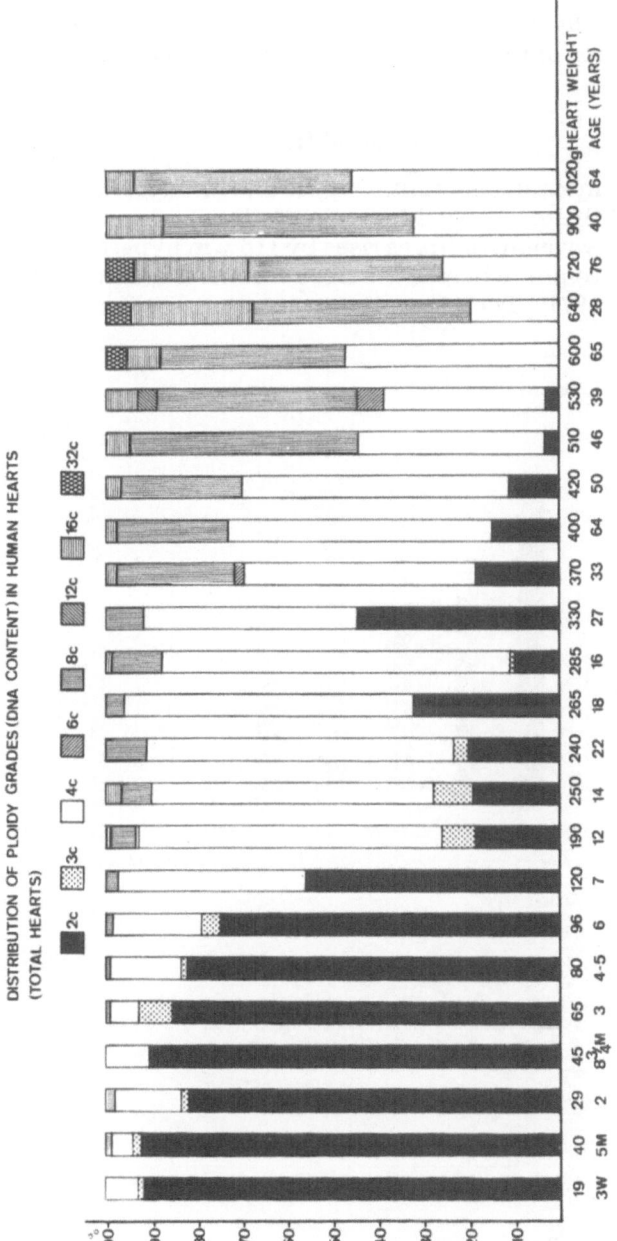

Fig. 1b. Percentage distribution of the ploidy grades of human heart muscle cell nuclei. With rising heart weight, there is an advanced polyploidisation of the heart muscle cells.

"swimming-training", we were able to detect an increase of 7% in the nuclear areas which may be regarded as nuclear swelling caused by an excessive functional activity of the heart. But in spite of this hyperfunction, the ratio of euchromatin and heterochromatin remains 4:1. After injections of *Strophanthin* no alterations of the ploidy grades and the chromatin structures of the heart muscle nuclei could either be observed.

C. Myoglobin

By means of combined historadiographic and interference microscopic determinations of the myocardial fibres in the *human hearts* we were able to show that the dry weight of fibres rises by 116% in hypertrophied hearts up to 600 g heart weight, whereas the fibre volume increases only by 79% (*Sandritter* et al., 1971). Therefore, the mass shows a more pronounced

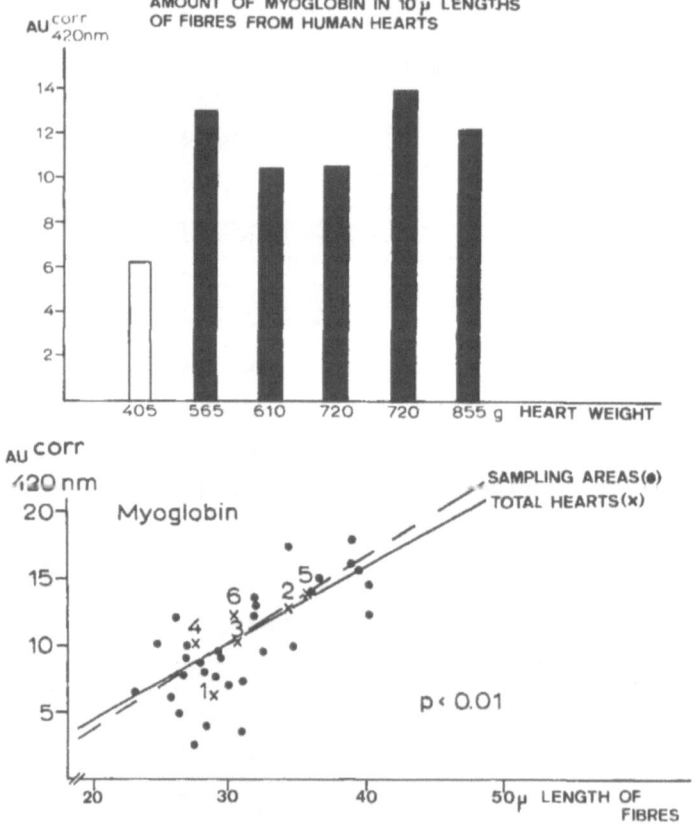

Fig. 2. Cytophotometrically estimated amount of myoglobin within the total human myocardium (above) and within single heart muscle fibres (below). In hearts weighing more than 500 g a significant higher amount of myoglobin is present. The rise of myoglobin is correlated with the width of the heart muscle fibres.

increase than the volume, which suggests that in the case of developing hypertrophy the concentration of the substrate of the individual fibres of the heart muscle has increased. In hearts with a higher weight, no significant increase in mass and volume could be seen, so this is not responsible for an increase in the weight of the heart. There are more likely other

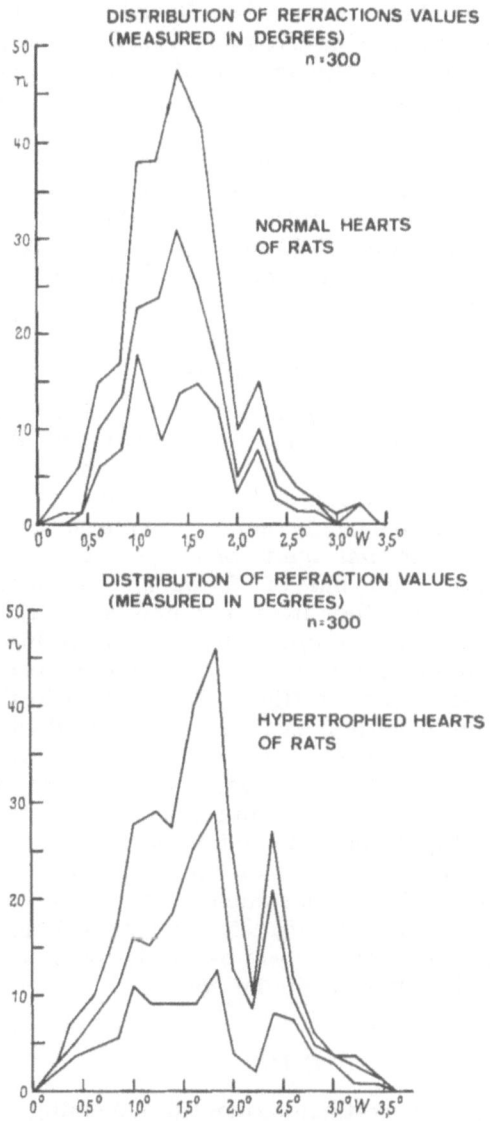

Fig. 3. Diagram of frequency of double refraction values in normal hearts (above) and hypertrophied hearts (below) of rats. The values are distributed normally in normal hearts (1.5°). In hypertrophied hearts there is a second maximum of double refraction at 1.0° and a third maximum at 2.4–2.6° indicating necrotic cells.

mechanisms involved, like an apposition of new sarcomeres, an interstitial edema and a numerical hyperplasia of the heart muscle cells.

The increase in mass of the heart muscle fibres results in particular from an augmentation and an enlargement of the myofilaments which has also been shown by means of investigations obtained with the electron microscope (*Onishi* et al., 1969). On the basis of quantitative ultraviolet-cytophotometric examinations we also observed an increased *amount of myoglobin* (fig. 2). In hearts of less than 500 g heart weight, the amount of myoglobin is 6 AU, and in hearts of more than 500 g weight it ranges from 10–14 AU. This shows that the amount of myoglobin varies greatly with differences of nearly 100% between normal and hypertrophied human hearts beyond the critical heart weight of 500 g. In hearts with a higher heart weight, however, no further increase in the amount of myoglobin of the myofibres is seen (*Adler*, 1973). Due to the measurement data obtained in correspondence with the width of fibres, the amount of myoglobin is correlated with the width of fibres (fig. 2), since hypertrophied heart muscle fibres contain a significantly larger amount of myoglobin than normotrophic fibres.

D. Myosin

By means of a polarisation microscope we investigated the *myosin structures* in heart muscle cells of rats (*Pilny* et al., 1969). They are characterized by a distinctive anisotropy which may be considered as "constant material". When measuring the double refraction of 300 sites chosen randomly within a single section, the measurement data is considerably scattered. In *normal hearts of rats* the estimated values cluster around a common median value of 1.5° (fig. 3). The shape of the frequency curve suggests that the values are distributed normally and that they may be considered as a collective unit. – In contrast to this, the values measured in experimentally induced *hypertrophied hearts* are not distributed according to a normal pattern (fig. 3). In addition to the principal maximum (1.5°), another class of measurements is found which show a secondary maximum with a phase difference of approximately 1.0°. A third maximum, with a phase difference varying from 2.4° to 2.0°, is most likely to originate from a group of heart muscle cells having a particularly high double refraction. Light microscopic investigations of these heart muscle cells reveal a strong predilection for eosin staining, indicating the presence of necrotic cells. Although some cells show a greater predisposition towards eosin staining and double refraction, morphologically they do not differ from normal cells. Probably one can ascribe this to an early stage of necrosis associated with intracellular edema.

E. Dry weight

We systematically investigated quantitative changes found in the substances of heart muscle fibres in both animal and human cases of cardiac hypertrophy. In an animal experiment cardiac hypertrophy was induced in guinea pigs by subjecting them to a period of "swimming-training", and the *dry weight* of heart muscle fibres measuring 10 μ was determined by means of X-ray historadiographs (*Sandritter* et al., 1971). One group of animals, which proved to be good swimmers, developed *concentric cardiac hypertrophy* after a total training period of 3 months. The hearts showed an average increase in weight of 43%. Here, the *volume* of the heart muscle fibres had increased by 75%. The average *dry weight* of the individual fibres was even greater, showing a percentage proportion of 110%.

The animals of a second group proved to be bad swimmers and could only be exposed to training every second day. These animals developed an *eccentric cardiac hypertrophy* having, however, an increase in heart weight of 55%. As compared with the controls, the *volume* of heart muscle fibres showed an average increase of only 49%. The *dry weight* of the fibres with only an increase of 36% in comparison with the intensively trained animals indicated a clear lessening in the increase of the mass weight.

A correlation between the fibre volume and the dry weight of the fibres became evident. Whereas, however, in concentric cardiac hypertrophy the mass concentration had increased by 20%, in hypertrophied and dilated hearts no significant increase of the mass per surface unit could be observed. The energetic insufficiency in eccentric hypertrophy, as opposed to concentric hypertrophy, thus expresses itself as a reduction of the mass and concentration of those structural elements of the myocardium, which are essential to functional activity of the heart.

F. Protein

It is principally the *protein* in these structural elements that are responsible for the dry weight of the fibres. By means of quantitative ultraviolet-cytophotometric investigations we determined the content of proteins in

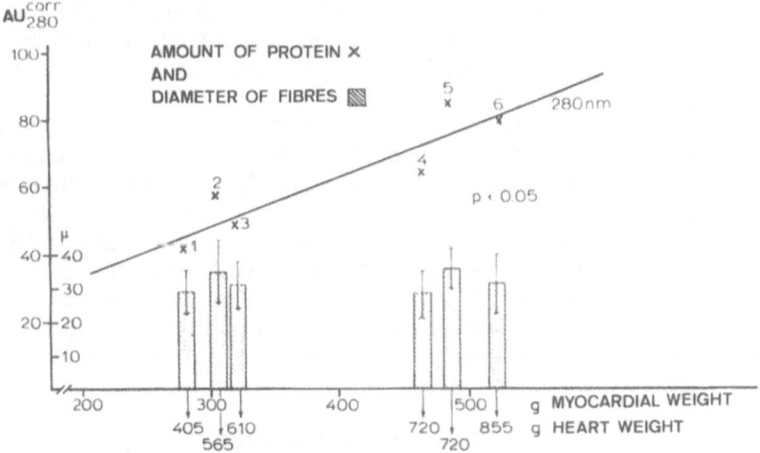

Fig. 4. Cytophotometrically estimated amount of protein within human hearts of different grades of hypertrophy. The increase of the amount of protein is correlated with the myocardial weight and the width of the single heart muscle fibres.

hypertrophied human hearts (*Adler*, 1973). These investigations showed that the *concentration of protein* within the heart muscle fibres increases significantly with the rising weight of the heart. This signifies an increase in the concentration of protein by 120%. – Also the *amount of protein* increases continuously during the process of cardiac hypertrophy (fig. 4). We found an increase in the protein amount of 90%, together with a simultaneous rise in the heart muscle weight by 84%.

If estimated values are made, based upon the width of fibres, they show that the amounts of proteins are correlated with the width of fibres. Hypertrophied heart muscle fibres contain a significantly larger amount of protein than normotrophic fibres. According to investigations carried out with an electron microscope this is due to an increase and enlargement of the myofibrils (*Poche*, 1969) which consist of the contractile proteins actin and myosin. *Nowy* et al. (1959) reported an increase of the actinomyosin concentration by 30%, and a decrease in the content of non-contractile proteins by 25% during experimental cardiac hypertrophy.

G. Influence of cytostatics

An alteration of substances within the heart muscle cells does not only occur in hypertrophied hearts caused by hyperfunction. Various drugs may also exert a corresponding influence on the heart muscle cells. In 42 growing hearts of rats we determined the *influence of cytostatics* which inhibit the DNA synthesis in relation to the growth period, to the DNA content of the myocardium and to the number of cells in the heart. In these animals the heart weight was reduced by 2–8% in comparison with controls. The administration of high doses of Cyclophosphamid diminished the *DNA concentration* of the myocardium by more than 17% and the total amount of DNA by 20%. The administration of Daunomycin and Vinblastin, on the other hand, did not exert any influence on the DNA content of the myocardium. The administration of Daunomycin results in a decrease of the *tetraploid heart muscle cells* from the norm of nearly 10% to 3.2%.

We have developed a method (*Adler*, 1971; *Sandritter* and *Adler*, 1972) whereby one can ascertain the *absolute number of cells* in hearts. By means of this method we established that 8.6×10^{0} muscle cells and 31.4×10^{6} connective tissue cells are found in the normal hearts of rats. No influence of cytostatics on the number of heart muscle cells could be observed. Under the influence of high doses of Cyclophosphamid (160 mg/kg), however, the number of connective tissue cells decreases by 26.5% compared with normal cells. In the Daunomycin-treated animals a decrease of connective tissue cells by 11.5% was seen. These findings proved that cytostatics which inhibit the DNA cause a decrease of the DNA content of the heart muscle, a reduction of the ploidy level of the heart muscle nuclei and a diminishing of the number of myocardial connective tissue cells.

H. Influence of Isoproterenol

The toxic effect of Isoproterenol on the heart muscle is well-known, in that it produces disseminated necroses of the myocardium when administered in high doses (*Pilny* et al., 1969). The administration of low doses results in cardiac hypertrophy (*Pfitzer* et al., 1972). We injected a single dose of 80 mg Isoproterenol/kg body weight to 50 female albino rats, and subsequently we observed a *polyploidisation of the heart muscle nuclei* (*Adler,* 1975). Within the first 48 hours following injection, the diploid heart muscle cells were reduced to 12% compared with a normal occurrence of 81%. 36% triploid cells could be seen, and tetraploid cells increased to nearly 30% compared with a normal occurrence of 10.5% (fig. 5a). This ploidy grade remains constant up to 3 weeks following the onset of the injury. Two months later, the diploid heart muscle cells dominated again showing a portion of 60%. However, 16.5% triploid and 19% tetraploid cells could still be seen. This indicates that an increased DNA synthesis is occurring within the regenerating myocardium.

Within the first 24 hours following the injury, the diploid nuclei decrease slightly from 81% to 70%, followed by a drastic reduction to 12%. Three weeks later, these cells again increase to 60%. The triploid nuclei, on the other hand, show an increase within the first three weeks from 8.5% to 63.5% followed by a drastic reduction to 16.5%. The tetraploid nuclei remain constant during the first 24 hours. On the second day after starting the experiment they show an increase of up to 30%. Even after two months the 4c-nuclei lie significantly above the norm at a value of 19%.

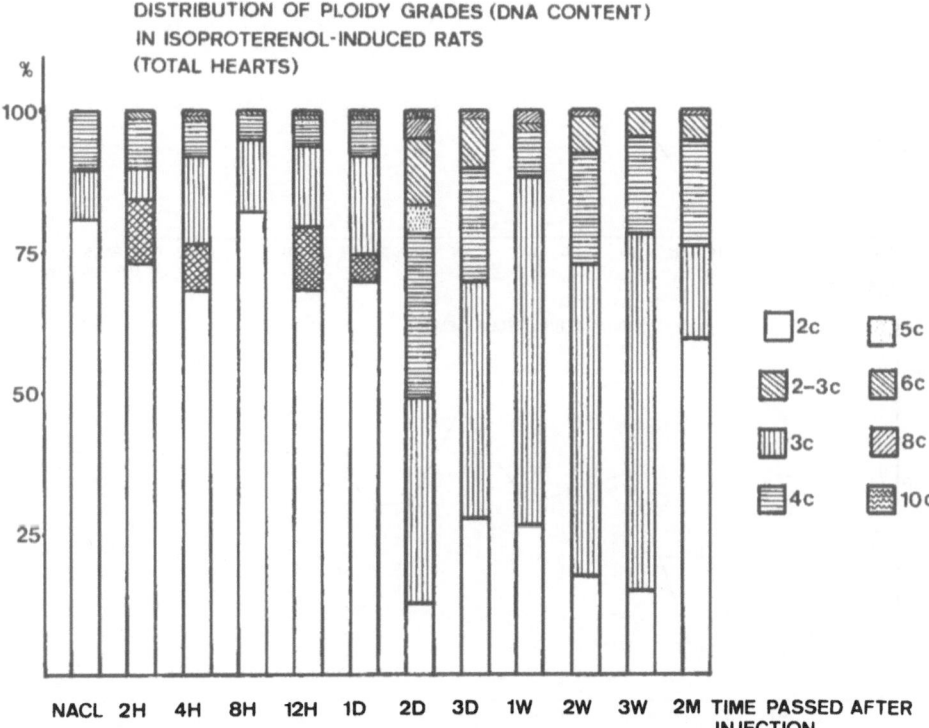

Fig. 5a. Percentage distribution of the ploidy grades of heart muscle cell nuclei of rats under the influence of Isoproterenol. A pronounced polyploidisation of the heart muscle nuclei can be seen.

Between 2 and 4 hours following the injection, the biochemically determined *amount of DNA* in the heart muscle is reduced from 660 µg to 240 µg. After 12 hours, an increase in the amount of DNA to approximately 1000 µg can be seen. The amount of DNA which originates exclusively from the heart muscle nuclei increases 24 hours following the administration of Isoproterenol from 1.4×10^{-9} g/200 nuclei to 2.3×10^{-9} g, which corresponds to an increase of the amount of DNA by approximately 70%. Later the curve sinks back to 1.6×10^{-9} g, but is still far beyond the initial level. Within a period of between 2–12 hours following the injection a loss of myocardial tissue must have occurred which caused the reduction of the amount of the biochemically measured DNA. The big increase of the DNA, 12 hours after the beginning of the experiment, is partly due to the increase of the DNA in the heart muscle nuclei.

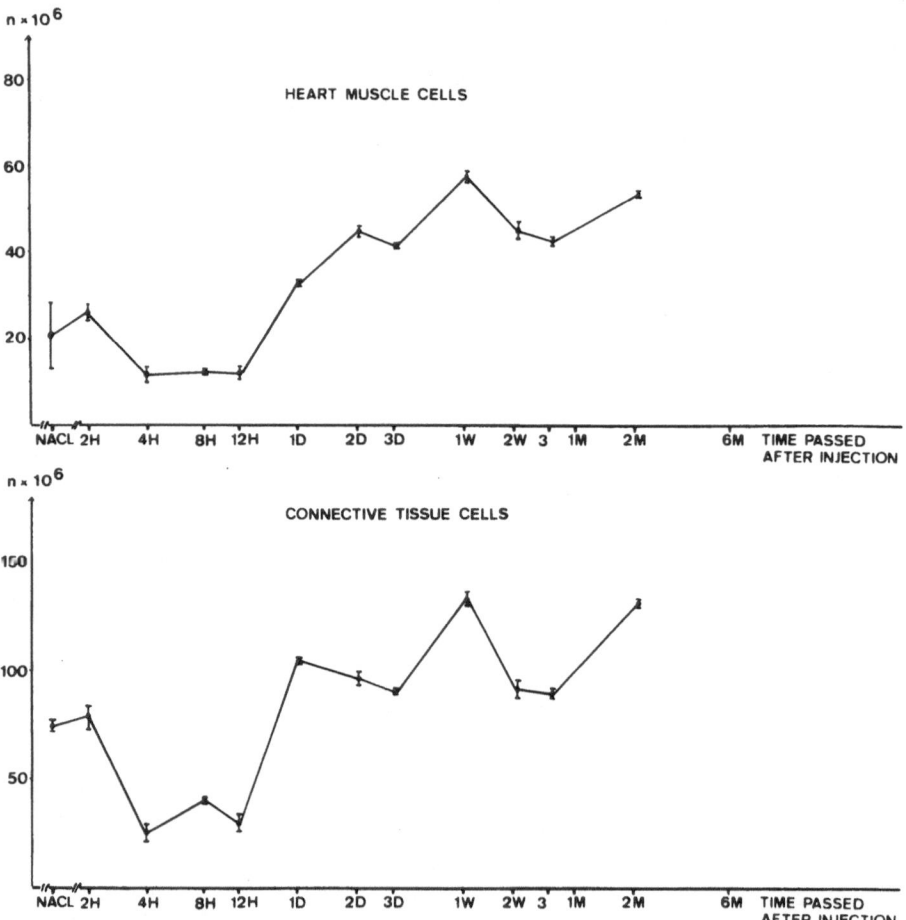

Fig. 5b. Cell number of the rat's myocardium under the influence of Isoproterenol. The pronounced increase of heart muscle cells as well as of connective tissue cells points to the regeneration capability of the myocardium.

The calculation of the *number of cells* in the hearts yielded the following results (fig. 5b): The number of connective tissue cells has been diminished from 75×10^6 to 26×10^6 within 4 hours following the administration of Isoproterenol. In a period ranging from 12 to 24 hours, an increase to $100\text{--}130 \times 10^6$ cells can be seen. The connective tissue remain therefore at an increased level of 33–37% compared with the norm. Two hours following the injection the number of heart muscle cells is reduced from 22×10^6 to 12×10^6. After 12 hours, their number reaches a maximum of 58×10^6, thus characterizing the regeneration capabilities of the myocardium.

Therefore cardiac hypertrophy caused by a prolonged functional activity of the heart occurs simultaneously with both quantitative and partly qualitative alterations seen in the substances of the heart muscle cells, as well as with an alteration of the absolute cell number. Due to these alterations the excessive strain put on the myocardium may be compensated to a certain degree, but, on the other hand, they may also lead to final heart failure.

Zusammenfassung

In wachsenden Menschenherzen nimmt die biochemisch bestimmte *Gesamtmenge an DNS* von 20 mg auf 50–100 mg zu, und in hypertrophierten Herzen kann die Zunahme der DNS das Dreifache gegenüber normalen Herzen betragen. Während die meisten Tierherzen fast ausschließlich diploide Muskelzellen besitzen, sind die meisten Muskelzellkerne in Menschenherzen polyploid. Entsprechend dem Hypertrophiegrad findet eine ausgeprägte *Polyploidisierung* der Herzmuskelzellen statt. Das quantitative Verhältnis nichtkondensiertes Chromatin/kondensiertes Chromatin bleibt bei allen Hypertrophiegraden konstant 4:1. Die *Menge an Myoglobin* beträgt in über 500 g schweren Herzen mehr als 100% gegenüber normalen Herzen und ist mit der Dicke der Herzmuskelfasern korreliert. In hypertrophierten Herzen läßt sich eine unregelmäßige und höhere *Doppelbrechung des Myosins* beobachten, die auf ein frühes Stadium der Nekrose hinweist. Bei der konzentrischen Herzhypertrophie hat das *Trockengewicht* der Muskelfasern mehr zugenommen als bei der exzentrischen Herzhypertrophie. Die *Proteinkonzentration* innerhalb der Muskelfasern nimmt mit steigendem Herzgewicht zu. Einige *Zytostatika* rufen eine Abnahme des myokardialen DNS-Gehaltes, eine Verminderung des Ploidieniveaus und eine Verringerung der Anzahl der Bindegewebszellen hervor. *Isoproterenol* bewirkt innerhalb der ersten 3 Wochen nach Verabreichung eine ausgeprägte Reduktion der Zellzahl; nach 2 Monaten findet eine erhebliche Polyploidisierung der Herzmuskelzellen statt, und die Zellzahl steigt wiederum über das Normalmaß an, was auf die Regenerationsfähigkeit des Myokards hinweist.

References

1. *Adler, C. P.:* Polyploidisierung und Zellzahl im menschlichen Herzen. Habilitationsschrift, Freiburg i. Br., 1971.
2. *Adler, C. P.:* Morphologische Grundlagen der Herzhypertrophie und des Herzwachstums. Med. Welt **23**, 477–484 (1972).
3. *Adler, C. P.:* Einfluß von Cytostatica auf den DNS-Gehalt und die Zellzahl in Herzen. Verh. Dtsch. Ges. Path. **56**, 656 (1972).
4. *Adler, C. P.:* Der Gehalt von Protein und Myoglobin in hypertrophierten Herzmuskelzellen. Mikrospektrophotometrische Untersuchungen an Menschenherzen. In: *H. Roskamm* und *H. Reindell* (ed.): Das chronisch kranke Herz. Grundlagen der funktionellen Diagnostik und Therapie, pp. 113–118 (Stuttgart–New York 1973).

5. *Adler, C. P.:* Myokardiale DNS und Zellzahl nach Isoproterenol-induzierten Herzmuskelnekrosen bei der Ratte. Verh. Dtsch. Ges. Path. **59**, 589 (1975).
6. *Adler, C. P.:* DNS in Kinderherzen. Biochemische und zytophotometrische Untersuchungen. Beitr. Path. **158**, 173–202 (1976).
7. *Adler, C. P., A. Hartz, W. Sandritter:* Form and Structure of Cell Nuclei in Growing and Hypertrophied Human Hearts. Beitr. Path. **161**, 342–362 (1977).
8. *Fanburg, B. L.:* Experimental cardiac hypertrophy. New Engl. J. Med. **282**, 723–732 (1970).
9. *Grove, D., R. Zak, K. G. Nair:* Mechanism of increase in myocardial DNA content during myocardial hypertrophy. Clin. Res. **16**, 231 (1968).
10. *Klinge, O.:* Karyokinese und Kernmuster im Herzmuskel wachsender Ratten. Virchows Arch. Abt. B. Zellpath. **6**, 208–219 (1970).
11. *Meerson, F. Z.:* Hyperfunktion, Hypertrophie und Insuffizienz des Herzens (Berlin 1969).
12. *Nowy, H., H. D. Frings, L. Tenderich:* Unterschiede der Eiweißzusammensetzung des normalen und des hypertrophischen Kaninchenherzens. Naturwiss. **46**, 18–19 (1959).
13. *Onishi, S., F. Büchner, M. Thermann, R. Zittel:* Das elektronenmikroskopische Bild des Herzmuskels bei experimenteller chronischer Hypertrophie in der Phase der Kompensation. Beitr. path. Anat. **140**, 38–53 (1969).
14. *Pfitzer, P.:* Nuclear DNA content of human myocardial cells. Current Topics Path. **54**, 125–168 (1971).
15. *Pfitzer, P., H. Kuhn:* DNS-Gehalt und DNS-Synthese in den Zellkernen normaler und hypertrophierter Rattenherzen. Verh. Dtsch. Ges. Path. **54**, 673 (1970).
16. *Pfitzer, P., H. J. Knieriem, H. Dietrich, G. Herbertz:* Hypertrophie des Rattenherzens nach Isoproterenol (morphometrische, elektronenmikroskopische, autoradiographische, cytophotometrische und biochemische Befunde). Virchows Arch. Abt. B Zellpath. **12**, 22–38 (1972).
17. *Pilny, J., G. Kiefer, W. Sandritter:* Quantitative und qualitative polarisationsoptische Untersuchungen am Myosin des Rattenherzens. Virchows Arch. Abt. B Zellpath. **3**, 359–364 (1969).
18. *Poche, R.:* Ultrastructure of heart muscle under pathological conditions. Ann. N.Y. Acad. Sci. **156**, 34 (1969).
19. *Rumyantsev, P. P.:* DNA synthesis and nuclear division in embryonal and postnatal histogenesis of myocardium (autoradiographic study). Fed. Proc. (Transl. Suppl.) **24**, 899–902 (1965).
20. *Sandritter, W., K. D. Grosser, H. G. Schiemer:* Trockengewichtsbestimmungen an normalen und pathologischen Herzmuskelfasern. Verh. Dtsch. Ges. Path. **44**, 192–194 (1960).
21. *Sandritter, W., G. Scomazzoni:* Deoxyribonucleic acid content (Feulgen photometry) and dry weight (interference microscopy) of normal and hypertrophic heart muscle fibres. Nature **202**, 100–101 (1964).
22. *Sandritter, W., K. D. Grosser, D. Rast, G. Schlüter, G. Beneke:* Trockengewichtsbestimmung an Herzmuskelfasern bei experimenteller Herzhypertrophie (Röntgenhistographische Untersuchungen). Beitr. Path. **143**, 261–270 (1971).
23. *Sandritter, W., C. P. Adler:* A method for determining cell number on organs with polyploid cell nuclei. Beitr. Path. **146**, 99–103 (1972).

For reprints:

Prof. Dr. med. *Claus-Peter Adler,* Institute of Pathology, University of Freiburg i. Br., Albertstr. 19, D-7800 Freiburg i. Br., Germany

Basic Res. Cardiol. **75**, 139–142 (1980)
© 1980 Dr. Dietrich Steinkopff Verlag, Darmstadt
ISSN 0300–8428

Paper, presented at the Erwin Riesch Symposium, Tübingen, April 3–7, 1979

Laboratoire de Physiologie Animale, Université Scientifique et Médicale, Grenoble

Increased uracil nucleotide metabolism during the induction of cardiac hypertrophy by β-stimulation in rats*)

Gesteigerter Uracil-Nucleotid-Metabolismus während der Erzeugung einer Herzhypertrophie durch β-Rezeptoren-Stimulierung bei der Ratte

A. Rossi, J. Olivares, J. Aussedat, and *A. Ray*

With 1 figure

Summary

The dynamics of uracil nucleotides was followed in the rat heart during the induction of cardiac hypertrophy by β-adrenoreceptor stimulation.

Isoproterenol (ISO) 5 mg · kg^{-1} was administered subcutaneously daily for 8 consecutive days. A significant increase in ventricular dry weight (40%) was observed on the 5th day of β-stimulation, thereafter no further increase occurred. A single dose of ISO increased uridine triphosphate (UTP) concentration and the whole uracil nucleotide pool (UN). The increase was maximal (80 and 100%) 12 hours after ISO administration. The ^{32}phosphate incorporation into the α-phosphate group of UN was increased by about a factor of 2 for the same period of time. Slight decrease in pool sizes (UTP and UN) and labelling occurred from 12 to 24 h after β-stimulation. Similar changes also occurred on the 8th day of ISO administration, however modifications in concentrations and labelling were attenuated. The results show that modifications in the synthesis of UN should also be taken into account when studying the early events leading to cardiac hypertrophy.

Alterations in the level and the synthesis of adenine nucleotides have been shown to occur during the genesis of cardiac hypertrophy (1–4). Lesser attention has been paid to the study of the metabolism of uracil nucleotides in hypertrophy. An expansion of the UN pool has been reported for the rat heart after constriction of the aorta (5), and an increased activity of uridine kinase was demonstrated under similar experimental conditions (6). It was of interest to further investigate whether changes could in fact occur using a different stimulus. Isoproterenol (ISO) was used for the induction of cardiac hypertrophy because of its early onset of action. Uridine triphosphate (UTP) and whole uracil nucleotide pool (UN) concentrations were monitored. Furthermore, by using the labelling technique with ^{32}phosphate, the turnover rates of UN were also studied.

---

*) Supported by a grant from the DGRST (n° 77. 7. 1023)

Methods

Female Wistar rats (220–260 g) were used in the present study. ISO (5 mg · kg⁻¹) was administered subcutaneously on each of the 8 days of the study period. Nucleotides were extracted from the ventricles with cold perchlorid acid. UTP was determined by the enzymatic method described by *Keppler* et al. (7). For the determination of the whole uracil nucleotide pool (UN) the nucleotides were alkaline-hydrolyzed to monophosphates and then separated by ion-exchange chromatography (8). The pool size was estimated either spectrophotometrically (8) or by the method of labelling (9), ^{3}H-Uridine being used as tracer. The turnover of UN was estimated by the rate of ^{32}phosphate (^{32}P) incorporation into α position of the nucleotides (10). For this purpose ^{32}P (4 µCi · g⁻¹) was injected into the femoral vein of slightly anesthetized rats by ether. The animals were killed 2, 4, 6 and 8 hours after the injection of radioactive phosphate. The nucleotides, extracted from the ventricles, were cleaved as monophosphates, then separated and purificated as previously described (8–10). The specific activity of both uridine monophosphate and inorganic phosphate (Pi) was calculated.

Results

Under our experimental conditions the dry weight of ventricles increased by about 40% on the 5th day. Ribonucleic acid concentration (expressed by g dry weight) increased by 39%. No further significant increase of weight and ribonucleic acid occurred later.

Figure 1 summarizes the main results of the present report.

UTP and UN levels

The first injection of ISO had a biphasic effect. A transient decrease in UTP content was followed by an increase of up to 80% above the control value 12 hours after injection. 20 hours after ISO injection a slight decrease of nevertheless 50% above control level was observed. Eight days following daily ISO administration, the pattern of UTP changes was similar to that seen during the first day, although less pronounced. Measurements of UN pool size 12 hours after the 1st and 8th ISO injection revealed that the enlargement of the whole UN pool parallels that of UTP.

^{32}Phosphate labelling

The kinetics of ^{32}P incorporation into the α-phosphate group (αP) showed that the dynamics of UN is modified in the same direction as pool sizes. The ^{32}P incorporation was increased by a factor of 2 in the period of time from the 7th to 13th hour after ISO administration. A slight decrease of this labelling was observed in the period from the 18th to 24th hour.

Discussion

The results reported in this paper demonstrate that the β-stimulation induces marked modifications both in pool size and rate of phosphorylation of cardiac uracil nucleotides. Since increased turnover rate of UN precedes enhanced synthesis of nucleic acids, it seems reasonable to assume that these two processes may be intimately related. In addition the

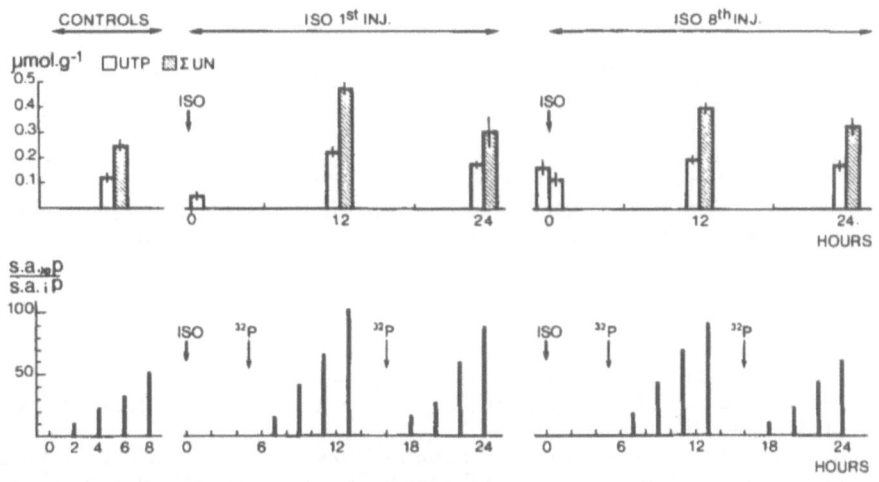

Fig. 1.

Upper panel. Effect of the administration of Isoproterenol (5 mg · kg⁻¹) on the levels of uridine triphosphate (UTP) and uracil nucleotide (Σ UN) pool sizes on the first and the eighth consecutive days. Values are presented in micromolar concentrations per gram wet weight (with appropriate corrections for constant water content). All values are significantly different (P = 0.05) from controls. Each measurement is the mean ± S.D. of at least 5 hearts for UTP and the mean ± S.D. of 3 measurements of 5 pooled hearts each for UN.

Lower panel. Incorporation of ³²phosphate (³²P) into α-position of uracil nucleotides. ³²P (4 µCi · g⁻¹) was injected into the femoral vein 5 or 16 hours after the first or the eighth ISO administration. Measurements were made 2, 4, 6 and 8 hours after ³²P injection. The values are expressed as ratio of specific activity of α-phosphate to the specific activity of inorganic phosphate (S.a. αP/S.a. iP) and given in percentages. Each value was obtained from pooled ventricles (5 animals).

simultaneous decrease in UN synthesis and the absence of any further increase of nucleic acid synthesis further support such an interrelationship.

A decrease in myocardial ATP level has been suggested as a triggering factor in the induction of cardiac hypertrophy by different stimuli (11). However, the results of the present study seem to suggest that increase both in pool size and turnover rate of UN may also play a role through increased synthesis of nucleic acids. In fact, an increase of UN level has already been observed in cardiac hypertrophy induced by aortic constriction in rats (5).

Zusammenfassung

Die Dynamik der Uracil-Nucleotide wurde im Rattenherzen während der Auslösung einer Herzhypertrophie durch Stimulierung β-adrenerger Rezeptoren verfolgt.

Isoproterenol (ISO) (5 mg · kg⁻¹) wurde an 8 aufeinanderfolgenden Tagen subkutan verabfolgt. Es wurde ein signifikanter Anstieg des Trockengewichtes des linken Ventrikels bis zum 5. Tag der β-Stimulation beobachtet, danach kam es zu keinem weiteren Anstieg. Eine einzelne Dosis von ISO erhöhte die Uridintriphosphat-(UTP)Konzentration und den Gesamtvorrat an Uracil-Nucleotiden (UN). Der

Anstieg war 12 Stunden nach der Verabfolgung von ISO maximal (80 bzw. 100%). Die Inkorporation von ^{32}Phosphat in der α-Phosphatgruppe von UN stieg während des gleichen Zeitraums um etwa einen Faktor 2. Ein leichter Abfall in der Größe der Vorräte (UTP und UN) sowie der Markierung war von der 12. bis zur 24. Stunde nach β-Stimulierung zu verzeichnen. Ähnliche Veränderungen traten auch am 8. Tag der Verabfolgung von ISO in Erscheinung, jedoch waren die Unterschiede in den Konzentrationen und der Markierung abgeschwächt. Die Ergebnisse zeigen, daß beim Studium der frühen Veränderungen, die zur Herzhypertrophie führen, auch Modifikationen in der Synthese von UN in Betracht gezogen werden sollten.

References

1. *Kako, K.:* Biochemical changes of the rat myocardium induced by iso-proterenol. Canad. J. Physiol. Pharmacol. **43**, 541–549 (1965).
2. *Fleckenstein, A., H. J. Döring, O. Leder:* The significance of high-energy phosphate exhaustion in the etiology of isoproterenol-induced cardiac necrosis and its prevention by iproveratril, compound D 600 or prenylamine. In: International Symposium on Drugs and Metabolism of Myocardium and Striated Muscle. *M. Lamarche, R. Royer.* Nancy 11–22 (1969).
3. *Fizel, A., A. Fizelova:* Cardiac hypertrophy and heart failure dynamics of changes in high-energy phosphate compounds, glycogen and lactic acid. J. Mol. Cell. Cardiol. **2**, 187–192 (1971).
4. *Zimmer, H. G., E. Gerlach:* Effect of beta-adrenergic stimulation on myocardial adenine nucleotide metabolism. Circulat. Res. **35**, 536–543 (1974).
5. *Koide, T., M. Rabinowitz:* Biochemical correlates of cardiac hypertrophy. II. Increased rate of RNA synthesis in experimental cardiac hypertrophy in the rat. Circulat. Res. **24**, 9–18 (1969).
6. *Matsushita, S., B. L. Fanburg:* Pyrimidine nucleotide synthesis in the normal and hypertrophying heart. Relative importance of the de novo and salvage pathways. Circulat. Res. **27**, 415–428.
7. *Keppler, D., J. Rudigier, K. Decker:* Enzymic determination of Uracil Nucleotides in tissues. Anal. Biochem. **38**, 105–114 (1970).
8. *Rossi, A., P. Mandel, G. Dessaux:* Cinétique de renouvellement du phosphate α des nucléotides libres dans le tissu myocardique du rat. Arch. int. Physiol. Biochem. **80**, 59–77 (1972).
9. *Rossi, A.:* Incorporation of uridine by the perfused rabbit heart. Life Sciences, **16**, 1121–1132 (1975).
10. *Rossi, A.:* ^{32}P labelling of the nucleotides in α-position in the rabbit heart. J. Mol. Cell. Cardiol. **7**, 891–906 (1975).
11. *Meerson, F. Z., V. D. Pomoinitsky:* The role of high-energy phosphate compounds in the development of cardiac hypertrophy. J. Mol. Cell. Cardiol. **4**, 568–578 (1972).

Authors' address:

Dr. *A. Rossi,* Laboratoire de Physiologie Animale, Université Scientifique et Médicale, BP. 53 X – 38041 Grenoble-Cedex (France)

Basic Res. Cardiol. **75**, 143–148 (1980)
© 1980 Dr. Dietrich Steinkopff Verlag, Darmstadt
ISSN 0300–8428

Paper, presented at the Erwin Riesch Symposium, Tübingen, April 3–7, 1979

U 127 INSERM, Hôpital Lariboisière, Paris (France)

Experimental systolic and diastolic overloading in rats: total proteins turnover rate. Enzymatic and structural properties of myosin

Experimentelle systolische und diastolische Überbelastung bei der Ratte: Umsatzrate der Gesamtproteine. Enzymatische und strukturelle Eigenschaften von Myosin

B. Swynghedauw, K. Schwartz, J. Bercovici, P. Bouveret, A. M. Lompre, N. V. Thiem, and *G. Lacombe*

With 1 table

Summary

The fractional turnover rate of the total cardiac proteins has been measured by using the continuous infusion technique with ^{3}H lysine. It augments by a factor of 3 in systolic as well as in diastolic overloading, but in the former the peak was reached within the first week after operation and in the later the peak was not reached until the 14th day.

The myosin structure and enzymatic properties have been studied in several huge hypertrophic hearts (around 100% hypertrophy). In this condition the burst size of myosin is normal, as well as its K^+ATPase, but there is a sharp decline in the Ca^{2+} ATPase activity. Moreover, antibodies against native or defolded heavy meromyosin exhibit, a vertical shift in microcomplement fixation when made to react with molecules extracted from hypertrophied hearts. The normal isozymic pattern of rat heart myosin, as shown in non dissociating electrophoresis, was reversed.

Systolic and diastolic overloading in rats were studied separately and then compared. They were also combined in such a way as to achieve gradual overloading capable of doubling heart weight.

Protein synthesis

This was studied by the continuous infusion flow technique (1) which allows measurement of turnover in a relative steady state without appreciable isotope recirculation.

Systolic and diastolic overloading were compared in an attempt to explain the slow increase in heart weight after aortic incompetence. The increase reached its peak between the 10th and 20th days, whereas in aortic stenosis, the plateau in hypertrophy was reached between the 5th and 8th days both in rabbits and rats (see further on).

Techniques

Unanesthetized restrained rats underwent continuous flow pump perfusion for 6 hours at a flow rate of 0.5 ml/hour with 10 μCi/ml of ^{3}H lysine dissolved in saline (1). The ventricles were frozen, ground and stirred for 5 min in water at + 100 °C (2) to extract free amino acids which were then separated by precipitation in 10% TCA. The pellet was washed several times and hydrolyzed once for 20 min in 0.83 N PCA at 90° to obtain DNA and RNA, and once again in 6N HCl at 120° for 18 h to obtain protein-bound amino acids. Free amino acids were desalted on AG 50 W X 8. Taurine and lysine were measured by high voltage electrophoresis. Radioactive lysine was eluted with methanol and counted in a scintillation counter (3). In some cases C^{14} tyrosine was infused and samples were treated with tyrosine decarboxylase for tyramine measurement by electrophoresis. The fractional turnover rate (Ks) was calculated according to *Millward* (1) using the specific radioactivity of free and bound lysine. Our ratio of bound to free total lysine ranged from 0.003 to 0.005 which is a little higher than the figures previously reported (1).

DNA was measured according to *Burton* (4) and RNA according to *Ceriotti* (5). We checked that i) extraction of free amino acid in boiling water did not affect RNA (in fact, it slightly increased RNA yield); ii) the *Schneider's* technique (6), essentially used here, produced the same results as *Munro*'s method (7) provided the former was corrected for DNA coloration (12%), and iii) the RNA yield was 25% higher than that obtained when the heart was treated with SDS and extracted with phenol.

Aortic abdominal stenosis was induced according to *Cutilletta* (8) with a Weck Hemoclip. Incompetence was obtained by forcing a n° 3 or 4 Biotrol polyethylene catheter through the sigmoid cusps. When both conditions were combined incompetence was induced two weeks after stenosis (9).

Results

In aortic stenosis, *ventricular weight* increased by the 2nd or 3rd day. By the 5th day, it reached a plateau of 30 to 45%. For aortic incompetence, the plateau was reached by the 10–15th day but the degree of hypertrophy was comparable. In some instances aortic stenosis or incompetence alone doubled ventricular weight, but such hypertrophy was usually obtained by the two-step overloading technique. The degree of hydration was unchanged, as others have also shown (10).

The normal fractional turnover rate Ks was 14 ± 3% of the total proteins renewed per day; in the controls the specific radioactivity of free lysine was 52 ± 15 dpm/nmole and of bound lysine 1.5 ± 0.4. Normal hearts contained 43 nmole/100 mg fresh tissue of free lysine and 4.1 μmole/100 mg f.t. of protein bound lysine. The control Ks did not correlate with heart weight, which is in contradiction with other results. In protein hydrolysates, 90% of the radioactivity was in the lysine, compared to 30% in the free amino acids.

The specific radioactivity of free amino acids was unchanged during overloading, but the radioactivity of protein-bound lysine, and consequently the Ks, both increased and were correlated ($R = 0.73$, $p < 0.01$). In *systolic overloading* the peak was reached during the first week (Ks = 33% and protein-bound lysine = 3.8 dpm per mole); in diastolic overloading, on the other hand, the peak was not reached until the 14th day (Ks = 32%; protein-bound lysine = 40 dpm/mole) (table 1). In addition, normalization was slower in diastolic than in systolic overloading. The Ks was of course not measured in a steady state, and the growth rate of the heart during the infusion period has to be substracted from Ks, which in fact did not alter the results. Using the same calculation as *Everett* we compared protein synthesis and growth rate, to ascertain whether a decrease in lysis was necessary to explain hypertrophy. As in the case of *Everett* rough calculations showed that lysis not only failed to diminish but increased.

The fractional turnover rate was normal in *compensatory hypertrophy,* whatever its origin, as well as in the few animals with more than 100% cardiac hypertrophy and/or failing hearts (table 1). This contradicts the results of *Meerson's* group.

The *RNA concentration* increased after overloading, but only slightly. The increase (from 2.81 to 3.37 µg/mg f.t.) was observed during the first week in systolic overloading and during the second (up to 3.40 µg) in diastolic overloading. *The DNA content* of the heart was not only enhanced in aortic stenosis (from 1.45 mg per heart to 2.40), as shown by others and in aortic stenosis incompetence (up to 2.94), but also in aortic incompetence alone (up to 2.10 mg), which was unexpected.

The taurine concentration remained within the normal range (1.76 µmole/100 mg f.t.) even after one month of systolic and diastolic overloading. The only exceptions were some of the bulky failing hypertrophic hearts in which the concentration doubled. This is in agreement with others who showed that the increase in taurine correlates more closely with failure than with hypertrophy.

Discussion

This comparative study throws some light on the trigger mechanism that stimulates protein synthesis in overloading. At some stages such a

Table 1. Fractional turnover rate Ks (in % of protein renewed per day) in experimental cardiac overloading in rats.

	Normal	1st week	2nd week	3rd week	1 month +
Aortic stenosis (A. S.)	14 ± 3 (N=15)	33±8 (N = 9)	22±3 (N = 8)	18±3 (N = 3)	13±3 (N = 5)
Aortic insufficiency (A. I.)		18±5 (N = 4)	20±2 (N = 4)	32±7 (N = 5)	14±4 (N = 5)
A. S. + A. I.					14±3 (N = 5)

mechanism necessarily affects both the initial mechanical and biochemical events which follow overloading.

The tension-velocity curve shows that systolic overloading intensifies power by increasing the afterload and by reducing the shortening velocity, whilst in diastolic overloading the same effect was obtained by altering the length and, therefore, by using another velocity-tension curve with a faster shortening velocity (the afterload was not changed). It is generally known that, for both cardiac and skeletal muscle, efficiency, i.e. unit of work per mole of ATP or work/work + heat, reaches its peak at a given shortening velocity. For most muscles, maximum efficiency is reached during exercise and decreases at rest. This supports the hypothesis that systolic overloading, which depressed velocity instantaneously, also depresses efficiency; whereas diastolic overloading, which increases velocity, raises efficiency to its maximum at rest. This is why, under the present conditions, we observed a decline in efficiency during exercise. It is, in fact, the only way of explaining the observed delay and suggests that a decline in efficiency was the real mechanism triggering hypertrophy, a hypothesis closely resembling that of *Meerson*.

Structure and enzymatic properties of myosin

In skeletal muscle, new functional requirements can induce changes both in contractile activity and the isozymic pattern of myosin and the glycolytic enzymes. The overloaded heart may also be connected with isozymic changes in lactate dehydrogenases, although these changes may be the result of an increase in the number of fibroblasts (11), and in myosin.

Techniques

Cardiac ventricular myosin was prepared essentially according to *Offer* with slight modifications (12). The early phosphate burst size and the steady-state ATPase specific activities were measured as previously published (12). The antibodies have been raised in guinea-pigs against purified rat ventricular heavy meromyosin either in a native form (13) or denatured by treatment with sodium dodecyl sulfate (SDS) (14). The excess in SDS was removed by gel filtration (14). Electrophoresis in a nondissociating medium was performed according to *Hoh* (15) or *d'Albis* (14) using native myosin.

Heart hypertrophy was induced as above and animals exhibiting 60 to 120% hypertrophy have been selected. They were compared to sham-operated animals.

Results

The myosins from normal hypertrophied hearts have the same burst size, between 0.7 and 0.8 mole of ATP per active site, which rules out the possible presence of denatured or aggregated molecules. Moreover, SDS gel electrophoresis visualized the heavy and light subunits as single bands.

The steady-state Ca^{2+}-dependent ATPase activity of myosin from hypertrophied hearts (1120 ± 50 nmole PO_4/min mg^{-1}) was significantly depressed when compared to that from sham-operated animals (820 ± 30 nmole/min mg^{-1}, $p < 0.01$). By contrast, the K^+-dependent ATPase was unchanged (640 and 700 mmole/min mg^{-1}) (14).

Antibodies raised against native (13) or SDS-denatured (14) heavy meromyosin were tested by microcomplement fixation. Compared to the controls, they both showed a vertical shift in the maximum amount of C complement fixed when made to react with myosin from hypertrophied hearts (13). Several papers have shown that such a change in phylogeny indicates amino acid substitutions (16).

Electrophoresis in a nondissociating medium has shown that there are differences between the respective charges of several skeletal myosin isozymes. In normal rat ventricles there are 3 isozymes containing diffe-rent amounts of ATPase with a relative ratio of $V3 < V2 \ll V1$ (15). As shown by *Hoh*, thyroxine intoxication was characterized by an enhance-ment of V1 (15). We found the opposite in hypertrophied hearts after prolonged overloading. In this case the diminished ATPase was associated with an elevation of V3 at the expense of the other isozymic forms (14).

Discussion

Such an isozymic modification is undoubtedly related to the diminished maximum speed of shortening since, in overloading, this speed was inversely proportional to heart weight as in phylogenic studies. This could be the first myocardial adaptational step observed in overload-ing. As such, it would precede the functioning of the peripheral compen-satory mechanisms.

Supported by grant AU 78-107 and 5266/387670 from INSERM and 76-7-1413 from DGRST.
We thank Mrs. *Albaret* and *Dreyfus* for typing and rereading this paper.

Zusammenfassung

Die Umsatzrate der kardialen Gesamtproteine wurde unter Verwendung der kontinuierlichen Infusionstechnik mit ^{3}H-Lysin gemessen. Es ergab sich eine Zunahme um einen Faktor 3 sowohl bei systolischer als auch diastolischer Überbe-lastung. Jedoch wurde bei der ersteren das Maximum innerhalb der ersten Woche, bei der letzteren nicht vor 14 Tagen nach Operation erreicht.

Struktur- und enzymatische Eigenschaften von Myosin wurden bei verschiede-nen extrem hypertrophierten Herzen untersucht (Hypertrophiegrad ca. 100%). Unter diesen Bedingungen sind die initiale Phosphatfreisetzung sowohl als auch die K^+-ATPase-Aktivität von Myosin normal. Es ergab sich jedoch ein scharfer Abfall der Ca^{2+}-ATPase-Aktivität. Darüber hinaus zeigten Antikörper gegen natives oder „entfaltetes" schweres Meromyosin eine vertikale Verschiebung bei der Mikrokomplementfixierung, wenn man sie mit Molekülen aus hypertrophierten Herzen reagieren ließ. Das normale Isoenzymmuster von Myosin aus Rattenherzen, wie es sich bei Elektrophorese unter nicht dissoziierenden Bedingungen ergibt, war umgekehrt.

References

1. *Millward, D. J., P. J. Garlick, R. J. Stewart, D. O. Nnanyelugo, J. C. Waterlow:* Skeletal muscle growth and protein turn-over. Biochem. J. **150,** 235–243 (1975).
2. *Scharff, R., I. G. Wool:* Accumulation of amino acids in muscle of perfused heart. Effect of insulin. Biochem. J. **97,** 257–271 (1965).
3. *Blackburn, S.:* The determination of amino acids by high-voltage electrophoresis. In: Methods in Biochemical Analysis, *Glick* ed., Interscience publ. vol. 13, p. 1–45 (New York 1965).
4. *Burton, K.:* Determination of DNA concentration with diphenylamine. In: Methods in Enzymology, *Grossman* et al. ed. Vol. 12 (B), p. 163–166 (New York 1968).
5. *Ceriotti, G.:* Determination of nucleic acids in animal tissues. J. Biol. Chem. **214,** 59–70 (1955).
6. *Schneider, W. C.:* Phosphorus compounds in animal tissues. J. Biol. Chem. **161,** 293–303 (1945).
7. *Munro, H. W., A. Fleck:* The determination of nucleic acids. In: Methods in Biochemical Analysis, *Glick* ed. Intersciences pub. Vol. 14, p. 113–176 (New York 1965).
8. *Cutiletta, A. F., R. Zak:* Regression of myocardial hypertrophy. 1. Experimental model, changes in heart weight, nucleic acids and collagen. J. Molec. Cell. Cardiology **7,** 767–781 (1975).
9. *Hatt, P. Y.:* Cellular changes in mechanically overloaded heart. Bas. Res. Cardiology **72,** 198–202 (1977).
10. *Mavroudis, C., S. A. Jester, S. Jacobs, P. A. Ebert:* Extra cellular space, water and ion concentration in the hypertrophied rat myocardium. Amer. J. Physiol. **236,** 79–83 (1979).
11. *Revis, N. W., A. J. V. Cameron:* The relationship between fibrosis and lactate deshydrogenase isozymes in experimental hypertrophic heart of rabbits. Cardiovascular Res. **12,** 348–357 (1978).
12. *Thiem, N. V., G. Lacombe, B. Swynghedauw:* Early phosphate burst of heart myosins. Phylogenic variations. Europ. J. Biochem. **91,** 243–248 (1978).
13. *Schwartz, K., P. Bouveret, J. Bercovici, B. Swynghedauw:* An immunochemical difference between myosins from normal and hypertrophied rat hearts. FEBS Letters **93,** 137–139 (1978).
14. *Lompré, A. M., K. Schwartz, A. Albis, G. Lacombe, N. V. Thiem, B. Swynghedauw:* Myosin isoenzymic redistribution in chronic heart overload. Nature, in the press.
15. *Hoh, J. F. Y., P. A. McGrath, P. T. Hole:* Electrophoresis analysis of multiple forms of rat cardiac myosin: effects of hypophysectomy and thyroxine replacement. J. Mol. Cell. Cardiology **10,** 1053–1076 (1977).
16. *Schwartz, K., P. Bouveret, C. Sebag, Joc. Léger, B. Swynghedauw:* Immunochemical evidence for the species specificity of heart myosin and heavy meromyosin. Bioch. Bioph. Acta **435,** 24–36 (1977).

Authors' address:

Dr. *B. Swynghedauw,* U 127 INSERM, Hôpital Lariboisière, 41 Bd de la Chapelle, 75010 Paris, France

Basic Res. Cardiol. **75**, 149–156 (1980)
© 1980 Dr. Dietrich Steinkopff Verlag, Darmstadt
ISSN 0300-8428

Paper, presented at the Erwin Riesch Symposium, Tübingen, April 3–7, 1979

Section of Cardiovascular Medicine, Department of Medicine, University of
California San Francisco, School of Medicine

Mechanism of physiologic versus pathologic ventricular hypertrophy process: Enhanced or depressed myosin ATPase activity and contractility governed by type, degree and duration of inciting stress*)

Mechanismus der physiologischen und pathologischen Ventrikelhypertrophie: Erhöhte oder verminderte Myosin-ATPase-Aktivität und Kontraktilität in Abhängigkeit von Typ, Grad und Dauer der auslösenden Belastung

J. Wikman-Coffelt, M. M. Laks, T. H. Riemenschneider,
and *D. T. Mason*

With 2 figures and 2 tables

Summary

Types of hypertrophy, such as the normal development of the left ventricle of new-born lambs, induction of hypertrophy following administration of subhypertensive doses of norepinephrine, and hypertrophy where moderate pulmonic stenosis is the inciting stimulus, are all of a physiologic nature, i.e., cardiac function is elevated and K^+ stimulated myosin ATPase activity is increased. The K^+/EDTA stimulated myosin ATPase activity, used as an index of physiologic versus pathologic hypertrophy, may reflect alterations in myosin heavy chains since a large amount of light chains are in the dissociated state with this kinetic system. In experimental conditions where light-chain deficient-myosin was employed there was no corresponding decrease in myosin ATPase activity with the dissociation of light chains, irrespective of the cation activator utilized; there was however a decrease in the enzymatic activity of actomyosin with the loss of light chains. Furthermore, this decrease in actomyosin ATPase activity was partially restored with the reassociation of light chains with light-chain-deficient-myosin. Where excessive hypertrophy occurred, e.g., with moderate pulmonic stenosis, where the right ventricular free wall weight increased 100%, there was a decrease in cAMP content. This may result from the subsequent decrease in stress per sarcomere following massive hypertrophy. Where there was a lesser degree of hypertrophy, e.g., with mild pulmonic stenosis, creating a transitory 30% increase in right ventricular free wall weight, there was no subsequent decrease in cAMP content.

---

*) This study was supported by NIH-ROI-HL-23518-01 from the National Institutes of Health, Bethesda, Maryland.

Myosin ATPase activity provides a valuable parameter capable of distinguishing physiologic from pathologic ventricular hypertrophy in advanced stages of cardiac diseases. Physiologic hypertrophy is defined as hypertrophy accompanied by normal or augmented myosin ATPase activity and contractile state, whereas pathologic hypertrophy is associated with depressed myosin ATPase activity and contractility without necessarily concordant heart failure. Furthermore we formulate the concept of the dependance of the type of hypertrophy, i.e., physiological versus pathological, on the interdigitation of a combination of a number of defined major determinants, which comprise the degree of ventricular wall stress, the duration of such stress, the nature of the inciting stimulus, as well as the species, age and health of the animal.

As example of physiologic hypertrophy, experimental hyperthyroidism serves as one prototype since all myocardial metabolic and mechanical indices are elevated, including contractility and myosin ATPase activity (1). In the study described here we define further examples of physiologic hypertrophy, namely normal development of the left ventricles of newborn lambs, development of the adult dog heart following subhypertensive doses of norepinephrine, and mild as well as moderate pulmonic stenosis. We have designated the varying degrees of pulmonic stenosis as mild, moderate and severe depending on whether the pressure overloaded right ventricle resulted in a transitory increase (2), a sustained increase (3), or a diminished myosin ATPase activity (2), respectively. Thus with mild pulmonary artery banding causing a 50 to 100% rise in right ventricular peak systolic pressure, right ventricular free wall weight increased 30% (2). Moderate elevation of right ventricular peak systolic pressure of 150% resulted in increase of right ventricular free wall weight of 100% (3), whereas severe right ventricular peak systolic pressure rise of 200% caused increased free wall muscle mass of 50% (2). The study of severe pulmonic stenosis indicates that factors other than wall stress determine the degree of hypertrophy.

It is important to emphasize that when the hypertrophying stimulus is particularly prolonged and intense, excessive cell growth is elicited with disproportionate biosynthesis of organelles and contractile proteins as well as other subcellular structures, thereby leading to the evolution of pathologic hypertrophy. Pathologic hypertrophy may not only occur in chronic situations but may take place immediately such as in severe experimentally induced pulmonic or aortic stenosis (2). Pathologic hypertrophy is characterized by decreased myosin ATPase activity (2), diminished cAMP content (3) and depressed contractile function (4) as observed with severe pulmonary artery or aortic banding. These metabolic and mechanical features of pathologic hypertrophy may be the result of tissue acidity (5) and thus increased tissue PCO_2 (6).

Methods

Left ventricular and atrial myosin were prepared from canine hearts according to the methods described by *Long* et al. (7). Rabbit skeletal muscle myosin was purified by procedures defined by *Fabian* and *Muhlrad* (8). Five to twenty percent gradient polyacrylamide slab gels were used for analyzing the purity of myosin (7). Actin was extracted from beef heart using an acetone dry powder and further purified following the procedures described by *Spudich* (9). Trinitrophenylation of myosin by 2, 4, 6-trinitrobenzenesulfonate was carried out as described by *Fabian* and *Muhlrad* (8). The number of moles of trinitrophenyllysine was assessed by the methods of *Okuyama* and *Satake* as described by *Fabian* and *Muhlrad* (8) based on the change in absorbance at 346 mμ ($\varepsilon = 1.45 \times 10^4$). The reaction conditions for K^+ and Ca^{2+}-activated ATPase activities of myosin have been described earlier (7). For Mg^{2+} and actin-activated ATPase activities, the reaction mixture contained 1 mM $MgCl_2$, 0.8 mM ATP, 20 mM imidizole pH 7.0, 10^{-7} M $CaCl_2$ (EGTA-buffered), and 0.03 M KCl. To optimize the number of actomyosin sites, a weight ratio of actin to myosin of 1:2.5 was mixed as described by *Pemrick* (10).

Results and discussion

Under various normal and experimental conditions the correspondence between the rate of myosin ATP hydrolysis (irrespective of the cation activator) and actin-stimulated ATPase activity, are not always directly related (table 1). For example, the K^+-stimulated ATPase activity of sheep atrial and ventricular myosins are similar, whereas actin stimu-

Table 1. Myosin ATPase activity (37 °C) (moles Pi/mg/min).

	K$^+$	Ca^{2+}	Mg^{2+}	Actin+Mg^{2+}
		Cation activator		
Myosin				
Rabbit skeletal	5.60	1.30*	0.02*	0.65*
Sheep ventricle	1.80	0.75	0.01	0.03
Sheep atria	1.80	1.50*	0.02*	0.07*
	(Percent change in activity)			
Rabbit skeletal 6 mole TNP	95% ↓	82% ↓	1100% ↑	60% ↓
Sheep ventricle 6 moles TNP	60% ↓	60% ↓	300% ↑	60% ↓
	(Percent change in activity)			
Rabbit skeletal light-chain deficient	–0–	–0–	–0–	25% ↓
Rabbit skeletal reassociated	–0–	–0–	–0–	8% ↓
Sheep ventricle light-chain deficient	–0–	–0–	–0–	25% ↓
Sheep ventricle reassociated	–0–	–0–	–0–	9% ↓

Decrease ↓   Increase ↑

Normal myosin ATPase activity values, where K^+, Ca^{2+} or Mg^{2+} are the cation activators, are shown as well as that for actomyosin; procedures are as described in Methods. Shown also are variations in specific myosin ATPase activity values following trinitrophenylation of myosin which have been recently described in detail (17). Alterations in myosin ATPase activity following dissociation and reassociation of myosin light chains with light chain deficient myosin are the results of techniques described in earlier reports (16), namely, myosin was dissociated at 0.5 mg/ml for 5 min at 35 °C using the K^+/EDTA kinetic system.

* These values are to be compared relative to myosin ATPase activity with Ca^{2+} or Mg^{2+} as the activators with actomyosin ATPase activity.

Solid squares indicate comparisons discussed in the text.

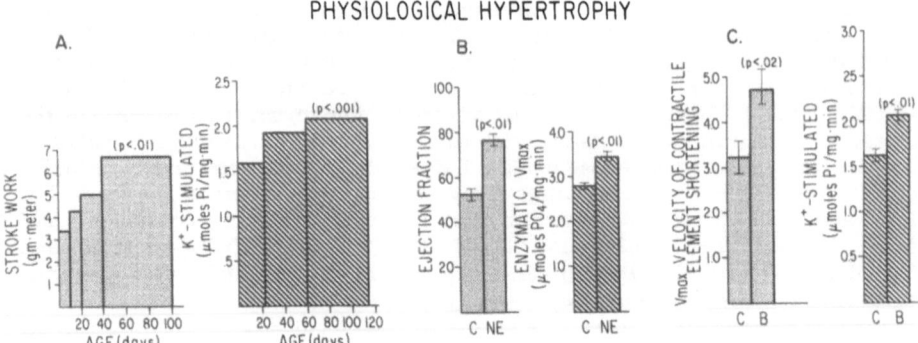

PHYSIOLOGICAL HYPERTROPHY

Fig. 1A. Thirty-five newborn lambs (ages 1 day to 120 days) were anesthesized with 40 mg/kg of alpha chloralose I.V., a left thoracotomy was performed and the animals were intrumented with Konigberg microtransducers, flow probes and catheters. Using resting conditions, recording of hemodynamics variables permitted calculation of ventricular stroke work. By 120 days the left ventricular free wall weight had increased to 300% over immediate postparturition weight. Myosin was purified from the isolated heart, and the rate of K+-stimulated ATPase activity analyzed.

Fig. 1B. A right atrial catheter was connected to a battery operated SAGE micro-infusion pump. The pump was set to deliver 2 ml of norepinephrine (0.5 µg/min) per day. After two weeks the dosage was increased to 0.9 µg/min; after another two weeks it was further increased to 1.4 µg/min and this dose was maintained for the remaining study. After three months there was a 15–20% increase in heart weight. Averages shown are for five dogs. Ejection fraction was calculated from single plane cineangiography, where end-diastolic volume, end systolic volume, and stroke volume were determined.

$$\frac{\text{Stroke Volume}}{\text{End-Diastolic Volume}} = \text{Ejection Fraction}$$

Infusion of norepinephrine continued for 3 months, after which time the animals were sacrificed. The K+-stimulated myosin ATPase activities, measured after sacrifice of the animal, are expressed as enzymatic V_{max} values.

Fig. 1C. Pulmonic stenosis utilizing the Jacobson cuff was performed as previously described (2, 3). There was a 100% increase in right ventricular free wall weight by three weeks postoperatively. The mechanical velocity of contractile element shortening (V_{CE}) was calculated based upon the three-component Hill model as we have delineated previously (3). In brief, a developed pressure-velocity curve was computed at 5 msec intervals by relating instantaneous V_{CE} to simultaneous developed ventricular pressure throughout the isovolumic phase of systole, with contractile state quantified as V_{CE} at 10 mm Hg developed pressure. The equation for V_{CE} constituted the quotient of instantaneous intraventricular rate of pressure rise (dP/dt) related to the product of developed isovolumic pressure (IP = instantaneous total pressure minus ventricular end-diastolic pressure) and the series elastic stiffness component of 32/muscle length. Thus the ordinate was $V_{CE} = (dP/dt) (32.IP)$ expressed in representative muscle lengths for the ventricle and the abscissa was simultaneous developed isovolumic pressure (IP). The intraventricular pressure was attained by a high-fidelity catheter system and several sequential beats were averaged to ascertain each pressure-velocity curve from which the peak V_{CE} was determined. Values shown are for five adult dogs. After the animals were sacrificed the heart was excised, myosin purified, and the K+-stimulated ATPase activity analyzed (3).

lated ATPase activity of sheep atrial myosin is twice as high as that of the ventricle. Both the Mg^{2+} and Ca^{2+}-stimulated ATPase activities of atrial myosin are greater than that of rabbit skeletal muscle myosin whereas the actin-activated ATPase activity is less. Relative to the light chains, they do not appear to be important for myosin ATPase activity but are important relative to actin-activated myosin ATPase activity. In assessing chemical modification of myosin with trinitrobenzene-sulfonate, following 6 moles of incorporation, the actin-activated myosin ATPase activity resembled that of Ca^{2+} and K^+ stimulation where the ATPase activity was depressed; on the other hand Mg^{2+} stimulated ATPase activity was augmented following such lysine modification with trinitrobenzenesulfonate (table I).

Series of studies are accumulating where, under experimental conditions, myosin expresses augmentated or depressed ATPase activity with defined cation activators but not with others. In two types of physiological hypertrophy described here (Fig. 1A and B), namely the normal development of newborn lamb hearts, and norepinephrine-induced hypertrophied hearts, there is an increase in K^+-activated myosin ATPase activity but not activation with other cations. With the K^+-activated myosin ATPase activity system a large percent of the myosin light chains are in a dissociated state (fig. 2); it is possible that some myosins may be more stable or labile under these dissociation conditions because of the type of heavy chain present, and thus K^+ stimulated myosin ATPase activity may reflect these variations. In the other type of physiological hypertrophy, namely pulmonic stenosis (fig. 1C) both K^+ and Ca^{2+}-stimulated ATPase activities are augmented (2).

It appears that with different types of hypertrophy we are observing variances in myosin modification which appear to be secondary to the hypertrophy process, and proposedly occur *de novo* protein biosynthesis.

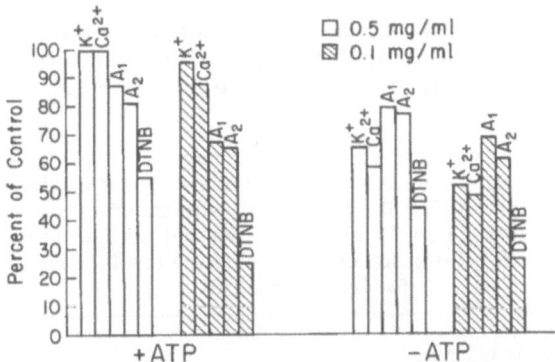

Fig. 2. The bar graphs marked with K^+ and Ca^{2+} indicate the rate of K^+ and Ca^{2+} activation of myosin following dissociation of the light chains as discussed in earlier reports (16). A_1 and A_2 indicate the percent of each of the respective alkali light chains following dissociation at the protein concentration indicated, and the bar graph marked DTNB indicates the amount of the calcium binding light chain present following dissociation. Dissociation was carried out using the K^+/EDTA kinetic system for 10 min at 37 °C as discussed earlier (16). Myosin was precipitated at the end of the incubation period and myosin subunit quantification carried out using polyacrylamide gradient slab gel electrophoresis (16).

It is proposed that increased systolic pressure, leading to increase in muscle fiber stretch (11) may act either directly (12) or indirectly on the nucleus causing alterations in transcription, and thus leading to such cellular changes as disparate turnover of light and heavy chains, induction of myosin isozymes, or alterations in myosin charge modification. In further substantiation that such variances in myosin could occur, isozymes of cardiac myosin have been shown to be present in atrial myosin. Sheep atrial myosin has twice the rate of actomyosin ATPase activity (table I), as sheep ventricular myosin. There are also structural differences between the light and heavy chains of atrial versus ventricular myosin (7, 13). The appearance of isozymes of myosin with thyroxine-induced hypertrophy has also been reported (14).

Since the early experiments of *Barany* (15) series of studies have been carried out relating the rate of myosin ATP hydrolysis with the velocity of muscle shortening. Further studies have correlated myosin ATPase activity with physiological parameters measured *in vivo*. Here we show in figure 1 that the K^+ stimulated ATPase activity of myosin correlates with cardiac output in hypertrophied hearts, induced by parturition, subhypertensive doses of norepinephrine and pressure overload (Figure 1). It is not shown here but all three types of hypertrophy demonstrated an increase in the V_{max} of the velocity of contractile element shortening. It is not known at this time whether these biochemical and mechanical correlates are only incidentally related or whether the mechanical alterations are a result of the biochemical alterations. We are also determining whether all or just restricted cation activation, i.e., K^+, Ca^{2+}, or Mg^{2+}-stimulation of myosin reflects alterations in actomyosin ATPase activity, and may be related to specific mechanical functions. We are looking into whether this specific analysis of myosin may be used as a meaningful index of mechanical function.

Where massive hypertrophy occurred, such as in moderate pulmonic stenosis, creating a right ventricular peak systolic pressure of 50 mm Hg at the time of sacrifice, there was a decrease in tissue cAMP content but

Table 2. With three weeks of moderate pulmonic stenosis as described in Figure 1 C there was a corresponding decrease in cAMP as described earlier (3) and normal cGMP levels. Procedures using the Schwartz/Mann radioimmunoassay for determining the concentration of cAMP and cGMP were described in earlier reports as well as normal values for the tissue cyclic nucleotide levels. Each set of values are for five animals (3).

$\dfrac{cGMP}{cAMP}$ Ratio in Canine Cardiac Tissue		
	S.E.	
Normal	1.12 ± 0.15	
3 Weeks Moderate Pulmonic Stenosis	2.20 ± 0.28	(p<.01)
3 Weeks Mild Pulmonic	1.38 ± 0.35	(N.D.)

S.E. = Standard error

N.D. = No significant difference

$\left(\dfrac{cGMP}{cAMP} \text{ Picomoles in 100 mg Tissue} \right)$

retention of normal cGMP levels (table II). This same alteration in cyclic nucleotide content was not observed when stenosis was mild and where there was a lesser degree of hypertrophy (table II). With increased tension on muscle fibers there is a subsequent release of norepinephrine from nerve endings and/or intracellular stores, leading to increases in cAMP content. With progression of hypertrophy and the laying down of more sarcomeres in series and parallel there is a decrease in tension and stress per sarcomere and thus a decrease in tissue levels of norepinephrine and cAMP. However, this decrease in tissue cAMP content ocours only with massive hypertrophy where there is also a reduction in tissue pO_2 levels (3). With advanced stages of moderate pulmonic stenosis in the dog there is a decrease in tissue pO_2 levels (3) and thus high energy phosphate levels; with a decrease in cAMP content there follows a decrease in glycogen breakdown and a subsequent reduction in the progression of tissue acidity. In the case of moderate stenosis (3) there is no decrease in contractility or myosin ATPase activity with this decrease in cAMP content. This may be due to some myofibrillar protein alteration.

We have described here types of physiologic hypertrophy in contrast to numerous reported examples of pathologic hypertrophy; the latter expresses a decrease in cardiac function and myosin ATPase activity. The metabolic and mechanical features of pathologic hypertrophy may be the result of tissue acidity. Nevertheless, there are factors secondary to the hypertrophy process occurring as a result of the various determinants discussed here and thus causing the development of such disparities. There appears to be a constellation of factors which determine the course of the hypertrophy process, causing it to result in physiologic versus pathologic hypertrophy. There exists a disparate tolerance to stress-induced hypertrophy according to animal species, age and health. As described in studies of pulmonary artery banded dogs (2, 3), the degree and duration of ventricular wall stress are also important to the development of physiologic versus pathologic hypertrophy, and as described here the nature of the inciting stimulus is also an important determining factor.

Zusammenfassung

Hypertrophietypen, wie die normale Entwicklung des linken Ventrikels neugeborener Lämmer, Hypertrophie nach Verabfolgung von Noradrenalin sowie bei mäßiger Pulmonalstenose, sind als physiologische Hypertrophie zu bezeichnen, d. h., die Herzfunktion ist gesteigert und die K^+-stimulierte Myosin-ATPase-Aktivität ist erhöht. Die K^+/EDTA-stimulierte ATPase-Aktivität wird als eine Möglichkeit zur Abgrenzung einer physiologischen Hypertrophie gegenüber einer pathologischen Hypertrophie gewertet und kann Änderungen der schweren Ketten des Myosins widerspiegeln, da die leichten Ketten zum großen Teil dissoziiert sind. In Experimenten, in denen Myosin ohne leichte Ketten benutzt wurde, kam es nicht zu einer korrespondierenden Abnahme der Myosin-ATPase-Aktivität mit der Dissoziation der leichten Ketten, unabhängig von dem jeweils benutzten kationischen Aktivator. Es kam jedoch mit dem Verlust von leichten Ketten zu einem Abfall in der enzymatischen Aktivität von Aktomyosin. Weiterhin wurde diese Minderung der Aktomyosin-ATPase-Aktivität teilweise rückgängig gemacht bei Reassoziierung der leichten Ketten mit dem restlichen Myosinmolekül. Wenn eine exzessive Hypertrophie zustande kam, z. B. bei mäßiger Pulmonalstenose mit einem Gewichtsanstieg der freien Wand des rechten Ventrikels um 100%, kam es zu einem

Abfall des cAMP-Gehalts. Dies könnte mit einer Hypertrophie-bedingten Minderung der mechanischen Spannung zusammenhängen. Bei geringeren Hypertrophiegraden, z. B. bei milder Pulmonalstenose mit transitorischem Gewichtsanstieg des rechten Ventrikels um 30%, war kein Rückgang des zyklischen AMP-Gehalts zu verzeichnen.

References

1. *Goodkind, M. J., G. E. Dambach, P. T. Thyrum, R. J. Luchi:* Effects of thyroxine on ventricular myocardial contractility and ATPase activity in guinea pigs. Amer. J. Physiol. **226**, 66–72 (1974).
2. *Wikman-Coffelt, J., C. Fenner, R. Walsh, A. Salel, T. Kamiyama, D. T. Mason:* Comparison of mild *vs* severe pressure overload on the enzymatic activity of myosin in the canine ventricles. Biochem. Med. **14**, 139–146 (1975).
3. *Stewart, D., D. T. Mason, J. Wikman-Coffelt:* Changes in cAMP concentrations during chronic hypertrophy. Basic Res. in Cardiol. **73**, 648–655 (1979).
4. *Meerson, F. Z.:* Contractile function of the heart in hyperfunction hypertrophy, and heart failure. Chapter 1. Circ. Res., 24 & 25, Suppl. II, 9–54 (1969).
5. *Poole-Wilson, P. A.:* Measurement of myocardial intracellular pH in pathologic states. J. Mol. Cell. Cardiol. **10**, 511–526 (1978).
6. *Wikman-Coffelt, J., T. Kamiyama, A. Salel, D. T. Mason:* Differential responses of canine myosin ATPase activity and tissue gases in the pressure overloaded ventricle dependent upon degree of obstruction: Mild versus severe pulmonic and aortic stenosis. In Recent Advances in Studies on Cardiac Structure and Metabolism, edited by *T. Kobayashi, Y. Ito, G. Rona,* Vol. 12, pp 367–372 (Baltimore 1978).
7. *Long, L., F. Fabian, D. T. Mason, J. Wikman-Coffelt:* A new cardiac myosin characterized from the canine atria. Biochem. Biophys. Res. Commun. **76**, 626–635 (1977).
8. *Fabian, F., A. Muhlrad:* Effect of trinitrophenylation of myosin ATPase. Biochim. Biophys, Acta **162**, 596–603 (1968).
9. *Spudich, J. A., S. Watt:* The regulation of rabbit skeletal muscle contraction. J. Biol. Chem. **246**, 4866–4871 (1971).
10. *Pemrick, S.:* Comparison of the calcium sensitivity of actomyosin from native and L$_2$-deficient myosin. Biochem. **16**, 4047–4054 (1977).
11. *Vanderburgh, H., S. Kaufman: In vitro* model for stretch-induced hypertrophy of skeletal muscle. Science **203**, 265–268 (1979).
12. *Schreiber, S. S., M. Oratz, M. A. Rothschild, F. Reff:* Effect of hydrostatic pressure on isolated cardiac nuclei: Stimulation of RNA polymerase II activity. Cardiovasc. Res. **12**, 265–268 (1978).
13. *Flink, I. L., J. H. Rader, S. K. Banerjee, E. Morkin:* Atrial and ventricular cardiac myosins contain different heavy chain species. FEBS Lett. **94**, 125–130 (1978).
14. *Flink, I. L., E. Morkin:* Evidence for a new cardiac myosin species in thyrotoxic rabbit. FEBS Lett. **81**, 391–394 (1977).
15. *Barany, M.:* ATPase activity of myosin correlated with speed of muscle shortening. J. Gen. Physiol. **50**, 197–199 (1967).
16. *Higuchi, M., F. Fabian, T. Wandzilak, Jr., D. T. Mason, J. Wikman-Coffelt:* Dissociation of light chains from cardiac myosin. Eur. J. Biochem. **92**, 317–323 (1978).
17. *Wikman-Coffelt, J., M. Higuchi, F. Fabian, and D. T. Mason:* Comparison of Mg^{2+} vs Ca^{2+}, K$^+$ and Actin-activation of myosin after trinitrophenylation. Res. Commun. in Chem. Path. & Pharmacol. (in press)

Authors' address:

Dr. *Joan Wikman-Coffelt,* Ph. D. Cardiovascular Research Institute 1197 Moffitt Hospital University of California, San Francisco, California 94143

Basic Res. Cardiol. **75**, 157–162 (1980)
© 1980 Dr. Dietrich Steinkopff Verlag, Darmstadt
ISSN 0300–8428

Paper, presented at the Erwin Riesch Symposium, Tübingen, April 3–7, 1979

Physiologisches Institut, Lehrstuhl II, Universität Tübingen

Cooperative effects of calcium on myofibrillar ATPase of normal and hypertrophied heart*)

Die kooperativen Effekte von Calcium auf die myofibrilläre ATPase aus normalen und hypertrophierten Herzen

H. Rupp

With 2 figures

Summary

The ATPase of myofibrils from normal and hypertrophied rat heart was studied in relation to the Ca^{2+}-dependence of the reaction. The experimental data were fitted to theoretical curves based on the Hill equation. A positive cooperativity (n = 1.6) was found for the activation curve of the ATPase from normal heart. For hypertrophied heart no significant change in either the cooperativity or the Ca^{2+}-sensitivity of troponin was detected. This indicates that the troponin-tropomyosin system is not altered during pressure-overload hypertrophy. However, it should be noted that no precautions were taken to control the state of phosphorylation of contractile proteins during the preparation of myofibrils.

The contractile process of cardiac muscle is activated by the binding of Ca^{2+} to troponin. It was found that the affinity of Ca^{2+} for the binding sites of troponin C is different for the complete contractile system compared to the isolated Ca^{2+} binding subunit (1). Furthermore, the degree of attachment of cross-bridges between actin and myosin filaments determines the cooperative properties and the number of binding sites. Thus, in the absence of cross-bridge attachments 3 mol Ca^{2+} are bound to troponin (1). Fibres with maximum filament overlap bound 4 mol Ca^{2+}/mol troponin and half of these binding sites exhibited a positive cooperativity. It should be noted that the number of cross-bridges were kept constant (rigor complexes) and were independent of Ca^{2+}. By contrast, in the presence of MgATP increasing Ca^{2+}-concentrations result in an increased number of cycling cross-bridges. If the ATPase reaction depends, at least partially, on a Ca^{2+}-binding site with cooperative interaction, then this cooperativity should be reflected also in the Ca^{2+}-activation curve of the ATPase. Changes in the cooperative interactions between the Ca^{2+}-binding sites are expected to result in different mechanical and chemical activities of the contractile system (2). A way of probing the Ca^{2+}-binding sites which influence ATPase activity is by studying the Ca^{2+}-activated ATPase of

---

*) Supported by the Deutsche Forschungsgemeinschaft

myofibrils. In this report, the ATPase activity vs. [Ca^{2+}] data were fitted to theoretical curves based on the Hill equation (3). Of particular interest was to compare the functioning of the troponin system of normal with that of hypertrophied heart.

Material and methods

Pressure-overload hypertrophy was induced in male Wistar rats by coarctation of the left renal artery (Goldblatt II). Myofibrils free of mitochondrial, sarcolemmal and sarcoplasmic reticular ATPase were prepared from rat heart as described by *Solaro* et al. (4). The isolation procedure involves the treatment of the myofibrils with Triton X-100. ATPase activity of myofibrils was determined at 25° C in 80 mM KCl, 4 mM $MgCl_2$, 40 mM imidazol, 4 mM ATP at pH 7.0. The assay medium contained in addition 2 mM EGTA and various amounts of $CaCl_2$. The apparent Ca-EGTA binding constant used for the calculation of free Ca^{2+}-concentrations was $10^{6.68}$. Reactions were initiated by the addition of ATP. Inorganic phosphate was determined by the method of *Fiske* and *Subbarow* (5) and protein concentration was measured according to *Lowry* et al. (6).

Reaction conditions were chosen so that ATPase activity could be assayed when less than 25% of the total ATP was hydrolyzed. The curves for ATPase stimulated by Ca^{2+} were fitted using a weighted least squares procedure to the equation $v = V_{max}/(1 + Q/[Ca^{2+}]^n)$. V_{max} and Q were treated as free parameters. The Hill coefficient n was derived from a linear regression of log $(v/(V_{max}-v))$ vs. log[Ca^{2+}] data. The pCa (i.e., $-log_{10}[Ca^{2+}]$) corresponding to 50% activity is given by $-(1/n)$ log Q. The curve fitting procedure was similar to that used for microwave power saturation studies (7, 8) and oxidation-reduction potential titrations (9). Theoretical curves were calculated and plotted using a Hewlett-Packard 9820A calculator and a HP 9862A calculator plotter.

Results and discussion

Ca^{2+} activated Mg^{2+}-ATPase of myofibrils from normal heart

The ATPase reaction of myofibrils was activated by free Ca^{2+} in the micromolar range. The activation followed a sigmoidal pattern which is indicative of cooperative interactions. As a diagnostic test, a 1/v vs. 1/[Ca^{2+}] plot was used. As expected for a positive cooperativity, a concave upward deviation was found. A similar effect of Ca^{2+} on the hydrolysis of ATP was observed employing cardiac and skeletal reconstituted actomyosins (10). By plotting log $(v/(V_{max}-v))$ vs. log[Ca^{2+}] the Hill coefficient was estimated to be 1.6 (fig. 1). A slope greater than 1.0 indicates positive cooperativity. Using the Hill coefficient of 1.6 the ATPase vs. [Ca^{2+}] data were fitted by treating V_{max} and Q as free parameters (fig. 2b). For comparative reasons a curve is also given (fig. 2a) which would be the best fit to experimental data assuming a non-cooperative system (n = 1.0). It is apparent also from the activation curve that a good fit to experimental data can be obtained only by assuming a positive cooperativity. The ATPase activity was 0.16 μmol of P_i/min per mg protein at saturating Ca^{2+} concentrations. Half-maximal activation occurred at pCa 6.87.

A consequence of the positive cooperativity is the smaller range of Ca^{2+} which is necessary for full activation of the ATPase. For force-generating systems the mechanical activity vs. [Ca^{2+}] slope is generally greater

(11–13). However, in the latter case the situation is more complex, since e.g. the force vs. $[Ca^{2+}]$ curves depend also on the concentration of free Mg^{2+} and MgATP. In this context it is worthwhile to consider some of the consequences of the cooperative interaction. Firstly, the positive feed back mechanism would promote the attachment of cross-bridges upon binding of Ca^{2+}. Secondly, the binding of additional Ca^{2+} to troponin would in turn be more favourable. Since the number of cross-bridges is related to the amount of Ca^{2+} bound to thin filaments, the magnitude of developed force would, therefore, also influence the time course of contraction. On the other hand, relaxation following an isotonic contraction would be delayed as the load is increased. These examples demonstrate that subtle changes in the Ca^{2+}-binding sites can result in drastic changes of mechanical activity.

Ca^{2+} activated Mg^{2+}-ATPase of myofibrils from hypertrophied heart

It is well documented that myofibrillar ATPase activity at saturating Ca^{2+} concentrations is decreased during hypertrophy induced by pressure-overload. By contrast, little is known as regards the activity at partial activation. This would be of particular interest, since the Ca^{2+} activation of myofibrillar ATPase reflects the functioning of the troponin-tropomyosin system. The ATPase activity vs. $[Ca^{2+}]$ data were fitted using

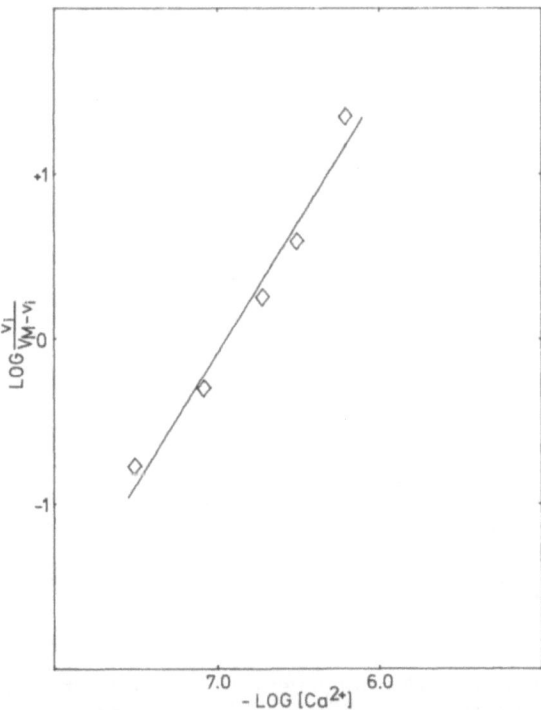

Fig. 1. Hill plot of the effect of Ca^{2+} on the hydrolysis of ATP by myofibrils from left ventricles of normal rats.

the Hill coefficient 1.6 as for normal heart. The good fit of the theoretical
curve to experimental data (fig. 2c) indicates that neither the Hill n value
nor the constant Q is altered significantly for hypertrophied heart. It
follows that also the pCa for 50% activation is not changed. Furthermore,
in the double reciprocal plot of ATPase activity and Ca^{2+} concentration a
curvilinear pattern was found for the ATPase both from normal and
hypertrophied myocardium. This indicates that in pressure-overload
hypertrophy the functioning of the regulatory proteins is not impaired as
related to the Ca^{2+}-sensitivity and the cooperativity of the contractile
system. The data agree well with the finding that the Ca^{2+}-tension relationship is not changed using chemically skinned muscle bundles from hypertrophied heart (14). As expected the myofibrillar ATPase activity is depressed at saturating Ca^{2+} concentrations (fig. 2c) reflecting most probably
an altered structure of myosin.

It should be pointed out that during the preparation of myofibrils no
precautions were taken to maintain the state of phosphorylation of troponin I, troponin T or myosin. This may be of importance, since the degree of
phosphorylation of the contractile proteins might be changed during
hypertrophy and insufficiency of the heart. For example, the functioning
of the sarcolemmal adenylate cyclase-cyclic AMP system is altered during

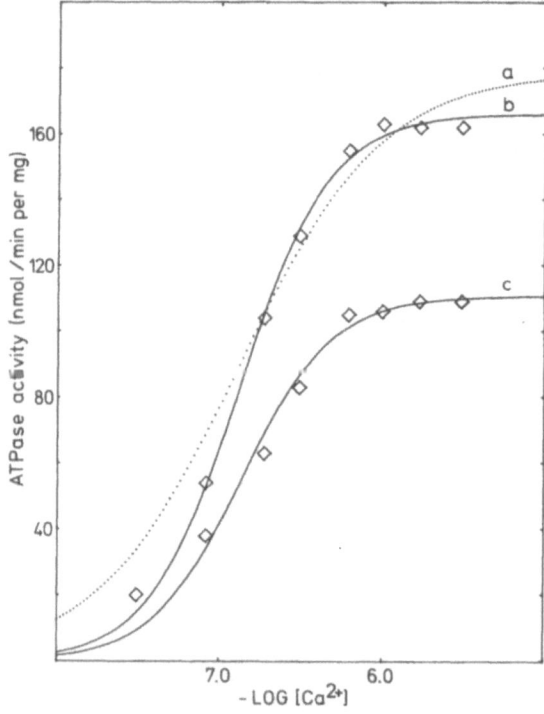

Fig. 2. $[Ca^{2+}]$-ATPase relationship for myofibrils from (b) normal and (c) hypertrophied rat left ventricles. The solid lines of (b) and (c) are computer fittings of
curves to means of the raw data as given by the symbols (n = 1.58, Q = 1.23×10^{-11}).
For curve (a) n = 1.0 was used.

different stages of heart failure (15). This would affect the cyclic AMP-dependent phosphorylation of troponin I, resulting in an altered Ca^{2+} sensitivity of the contractile system (16, 17). Obviously, the possibility that changes in phosphorylation reactions contribute to the mechanochemical properties of hypertrophied heart have to be considered before attributing e.g. changes of mechanical activity solely to a structural change of the myosin molecule. Work is in progress to elucidate the possible action of phosphorylation reactions during pathological changes of cardiac function.

Zusammenfassung

Die myofibrilläre ATPase aus normalen und hypertrophierten Herzen wurde untersucht in bezug auf die Aktivierung der Reaktion durch Ca^{2+}. Die experimentellen Daten wurden mit theoretischen Kurven auf der Grundlage der Hill-Gleichung angenähert. Es wurde eine positive Kooperativität (n = 1,6) für die Aktivierungskurve der ATPase aus normalen Herzen gefunden. Für das hypertrophierte Herz wurde weder eine signifikante Veränderung der Kooperativität noch der Ca^{2+}-Sensitivität von Troponin beobachtet. Dies bedeutet, daß bei der druckinduzierten Hypertrophie das Troponin-Tropomyosin-System nicht verändert ist. Nicht berücksichtigt wurden jedoch mögliche Änderungen im Phosphorylierungsgrad der kontraktilen Proteine bei der Präparation der Myofibrillen.

References

1. *Fuchs, F.:* Cooperative interactions between calcium-binding sites on glycerinated muscle fibers. The influence of cross-bridge attachment. Biochim. Biophys. Acta **462**, 314–322 (1977).
2. *Weber, A., J. M. Murray:* Molecular control mechanisms in muscle contraction. Physiol. Rev. **53**, 612–673 (1973).
3. *Koshland, D. E.,* Jr.: The molecular basis for enzyme regulation. In: The Enzymes, vol. 1, 3rd ed., *Boyer, P. D.,* (ed.) 341–396 (New York 1970).
4. *Solaro, R. J., D. C. Pang, F. N. Briggs:* The purification of cardiac myofibrils with Triton X-100. Biochim. Biophys. Acta **245**, 259–262 (1971).
5. *Fiske, C. H., Y. Subbarow:* The colorimetric determination of phosphorus. J. Biol. Chem. **66**, 375–400 (1925).
6. *Lowry, O. H., N. J. Rosebrough, A. L. Farr, R. J. Randall:* Protein measurement with the folin phenol reagent. J. Biol. Chem. **193**, 265–275 (1951).
7. *Rupp, H., K. K. Rao, D. O. Hall, R. Cammack:* Electron spin relaxation of iron-sulphur proteins studied by microwave power saturation. Biochim. Biophys. Acta **537**, 255–269 (1978).
8. *Rupp, H., A. L. Moore:* Characterization of iron-sulphur centres of plant mitochondria by microwave power saturation. Biochim. Biophys. Acta **548**, 16–29 (1979).
9. *Rupp, H., R. Cammack, H.-J. Hartmann, U. Weser:* Oxidation-reduction reactions of yeast Cu-Thionein (Metallothionein). Biochim. Biophys. Acta **578**, 462–475 (1979).
10. *Bailin, G., M.-J. Shen, A. Katz:* Cooperative interactions between the contractile proteins of cardiac and skeletal muscle. Biochim. Biophys. Acta **480**, 469–478 (1977).
11. *Schädler, M.:* Proportionale Aktivierung von ATPase-Aktivität und Kontraktionsspannung durch Calciumionen in isolierten contractilen Strukturen verschiedener Muskelarten. Pflügers Archiv **296**, 70–90 (1967).

12. *Solaro, R. J., F. N. Briggs:* Calcium and the control of enzymatic and mechanical activity in muscle. In: Calcium Binding Proteins, *Drabikowski, W., H. Strzelecka-Golaszewska, E. Carafoli,* (eds.) 587–607 (Warszawa 1974).
13. *Levy, R. M., Y. Umazume, M. J. Kushmerick:* Ca^{2+} dependence of tension and ADP production in segments of chemically skinned muscle fibers. Biochim. Biophys. Acta **430**, 352–365 (1976).
14. *Maughan, D., E. Low, R. Litten, III, J. Brayden, N. Alpert:* Calcium-activated muscle from hypertrophied rabbit hearts: Mechanical and correlated biochemical changes. Circulat. Res. **44**, 279–287 (1979).
15. *Dhalla, N. S., P. K. Das, G. P. Sharma:* Subcellular basis of cardiac contractile failure. J. Mol. Cell. Cardiol. **10**, 363–385 (1978).
16. *Ray, K. P., P. J. England:* Phosphorylation of the inhibitory subunit of troponin and its effect on the calcium dependence of cardiac myofibril adenosine triphosphatase. FEBS Lett. **70**, 11–16 (1976).
17. *Perry, S. V.:* The regulation of contractile activity in muscle. Biochem. Soc. Transactions **7**, 593–617 (1979).

Author's address:

Dr. *H. Rupp,* Physiologisches Institut, Lehrstuhl II, Universität Tübingen, Gmelinstraße 5, D-7400 Tübingen 1

Basic Res. Cardiol. **75**, 163–170 (1980)
© 1980 Dr. Dietrich Steinkopff Verlag Darmstadt
ISSN 0300–8428

Paper, presented at the Erwin Riesch Symposium, Tübingen, April 3–7, 1979

Physiologisches Institut II, Universität Tübingen

The myofibrillar ATPase activity and the substructure of myosin in the hypertrophied left ventricle of the rat*)

Myofibrilläre ATPase-Aktivität und Substruktur von Myosin im hypertrophierten linken Rattenmyokard

I. Medugorac

With 1 figure and 3 tables

Summary

The aim of the present study was to seek a possible correlation between changes in enzymatic activity of myofibrils, on the one hand, and the substructure of myosin in hypertrophied myocardium, on the other hand. The myofibrillar ATPase activity and relative quantity of single myosin subunits were investigated in the hypertrophied left ventricle of 10 old male rats with spontaneous hypertension (SHR) and 12 Goldblatt rats (6 months after coarctation of one renal artery) (GBR).

In SHR and GBR the weight of the left ventricle was 47% and 58% greater in comparison with control rats of the same age (WCR and CR respectively). The concentration of myofibrillar proteins was increased by 33% in SHR and GBR respectively. The myofibrillar ATPase activity (μmol $P_i \times mg^{-1} \times min^{-1}$) was decreased by 50% in SHR and 30% in GBR. The results of investigation of the relative amount of left ventricular myosin subunits show that the decrease in myofibrillar ATPase activity was associated with a slight decrease in the relative amount of myosin heavy chains (HC) over the amount of light chains 1 and 2 ($LC_{(1+2)}$) in the left ventricle of SHR (16%) and GBR (14%) as compared to control values. The relative amount of myosin light chain 1 to light chain 2 (LC_1 to LC_2) was decreased by 23% and 6% respectively.

On the basis of these results the control mechanism of the synthesis of individual myosin components cannot be ruled out as the regulatory mechanism of specific ATPase activity of contractile proteins of the left ventricle of the rat. A final positive answer to the question of a causal correlation between the structural and enzymatic alteration of myosin will require further biochemical investigation, however.

The myosin of different types of adult striated muscle in vertebrates possesses different ultrastructural and enzymatic properties. The subunits of myosin have been found with different patterns and with variable stoichiometry in the course of development (1–4) and in distinct physiological (5) and pathological (6) states of the same striated muscle type. The specific ATPase activity of contractile proteins also changes under

---

*) Supported by the Deutsche Forschungsgemeinschaft.

these conditions. It seems that at least the changes in enzymatic activity of contractile proteins in the course of development closely correlate with the changes in the ultrastructure of the myosin molecule (1).

It is not known whether a causal relation actually exists between the changes in the stoichiometry of myosin subunits and specific ATPase activity.

In order to seek further correlation between enzymatic and structural alterations in myocardial myosin, we investigated the relative stoichiometry of myosin subunits and myofibrillar ATPase activity in hypertrophied left ventricles from Goldblatt rats (GBR) and rats with spontaneous hypertension (SHR) in comparison to nonoperated control rats (CR) and normotensive Wistar control rats (WCR) respectively.

Methods

Hydroxyproline and protein determination

The hydroxyproline concentration was measured in samples of 10 mg of dry tissue. The samples were prepared according to *Medugorac* (8), the hydroxyproline concentration determined according to *Stegemann* (9).

The biuret and folin method was used for protein determination.

Assay of myofibrillar ATPase activity

A myofibrillar preparation was made from each single left ventricle. Each preparation was checked for purity using SDS-polyacrylamide (SDS-PAA 10%) gel electrophoresis (fig. 1).

The ATPase activity was assayed in a final volume of 2 ml. Incubating solution: 5.0 mM $MgCl_2$, 0.2 mM $CaCl_2$, 50 mM Tris/HCL buffer (pH 7.6), 2.5 mM ATP, 5 mM NaN_3 and 0.2–0.4 ml myofibril solution (0.3–0.6 mg protein). The reaction was started upon the addition of ATP and terminated after 5 min by the addition of 25% TCA.

Relative quantification of myosin subunits

Purified actomyosin was used for the relative quantification of myosin chains. Considerations on the use of actomyosin for SDS-PAA electrophoresis have already been discussed (10).

The complete dissociation of actomyosin and electrophoretical separation of its single subunits in SDS-PAA-gels was performed as reported earlier (10).

The relative quantity of myosin subunits was obtained on the basis of densitometry and the elution method applied to fast green-stained PAA-gels. The densitometer tracings were quantitated by planimetry. Following densitometry, the fast green dye from the gels was eluted and analyzed for absorbance at 623 nm. The staining intensities of the single myosin components in gel patterns determined by both methods were converted into relative protein content ratios on the basis of standardization with highly purified left ventricular myosin components (10). The results obtained by both methods were very similar.

Results and discussion

Table 1 shows the blood pressure and weight relationships between the SHR and WCR studied. As expected, under the increased systolic blood

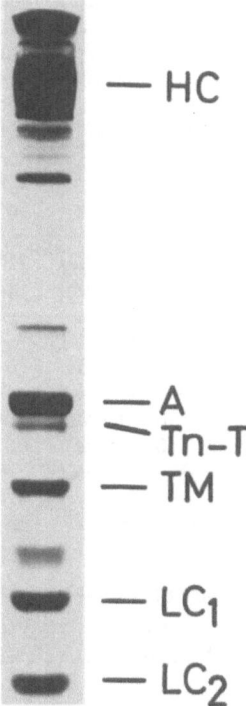

Fig. 1. Sodium dodecylsulfate polyacrylamide electrophoresis of highly purified myofibrils from the rat left ventricle. HC, LC_1 and LC_2 = myosin heavy chains, light chain 1 and 2, respectively; A = actin, Tn-T = troponin-T, TM = tropomyosin. Troponin-I (mol. wt. 28,000) and troponin-C (mol. wt. 18,000) are probably covered by LC_1 and LC_2.

pressure the ventricular overload was associated with an increase in ventricular weight, both absolutely and in relation to body weight. The gain in body weight in the SHR was markedly reduced (31%). Therefore a considerably greater increase was observed in the ventricular weight/body weight ratio (114%) than in the absolute left ventricular weight increase in comparison to ventricular weight of control animals of the same age (47%).

The concentration of hydroxyproline of SHR in the hypertrophied left ventricular tissue was increased by 33%.

As reported earlier (7), the left ventricle and right ventricle (54% and 32% respectively) were hypertrophied in the GBR 6 months after surgery. The concentration of hydroxyproline in left ventricular tissue of GBR was increased by 22%.

Changes in ATPase activity and concentrations of myofibrillar proteins

The specific myofibrillar ATPase activity in left ventricles of SHR and GBR was decreased by 50% and 30% respectively as compared with control rats of the same age (table 2). Simultaneous with the decrease in the ATPase activity, the concentration of myofibrillar proteins in wet

Table 1. Blood pressure and body and ventricular weights in rats with left ventricular
pressure overload in comparison to control rats of the same age. SHR = spontaneously
hypertensive rats; WCR = Normotensive Wistar control rats; GBR = Goldblatt rats
(6 months after coarctation of one arteria renalis); CR = nonoperated control rats; BW,
LVW and RVW = body, left and right ventricular weight, respectively.
Statistical values are ($\bar{x}$) ($\pm S_{\bar{x}}$). N.S. = $p > 0.05$.

Experimen- tal group	n	Blood pressure (mm Hg)	BW (g)	LVW (mg)	RVW (mg)	LV/BW (mg/g)
SHR	10	145–235	348 ($\pm$ 62)	1268 ($\pm$ 250)	285 ($\pm$ 46)	3.64
WCR	10	105–125	508 ($\pm$ 98)	863 ($\pm$ 101)	266 ($\pm$ 31)	1.70
SHR/WCR % change			−31 ($p < 0.05$)	+ 47 ($p < 0.01$)	+ 7 (N.S.)	+ 114
GBR	12	130–195	374 ($\pm$ 71)	1046 ($\pm$ 201)	233 ($\pm$ 37)	2.80
CR	12	105–115	368 ($\pm$ 40)	681 ($\pm$ 70)	177 ($\pm$ 22)	1.85
GBR/CR % change			+ 2 (N.S.)	+ 54 ($p < 0.01$)	+ 32 ($p < 0.01$)	+ 51

ventricular tissue increased by 33% (SHR) and 20% (GBR). In this way the
loss in the capacity of ventricular tissue to hydrolyze ATP, which occurred
because of the reduction in the specific ATPase activity was compensated
to a large extent.

Changes in relative content of myosin subunits

In the myosin of hypertrophied ventricular tissue (SHR and GBR) the
relative amount of light chains in relation to heavy chains decreases by
16% and 14% respectively in comparison to control values. The ratio of
LC_1 to LC_2 decreases in SHR by 23% and in GBR by 6% (table 3).
Taking a molecular weight for heavy chains of 210,000 (11), and for LC_1
and LC_2 of 26,000 and 18,500 (5) respectively, those polypeptides are
present in a molar ratio of: 2.00:1.25:1.70 in SHR and 2.00:1.37:1.41 in GBR,
and 2.00:1.16:1.23 and 2.00:1.22:1.18 in control rats respectively (table 3).
According to the results of *Pelloni-Müller* et al. (4) and *Medugorac*
(unpublished data) the relative quantity of myosin heavy chains to light
chains also changes during the development of cardiac and skeletal muscle. With advancing ontogenesis the relative amount of heavy chains to
light chains increases gradually. The specific ATPase activity of contractile proteins also increases in correlation with these changes in the
stoichiometry of myosin subunits. *Wikman-Coffelt* et al. (11) found a
remarkable decrease in myosin enzymatic activity and in the relative
amount of HC to $LC_{(1+2)}$ in the hypertrophied right ventricle (pulmonic
insufficiency) of the dog.
According to our findings the specific myofibrillar ATPase activity in
the hypertrophied left ventricle of SHR and GBR was vigorously reduced
(by 50% and 30% respectively). The concurrent relative heavy-chains-to-
light-chains ratio decreases only slightly both in hypertrophied ventricles
of SHR (15%) and GBR (14%).

Table 2. ATPase activity (per mg of myofibrils and per g of ventricular wet tissue) and concentration of myofibrillar proteins in SHR and GBR in comparison to control values. See also legend to table 1.

Experimental group	n	Concentration of myofibrillar proteins in mg/g of fresh left ventricular tissue	Myofibrillar ATPase activity (μmol $P_i \times$ min^{-1}) in	
			mg of myofibrils	g of fresh ventricular tissue
SHR	10	64 ($\pm$ 11)	0.155 ($\pm$ 0.028) ($p < 0.001$)	0.992
WCR	10	48 ($\pm$ 9)	0.312 ($\pm$ 0.031)	1.498
SHR/WCR % change		+33 ($p < 0.05$)	−50 ($p < 0.001$)	−34
GBR	12	55 ($\pm$ 10)	0.192 ($\pm$ 0.0030)	1.018
CR	12	45 ($\pm$ 7)	0.274 ($\pm$ 0.0023) ($p. < 0.001$)	1.206
GBR/CR % change		+22 ($p < 0.05$	−30 ($p < 0.05$)	−16

Table 3. Quantitative evaluation of myosin subunits from electrophorized ventricular actomyosin of hypertrophied left ventricles (SHR and GBR) in comparison to values in control ventricles. The amounts of single myosin chains were calculated as a percentage of total myosin content. An actomyosin preparation was made from each single rat left ventricle. From each actomyosin preparation 6–10 samples with four different concentrations were electrophoretically analyzed in SDS-PAA gels. The fast green-stained gels were evaluated by densitometry and the elution method (10). HC = heavy chains; LC_1 and LC_2 = light chains 1 and 2 of ventricular myosin. See also legend to table 1.

Experimental group	Amounts of single myosin chains as percentage of total myosin content					Molar ratio
	HC	LC_1	LC_2	HC/LC$_{(1+2)}$	LC_1/LC_2	HC:LC_1:LC_2
SHR	86.8 $\pm$ 12.0	6.7 $\pm$ 0.98	6.5 $\pm$ 0.83	6.6	1.03	2.00:1.25:1.70
WCR	88.8 $\pm$ 11.2	6.4 $\pm$ 0.83	4.8 $\pm$ 0.67	7.9	1.33	2.00:1.16:1.23
SHR/WCR % change	−2 (N.S.)	+5 (N.S.)	+35 $p < 0.05$	−16	−23	
GBR	87.2 $\pm$ 11.3	7.4 $\pm$ 1.25	5.4 $\pm$ 0.73	6.8	1.37	2.00:1.37:1.41
CR	88.8 $\pm$ 10.6	6.7 $\pm$ 0.92	4.6 $\pm$ 0.61	7.9	1.46	2.00:1.22:1.18
GBR/CR % change	−2 (N.S.)	+10 (N.S.)	+17 (N.S.)	−14	−6	

However, we found that the positive trend of the correlation between remarkable changes in ATPase activity of myofibrils and slight changes in the relative amount of myosin heavy chains to light chains as well as in the

LC_1-to-LC_2 ratio (table 3) was persistent. Furthermore, the trend was in the same direction as found in the hypertrophied right ventricle of dog (12), in developing rabbit (4) and rat (*Medugorac*, unpublished data) cardiac muscle, and in rabbit skeletal muscle (4). In contrast to these findings, no differences between stoichiometry of myosin subunits in hypertrophied and normal cardiac muscle were found in some other studies (13–15). This discrepancy could be explained if the changes in the relative amount ratios of myosin components in hypertrophied ventricular tissue are very inconspicuous and only demonstrable by comprehensive systematic analysis. It should also be noted, however, that these other studies did not take into account possible differences in the staining intensities of different proteins.

Therefore it is possible that the ATPase activity of contractile proteins can be controlled by changes in the ultrastructure of the myosin molecule. As reported earlier, we found a simultaneous increase in specific ATPase activity and the relative amount of LC_1 to LC_2 in myosin of slightly hypertrophied left ventricles from swimming rats. In skeletal fast muscle the amount of the smallest myosin light chain (LC_{3f}) increases markedly in the course of ontogenesis (1–3). This increase in the relative amount of LC_{3f} is closely correlated with the increase in actomyosin ATPase activity of corresponding muscle (1). The same trend in enzymatic and structural changes was reported in hypertrophied skeletal muscle of running rats (16). It is still unclear, however, as to whether the enzymatic activity of contractile proteins can be regulated by alterations in the relative amount of myosin subunits to each other, through alterations in the primary structure of individual myosin subunits, or as a result of both phenomena.

In any case, the present results indicate that the control mechanism of the synthesis of individual myosin components could be the regulative mechanism for specific ATPase activity of contractile proteins in the left myocardium of the rat.

However, final clarification of the question of causal correlation between the enzymatic and structural properties of myosin will require further biochemical investigation of the significance of the individual myosin subunits and their stoichiometry with regard to the ATPase activity of myosin.

Zusammenfassung

Ziel der vorliegenden Arbeit war, eine mögliche Beziehung zwischen den Änderungen der enzymatischen Aktivität der Myofibrillen und der Substruktur von Myosin im hypertrophierten Myokard nachzuprüfen. In hypertrophierten linken Ventrikeln von 10 alten männlichen Ratten mit spontaner Hypertension (SHR) und 12 Goldblatt-Ratten (6 Monate nach Stenosierung von einer Renalarterie) (GBR) wurden die spezifische ATPase-Aktivität der Myofibrillen und die relativen Mengen der Myosinuntereinheiten untersucht. In SHR war das Ventrikelgewicht um 47% und in GBR um 54% größer als bei gleichaltrigen Kontrolltieren (WCR bzw. CR). Die Konzentration der myofibrillären Proteine war um 33% (SHR) bzw. um 22% (GBR) gestiegen. Die myofibrilläre ATPase-Aktivität ($\mu molP_i \times mg^{-1} \times min^{-1}$) war um 50% (SHR) bzw. um 30% (GBR) vermindert. Die erhebliche Abnahme der myofibrillären ATPase-Aktivität war von einer leichten Abnahme (16% bzw. 14%) der relativen Mengen der schweren Ketten (HC) gegenüber den leichten Ketten 1 und 2 (LC_{1+2}) begleitet. Die relative Menge der leichten Kette 1 zur leichten Kette 2 ($LC_1:LC_2$) war um 23% bzw. um 6% vermindert.

Aufgrund dieser Ergebnisse ist es nicht auszuschließen, daß der Kontrollmechanismus für die Synthese der einzelnen Komponenten von Myosin auch der regulatorische Mechanismus für die spezifische ATPase-Aktivität der kontraktilen Proteine des linken Ventrikels sein könnte. Jedoch bedarf die endgültige Klärung der Frage nach einem kausalen Zusammenhang zwischen enzymatischen und strukturellen Eigenschaften von Myosin weiterer biochemischer Untersuchungen, besonders bezüglich der Bedeutung einzelner Myosinuntereinheiten und ihrer Stöchiometrie für die ATPase-Aktivität.

References

1. *Takahashi, M., Y. Tonomura:* Developmental changes in the structure and kinetic properties of myosin adenosine-triphosphatase of rabbit skeletal fast muscle. Biochem. J. **78**, 1123–1133 (1975).
2. *Rubinstein, N. A., F. Pepe, H. Holtzer:* Myosin types during the development of embryonic chicken fast and slow muscles. Proc. nat. Acad. Sci. (Wash.) **74**, 4524–4527 (1977).
3. *Syrový, I., E. Gutmann:* Differentiation of myosin in soleus and extensor digitorum longus muscle in different animal species during development. Pflügers Arch. **369**, 85–89 (1977).
4. *Pelloni-Müller, G., M. Ermini, E. Jenny:* Changes in myosin light and heavy chain stoichiometry during development of rabbit fast, slow, and cardiac muscle. FEBS Lett. **70**, 113–117 (1976).
5. *Medugorac, I., A. Kämmereit, R. Jacob:* Einfluß eines chronischen Schwimmtrainings auf Struktur und Enzymaktivität von Myosin beim Rattenmyokard. Hoppe-Seyler's Z. Physiol. Chem. **356**, 1161–1171 (1975).
6. *Lobley, G. E., S. V. Perry, D. Stone:* Structural changes in myosin induced by Vitamin E dystrophy. Nature **231**, 317–318 (1971).
7. *Medugorac, I.:* Characteristics of the hypertrophied left ventricular myocardium in Goldblatt rats. Basic Res. Cardiol. **72**, 261–267 (1977).
8. Medugorac, I., R. Jacob: Concentration and adenosine-triphosphatase activity of left ventricular actomyosin in Goldblatt rats during the compensatory stage of hypertrophy. Hoppe-Seyler's Z. Physiol. Chem. **357**, 1495–1503 (1976).
9. *Stegemann, H.:* Mikrobestimmung von Hydroxyprolin mit Chloramin-T und p-Dimethylaminobenzaldehyd. Hoppe-Seyler's Z. Physiol. Chem. **311**, 41–45 (1958).
10. *Medugorac, I.:* Quantitative determination of cardiac myosin subunits stained with fast green in SDS-electrophoresis gels. Basic Res. Cardiol. **74**, 406–416 (1979).
11. *Wikman-Coffelt, J., R. Zelis, C. Fenner, D. T. Mason:* Myosin chains of myocardial tissue – I. Purifications and immunological properties of myosin heavy chains. Biochem. biophys. Res. Commun. **51**, 1097–1104 (1973).
12. *Wikman-Coffelt, J., R. Walsh, C. Fenner, T. Kamiyama, A. Salel, D. T. Mason:* Activity and molecular changes in right and left ventricular myosins during right ventricular volume overload. Biochem. Medicine **13**, 33–41 (1975).
13. *Siemankowski, R. F., P. Dreizen:* Canine cardiac myosin with special reference to pressure overload cardiac hypertrophy. I. Subunit composition. J. Biol. Chem. **253**, 8648–8658 (1978).
14. *Shiverick, K. T., B. B. Hamrell, N. R. Alpert:* Structural and functional properties of myosin associated with the compensatory cardiac hypertrophy in the rabbit. J. Mol. Cell. Cardiol. **8**, 837–851 (1976).

15. *Katagiri, T., E. Morkin:* Studies on the substructure of myosin in cardiac hypertrophy. Characterization of light chains. Biochim. Biophys. Acta **342**, 262–274 (1974).
16. *Yamaguchi, M., K. Nagakura, M. Yoshida, T. Sekine:* Effect of exercise on the skeletal myosin of growing rat. Jap. J. Physiol. **27**, 367–377 (1977).

Author's address:

Dr. *T. Medugorac,* Physiologisches Institut II der Universität Tübingen, Gmelin-straße 5, 7400 Tübingen

Basic Res. Cardiol. **75**, 171–178 (1980)
© 1980 Dr. Dietrich Steinkopff Verlag, Darmstadt
ISSN 0300–8428

Paper, presented at the Erwin Riesch Symposium, Tübingen, April 3–7, 1979

*Cardiology Section of the Department of Medicine, the Department of
Biochemistry, and The Franklin McLean Memorial Research Institute,
The University of Chicago, Chicago, Illinois 60637*

Mitochondrial Proliferation in Cardiac Hypertrophy*)

Proliferation der Mitochondrien bei Herzhypertrophie

R. Zak, M. Rabinowitz, C. Rajamanickam, S. Merten,
and *B. Kwiatkowska-Patzer*

With 3 figures and 2 tables

Summary

Mitochondrial proliferation was studied in mature female rats following aortic
constriction. Mitochondrial DNA (mtDNA) was assayed by a fluorometric method.
The conditions for removal of nuclear DNA were developed and verified by assessment of molecular conformation of DNA. The mtDNA concentration in mitochondria increased 2,4, and 7 days post-operatively by 11, 72 and 117% respectively.
Comparison with the rates of accumulation of cytochrome c, b, and aa$_3$ indicates
that during the first 24 hours of cardiac enlargement the inner mitochondrial
components accumulate faster then mtDNA, but during the six subsequent days
the rate of mtDNA increment far outstrips that of the cytochromes. These data
indicate that the amount of available mtDNA template is not the only factor
regulating the transcriptional and translational processes in the enlarging myocardium.

The analysis of population of replicative intermediates of mtDNA have shown
dramatic decrease in the frequency of D-loops in preparations obtained from
hypertrophied hearts. This observation indicates that the increase in replicative
flux of mtDNA is associated with the removal of a block in the conversion of D-
loops to other intermediates.

The cardiac growth induced by hemodynamic overload is reflected in
increased incorporation of labeled amino acid into cardiac subcellular
fractions, including mitochondria (1). Quantitative electron microscopic
analysis (6) and measurements of mitochondrial cytochromes (3) indicate
that, in early hypertrophy, mitochondria accumulate in preference to
other organelles. The study of processes leading to mitochondrial prolifer-

*) This work was supported in part by USPHS Grants HL09172, HL04442,
HL16637, and 1-p-17-HL17649 (Specialized Center of Research in Ischemic Heart
Disease), from the National Heart and Lung Institute, grants from the Muscular
Dystrophy Association of America, the Chicago and Illinois Heart Association, and
the Louis Block Fund of The University of Chicago. The Franklin McLean Memo-
rial Research Institute is operated by The University of Chicago for the U.S.
Department of Energy under Contract No. EY-76-C-02-0069.

ation may thus provide clues about the processes that couple hemodynamic load with biosynthetic pathways.

It is of considerable interest that the amount of mtDNA expressed per unit of mitochondrial protein is increased in rapidly growing cells, such as embryonic tissues, tumor cells or cells grown in culture (see Table 1). Moreover, mtDNA was found to be increased in myocardium enlarging secondary to aortic constriction (5). The quantitation of mtDNA, however, is technically very difficult, since the amount of nuclear DNA vastly exceeds that of mtDNA. Thus, minor contamination with nuclear fragments can lead to erroneous results. Accurate determination of the mtDNA present per unit mass of mitochondria is important for an assessment of the coding capacity of mtDNA in relation to induced cardiac growth.

Mitochondria isolated by procedures available so far yields DNA preparation which contains large quantities of nuclear DNA as can be demonstrated by analysis of molecular conformation and by renaturation-kinetic studies. Nuclear DNA can be removed by treatment of the isolated mitochondria with DNAse. In order to develop this procedure into a quantitative assay, it must be first demonstrated that the mitochondria have intact membranes capable of effective exclusion of DNAse, whereas the nuclear DNA, associated with contaminating nuclear fragments, is freely accessible to the action of DNAse.

Material and Methods

Mature female Sprague-Dawley rats were used for experiments. The constriction of ascending aorta to approximately 30% of its original lumen diameter was performed as described by us previously (3). Mitochondria were isolated from hearts pooled from three animals by the method of *Albin* et al. (3). To remove contaminating nuclear DNA, the mitochondria were digested with 100 µg DNAse/ml for 30 minutes at 24 °C in a final volume of 2.0 ml of 0.25 M sucrose containing 5 mM Tris-HCl buffer pH 7.4, 50 mM NaCl, and 10 mM $MgCl_2$. After digestion the mitochondria were cooled in ice and diluted with 0.25 M sucrose containing 25 mM EDTA. For electrophoretic analysis, the DNAse-treated mitochondria from pooled hearts were lysed by addition of 0.1 volume of 20% SDS and allowed to stand at room temperature for 30 minutes with occasional gentle stirring. Pronase, predigested for 2 hours at 37 °C, was then added (75 µg/ml). After 5 minutes, CsCl was added to a final concentration 1.0 M, and the lysate was immediately frozen. After one hour, the lysate was thawed and centrifuged for 10 minutes at 12,100 × g. The RNA and SDS were separated from DNA by Agarose BioGel A150 column chromatography. The agarose gel electrophoresis in the presence of ethidium bromide (4 µg/ml) was carried out at room temperature in glass tubes with a current of 5 mM/gel for 6 hours. For electron microscopy the mitochondrial pellets were lysed, and the lysates were deproteinized in CsCl as described above. After centrifugation, additional CsCl was added to adjust the refractive index to 1.39. Ethidium bromide was then added (100 µg/ml). The density gradient was produced by centrifugation at 36,000 rpm for 60–72 hours at 20–24 °C. Two bands were observed; the upper band corresponding to nuclear DNA and open circular mtDNA; the lower band contained covalently closed circular mtDNA molecules. The mtDNA was determined by modification of the fluorometric method of *Kissane* and *Robins* (6).

The details of experimental procedures are given by *Rajamanickam* et al. (10).

Results

In order to measure the amount of mtDNA per unit mass of mitochondria we have examined the conditions necessary for removal of nuclear DNA. Treatment of mitochondria with DNAase at 4°C did not cause any significant decrease of DNA. In contrast, increasing the temperature to 24 °C resulted in loss of 20–30% of the DNA.

To determine the conditions under which nuclear DNA is removed without loss of mtDNA, we analyzed the structure of DNA isolated from

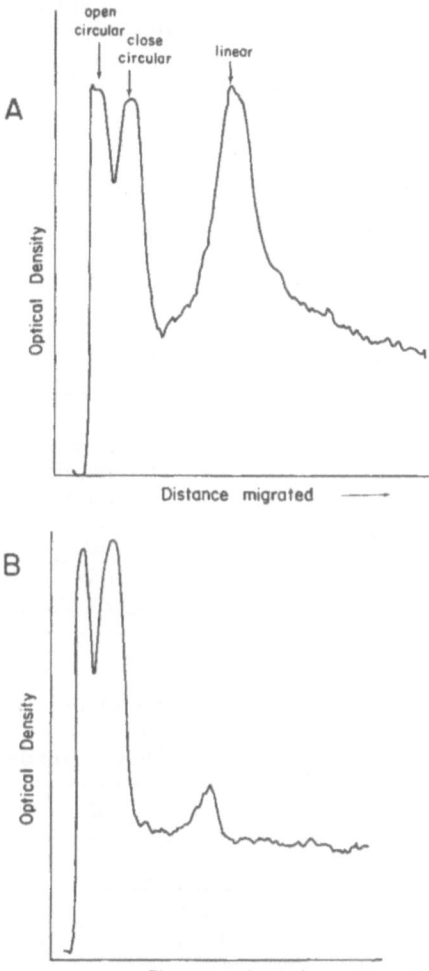

Fig. 1. Agarose gel electrophoresis of mtDNA isolated from DNAse treated and untreated mitochondria. Densitometric tracing of negatives of ethidium bromide fluorescence of 2% agarose gels are shown.
A: DNA extracted from mitochondria not subjected to DNAse treatment.
B: Same as A, except that the mitochondria were digested with 100 µg DNAse/mol for 30 minutes at 4 °C. (From ref. 10.)

DNAse-treated mitochondria. The purity of mtDNA can be assessed from its molecular conformation. In mammalian cell the nuclear DNA is linear, whereas mtDNA is predominantly in open or closed circular configuration. The three configurational species of DNA can be visualized by electrophoresis on 2% agarose gels. Linear molecules migrate more rapidly than closed circular and open circular DNA molecules (fig. 1) irrespective of size; closed circular molecules, in turn, migrate faster then open circular molecules. Photographs of ethidium bromide fluorescence in DNA electrophoreograms traced densitometrically are shown in figure 1. Large amounts of linear DNA is present when mitochondria are undigestes with DNAse. If mitochondria are digested with DNAse at 4 °C, the DNA has predominantly open and closed circular configuration with a small quantity of linear molecules.

Table 1. Rate of cellular growth and DNA content of mitochondria.

Tissue or cell type	mtDNA µg DNA/mg protein)	Author
Adult tissues		
Heart (beef)	0.24	*Schatz* et al., 1964 (4)
Heart (rat)	0.45	*Meerson* and *Pomoinitsky,* 1972 (5)
Liver (rat)	0.65	*Nass* et al., 1965 (6)
Growing cells		
L cells (culture)	1.1	*Borst* et al., 1966 (7)
Whole embryo (rat)	1.8	*Wunderlich* et al., 1966 (8)
Hypertrophic heart (rat)	2.7	*Meerson* and *Pomoinitsky,* 1972 (5)
Tumors		
Hepatoma (rat)	5.3	*Wunderlich* et al., 1966 (8)
Sarcoma (mouse)	4.7	*Wunderlich* et al., 1966
Ascites tumor	2.5	*Nass,* 1969 (6)

Table 2. Changes in mitochondrial DNA content after aortic constriction in the rat.

Experiment	DNA (µg/nmole cytochrome a)		
	Days after surgery		
	2	4	7
Sham operation	0.501	0.497	0.455
± S. D.	0.003	0.010	0.020
# of preparations (5 rats each)	4	3	3
Aortic constriction	0.555	0.853**	0.986**
± S. D.	0.002	0.041	0.062
# of preparations (5 rats each)	3	3	3
% Increase in constricted rats	11	72	117

 * P < 0.02
 ** P < 0.001

If an assay for mtDNA is to be valid, it is necessary to determine whether there was any loss of mtDNA due to DNAse digestion. For that purpose, the DNA content of mitochondrial preparation was measured after varying periods of DNAse digestion at 24 °C. The DNA content reached a minimal value after 30 minutes of digestion and remained unchanged during subsequent hour of DNAse treatment. From this data it is concluded that digestion of mitochondria with DNAse at 24 °C is suitable for elimination of contaminating nuclear DNA.

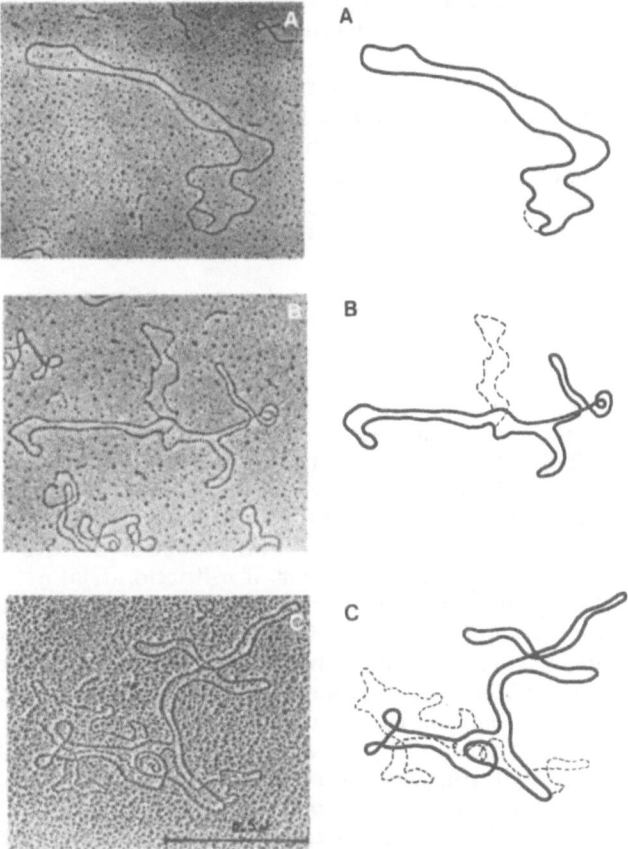

Fig. 2. Electron micrographs and schemes of intermediates of mtDNA replication. A: D-loop. B, C: Different stages of expanded D-loop molecule. The interrupted lines on schemes represent single strand regions. The mtDNA molecules were spread according to the formamide-urea technique. The spreading mixture, containing 50% formamide, 2 M urea, 100 mM Tris buffer pH 8.2, 10 mM EDTA, 50 µg/ml cytochrome c, and 1 µg/ml of DNA, was delivered slowly onto a water hypophase. The DNA-cytochrome c film was allowed to stand for only a few seconds before being picked up on a parlodion coated grid. The grids were stained with uranyl acetate and rotary-shadowed with platinum-palladium. The electron micrographs were taken at magnifications of 8,000 to 12,000 with a Siemens model 101 electron microscope. (From ref. 10.)

Next we have examined changes in mtDNA during development of cardiac hypertrophy. Constriction of the ascending aorta in mature rats resulted in cardiac enlargment of 15, 26, and 38% above the size in sham-operated controls 2, 4, and 7 days, respectively, after the surgery (table 2). The mtDNA content, expressed per nmole of cytochrome *a* was found increased by 11% two days after aortic constriction, whereas the maximal increment (117%) was observed after 7 days. Similar results were obtained when mtDNA content was expressed in unit of mitochondrial protein.

The increased rate of mtDNA synthesis should allow us to analyze the replicative forms of the mtDNA population in hypertrophied hearts. Electron micrographs of various molecular forms of rat cardiac mtDNA are shown in Figure 2. The mtDNA population of hearts from normal and sham-operated rats contained a high frequency of D-loops (42–49%). Intermediates of replication, other than D-loops, were rare. In mtDNA preparations from hypertrophied hearts, the frequency of mtDNA molecules containing D-loops was markedly reduced, from about 45% to 5 to 7% of the population, in all samples analyzed. In contrast, the frequency of expanded D-loops increased substantially in hearts undergoing hypertrophy.

Discussion

One of the earliest changes in the myocardium subjected to acute pressure overload is an increase in the cellular volume occupied by mitochondria. The preferential accumulation of mitochondria is only transient, however, during the last phase of developing hypertrophy, myofibrils accumulate more rapidly than mitochondria (2, 3). As a consequence, there is a progressive decrease in the fraction of mitochondria per unit of myofibrillar mass. The synthesis of mitochondrial cytochromes is increased in developing hypertrophy and as a consequence their content per unit of mitochondrial protein is increased. The changes in cytochromes c, b and aa₃ are in parallel. In contrast, our present measurements indicate, that the mtDNA content increased proportionately more than the content of cytochromes. The time sequence of changes in mtDNA agrees with the earlier observations by *Meerson* and *Pomoinitsky* (5) but they differ quantitatively, in that we observed only about 20% of the increment in mtDNA reported by these investigators.

The increased synthesis of mtDNA is accompanied by marked reduction in D-loop forms of mtDNA during developing hypertrophy. The D-loop is usually present with extraordinarily high frequency (up to 50%) as in other differentiated non-growing tissues (11). The D-loop frequency falls when mitochondrial replication is stimulated. For example, in regenerating liver the percent of D-loops drops to about 50% of values found in non-growing rat liver (12). Our results show an even more striking decrease in D-loop frequency in hypertrophied rat heart in which mtDNA synthesis is elevated. The marked depletion of the D-loop population during hypertrophy and the increase in number of expanded D-loops indicates removal of a block in replication at this site when the replicative flux through the cycle is increased.

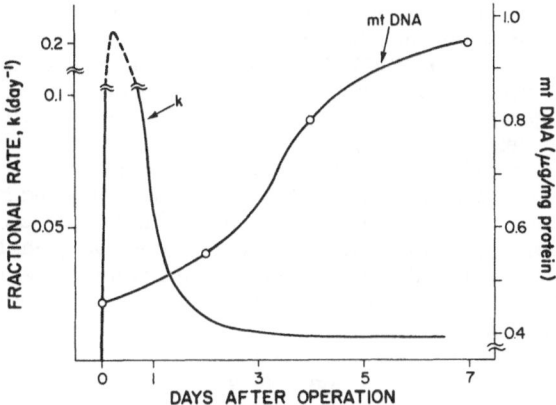

Fig. 3. Relation between the rate of cytochrome c accumulation and mitochondrial DNA content after aortic constriction. Cytochrome c accumulation is expressed as a fractional rate which corresponds to the rate of cytochrome c accumulation expressed as a fraction of the mean cytochrome c content for a particular time interval. (From ref. 10.)

Of considerable interest is the comparison of mitochondrial cytochromes with the changes in mtDNA content. It may be postulated that mtDNA must increase during active growth to provide additional template for the transcription of mtDNA required to support enhanced protein synthesis. Since there is probably only one promoter per DNA strand, and selective transcription of the mitochondrial genome does not occur, it was postulated by *Meerson* and *Pomoinitsky* (5) that the rate of mitochondrial RNA transcription depends on the amount of available template. Comparison of the rates of cytochrome c accumulation with the levels of mtDNA (Fig. 3), however, indicates that there is clearly a different temporal pattern in the increase of mtDNA, and in the accumulation of mitochondrial protein. During the first 24 post-operative hours, the inner mitochondrial components accumulate much faster than mtDNA. During the subsequent six days, however, the rate of mtDNA increment far outstrips that of the cytochromes. It is during this period when the cell volume occupied by mitochondria begins to show a decrease (2, 3). It must therefore be concluded that the regulation of mitochondrial replication, transcription, and translation is complex, and that the relationship between the amount of mtDNA and the synthesis of RNA and protein is not a simple one.

Zusammenfassung

Bei erwachsenen weiblichen Ratten wurde die Proliferation der Mitochondrien nach experimenteller Aortenkonstriktion untersucht. Die mitochondriale DNA (mtDNA) wurde fluorometrisch bestimmt. Die methodischen Voraussetzungen für eine Beseitigung der Zellkern-DNA wurden entwickelt und überprüft durch Bestimmung der molekularen Konformation der DNA. Die Konzentration an mtDNA in den Mitochondrien war 2,4 und 7 Tage nach der Operation um 11, 72 bzw. 117% erhöht. Bei Vergleich mit der Akkumulationsgeschwindigkeit von Cytochrom c, b und aa₃ ergaben sich Hinweise dafür, daß während der ersten 24 Stunden der Herzerweiterung die inneren Komponenten der Mitochondrien schneller akkumulieren als mtDNA. Jedoch überholt der mtDNA-Anstieg während der 6 folgenden Tage die Geschwindigkeit des Anstiegs der Cytochrome bei weitem. Diese Ergebnisse weisen darauf hin, daß die Menge verfügbarer mtDNA „templates" nicht den einzigen regulierenden Faktor für die Transkriptions- und Translationsprozesse während der Herzerweiterung darstellt.

Die Analyse der Zusammensetzung replikativer Intermediärprodukte von mtDNA zeigte einen dramatischen Rückgang in der Frequenz der D-loops bei Präparaten, die von hypertrophierten Herzen gewonnen wurden. Diese Beobachtung zeigt, daß der Anstieg des replikativen Fluxes von mtDNA mit der Beseitigung eines Blocks in der Umwandlung von D-loops zu anderen Intermediärprodukten verknüpft ist.

References

1. *Rabinowitz, M., R. Zak:* Mitochondria and cardiac hypertrophy. Circ. Res. **36**, 367 (1975).
2. *Page, E., P. I. Polimeni, R. Zak, J. Early, M. Johnson:* Myofibrillar mass in rat and rabbit heart muscle. Circ. Res. **30**, 430 (1972).
3. *Albin, R., R. T. Dowell, R. Zak, M. Rabinowitz:* Synthesis and degradation of mitochondrial components in hypertrophied rat heart. Biochem. J. **136**, 629 (1973).
4. *Schatz, G., E. Haselbrunner, H. Tuppy:* Mschr. Chem. **95**, 1135 (1964). (Quoted in ref. 6).
5. *Meerson, F. Z., V. D. Pomoinitsky:* The role of high-energy phosphate compounds in the development of cardiac hypertrophy. J. Molec. Cell. Cardiol. **4**, 571 (1972).
6. *Nass, M. M. K.:* Mitochondrial DNA: Advances, problems and goals. Science **165**, 25 (1969).
7. *Borst, P., G. J. C. M. Ruttenberg, A. Kroon:* Preparation and properties of mitochondrial DNA. Biochim. Biophys. Acta **149**, 140 (1967).
8. *Wunderlich, V., M. Schutt, A. Graffi:* Acta Biol. Med. German. **17**, K27 (1966). (Quoted in ref. 6).
9. *Kissane, J. M., E. Robins:* The fluorometric measurement of deoxyribonucleic acid in animal tissues with specific reference to the central nervous system. J. Biol. Chem. **233**, 184 (1958).
10. *Rajamanickam, C., S. Merten, B. Kwiatkowska-Patzer, C-H. Chuang, R. Zak, M. Rabinowitz:* Changes in mitochondrial DNA in cardiac hypertrophy in the rat. Circulat. Res. **45**, 505 (1979).
11. *Kasamatsu, H., L. I. Grossman, D. L. Robbertson, R. Watson, J. Vinograd:* The replication and structure of mitochondrial DNA in animal cells. Cold Spring Harbor Symp. Quant. Biol. **38**, 281 (1973).
12. *Gilbert, W., D. Dressler:* DNA replication: The rolling circle model. Cold Spring Harbor Symp. Quant. Biol. **33**, 473 (1968).

Authors' address:

Prof. *Radovan Zak,* Department of Medicine Box 407, University of Chicago, 950 East 59 Street, Chicago, Illinois 60637

Basic Res. Cardiol. **75**, 179–184 (1980)
© 1980 Dr. Dietrich Steinkopff Verlag, Darmstadt
ISSN 0300–8428

Paper, presented at the Erwin Riesch Symposium, Tübingen, April 3–7, 1979

*University of Vermont College of Medicine, Department of Physiology and
Biophysics, Burlington, Vermont 05405*

The functional significance of altered tension dependent heat in thyrotoxic myocardial hypertrophy*)

Über die funktionelle Bedeutung der veränderten
spannungsabhängigen Wärmeproduktion bei der
thyreotoxischen Herzhypertrophie

N. R. Alpert and *L. A. Mulieri*

With 3 figures and 1 table

Summary

Enlargement of the heart secondary to 14 daily injections of L-thyroxine (0.2 mg/
kg) in the male albino rabbit results in an increase in actin-activated myosin
ATPase, velocity of unloaded shortening and rate of isometric tension development. The contribution of the altered myosin to contractile efficiency is assessed by
making temperature measurements on right ventricular papillary muscles from
these hearts during isometric contraction. Measurement of tension dependent heat
per unit of tension is derived from rapid myothermal measurements of initial heat,
tension independent heat and isometric force. The tension dependent heat measurement is used to evaluate the crossbridge cycling *in vivo* and the contribution of
the changes in the pattern of crossbridge cycling to the efficiency of tension
development. In the thyrotoxic heart the peak twitch tension is 72% of normal
while the tension dependent heat per unit tension is 175% of normal. This *in vivo*
measurement correlates well with changes in *in vitro* actin-activated myosin
ATPase measurements. Analysis of the data in terms of a model derived from rapid
enzyme kinetics and mechanical transient analysis indicates that crossbridges from
the thyrotoxic hypertrophy myosin cycle faster and stay attached to actin for a
shorter period of time than normal myosin. This alteration in cycling pattern may
be the basis for the inverse relationship between myosin ATPase activity and the
efficiency of tension development.

When the heart enlarges in response to a thyroid stress there is an
increase in actin-activated myosin ATPase activity (1, 2). It is important to
know if the in vitro change in the splitting of ATP by actomyosin is a
reflection of the in vivo behavior of the myosin molecules when they are
present in thick filaments associated with actin in an organized pattern.
Furthermore analyses which provide data relating to the *in vivo* splitting
of ATP by actomyosin during tension development should provide infor-

---

*) This work was supported in part by NIH grants 1 R01 HL22845-01, T32
HL07073 and R01 HL 17592.

mation concerning the myosin crossbridge cycling pattern and its contribution to the energetics of tension development.

The strategy is to evaluate the intracellular behavior of myosin by using rapid myothermal methods on normal rabbit hearts and those with thyrotoxic hypertrophy. With these techniques the initial heat can be partitioned into a tension dependent and a tension independent portion. The former is a measure of ATP splitting by actomyosin during tension development and reflects myosin crossbridge cycling. It thus should provide information about *in vivo* myosin ATPase activity and energetics during tension development.

Methods

Animal model

All experiments are performed on right ventricular papillary muscle preparations from male albino rabbits. Thyrotoxic hypertrophy is induced by 14 daily injections of L-thyroxine (0.2 mg/kg) after which the rabbits are sacrificed, the hearts removed, placed in oxygenated Krebs-Ringer, and the papillary muscle is isolated and mounted on the thermopile as described below.

Myothermal and force measurements

Right ventricular papillary muscles are excised and mounted on vacuum deposited thermopiles as previously described (3). The cut end of the muscle is attached to an isometric force transducer while the tedinous end is anchored to a stationary hook. Close contact with the thermopile elements is insured by a tether. The thermopile assembly is placed inside a chamber allowing the muscle to be bathed in oxygenated Krebs-Ringer solution or surrounded by moist gas. The entire myothermal assembly is placed in a 70 liter constant temperature bath where equilibration is carried out at 21 °C for two hours. The muscle is stimulated at 0.2 Hz and the

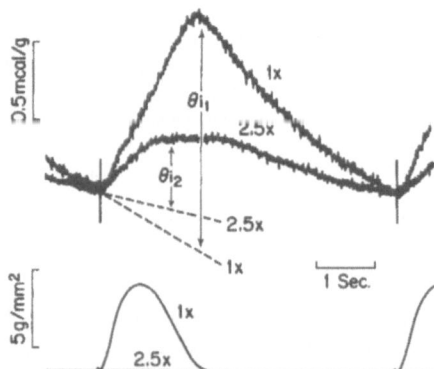

Fig. 1. Temperature and force changes in a control papillary muscle incubated in normal Krebs solution (1X) and hyperosmotic mannitol-Krebs solution (2.5X). The upper trace is the temperature and the lower trace the force records. The stimulus marker is indicated in the temperature record by the vertical line preceding the temperature change and in the force record by the deflection preceding the force change. See text for a description of the method used to calculate the initial, tension dependent and tension independent heats.

experiments are accepted only if the muscle heat and tension performance are stable over the entire experimental period and isometric twitch tension is at least four times greater than resting tension.

Tension dependent heat measurements

The temperature of a contracting muscle is determined by evolution of resting heat, initial heat and recovery heat. When rapid myothermal techniques are used the temperature oscillation which occurs with each beat is made up of the initial heat and the recovery heat (fig. 1). Temperature changes associated with the initial heat liberation are corrected for heat loss by the extrapolation procedures shown by the dashed line in figure 1 labeled 1X. The dashed line is obtained by translating the cool off curve which occurs upon cessation of stimulation. The corrected temperature change, θ_{i1}, is converted to the corresponding heat evolution by multiplication with the effective heat capacity of the muscle plus adhering Krebs solution determined as previously described (3). The initial heat consists of the sum of the tension dependent and tension independent heats. The former represents crossbridge cycling during tension development and hence *in vivo* actomyosin ATPase activity. The latter represents the initial energy cost of excitation and the translocation of calcium during contraction and relaxation. Tension independent heat is obtained by measuring the triggerable heat output when tension is eliminated by incubating the muscle in hyperosmotic (2.5 X N) mannitol-Krebs solution (θ_{i2}, fig. 1) and multiplying this temperature by the effective heat capacity of the muscle and adhering *Krebs* solution. The tension dependent heat is the difference between initial heat and tension independent heat.

Results
General

The right ventricular heart weight : body weight ratio increased by 197% in the thyrotoxic hypertrophy (table 1). There was no significant change in the cross-sectional area of the papillary muscles or in the dry wet weight ratios of the papillary muscle and liver (table 1).

Mechanical and thermal measurements

The peak isometric twitch tension was 5.8 ± .3 (SEM) g/mm² for the control muscles. The thyrotoxic preparations had an isometric twitch tension which was 72% (p < .05) of the control. The tension dependent heat per unit of tension developed was 2.08 ± .21 and 3.65 ± .18 μCal/g cm for the control and thyrotoxic preparations, respectively (N = 8).

Discussion

Hypertrophy of the myocardium which occurs following prolonged thyrotoxic stress permits the heart to meet the additional demands for

Table 1. Thyrotoxic hypertrophy.

	RV/Body wt g/kg	X Sec RV PAP M mm²	Dry/wet wt PAP M	liver
Normal	0.31 ± .01	0.59 ± .04	0.23 ± .006	0.28 ± .01
Thyrotoxic	0.61 ± .02	0.66 ± .06	0.24 ± .005	0.25 ± .01
	p < .002	N. S.	N. S.	N. S.

increased cardiac output placed on it. The change in performance is not simply the result of arithmetic addition of muscle mass. There is an alteration in the quality of performance of each muscle unit. In previous studies of pressure overload hypertrophy we reported a depression in mechanical V_{max} (4), an increase in time to peak tension (4), a depressed myosin ATPase activity (5, 6) and a depressed heat production per unit of tension (7). The present studies on thyrotoxic hypertrophy are a logical extension of the pressure overload experiments in that the changes are generally in the opposite direction. Thus the velocity of unloaded shortening and rate of isometric tension development increase while the time to peak tension decreases. In addition the actin-activated myosin ATPase from these hearts is increased (1, 2). The goal of these experiments is to use high speed myothermal measurements to analyze the contribution of the altered contractile proteins to the energetics of force development. The tension dependent heat results from the splitting of ATP during crossbridge cycling and the associated tension development. In the thyrotoxic preparation the tension dependent heat rate is 175% of control.

These results can be interpreted in terms of the rapid enzyme kinetic (8) and mechanical tension transient (9) hypotheses of crossbridge cycling rates and tension development (fig. 2). At rest myosin crossbridges and actin do not interact with each other. In the activated tension producing part of the cycle the actomyosin crossbridge system exists in two distinct states, where the actin and myosin crossbridges are dissociated (fig. 2, top) or associated (fig. 2, bottom). In the former, i.e., the dissociated or "off" state, there is a rate limiting step at arrow 1 between the two conformational states M^{**} ADPPi and M^{+}ADPPi. This rate limiting step probably plays the major role in determining the overall cycling rate and is characteristic of each type of myosin. In the associated or "on" state, force is believed to be generated when the crossbridge head rotates from the 90° (AM^{+}ADPPi) to the 45° (AM ADPPi) position stretching the compliant elements in the myosin molecule. In this scheme the length of time during which the myosin head is attached in a position less than 90° (i.e. between 90° and 45°) and the stiffness of the compliant element determine the integrated force developed during a single cycle. The time course of the

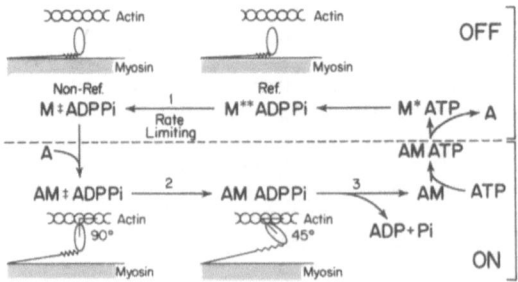

Fig. 2. Actin-activated myosin kinetics and crossbridge behavior. The following symbols are used: M, myosin; A, actin; ATP, adenosine triphosphate; ADP, adenosine diphosphate; Pi, inorganic phosphate; M^{+}, M^{**}, different conformational states of myosin (redrawn from *Eisenberg* and *Hill,* 1978 (8)).

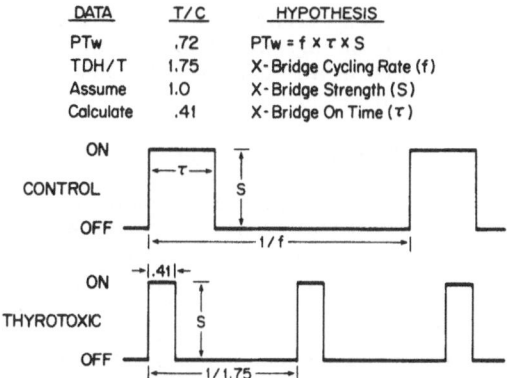

Fig. 3. The "on-off" cycle of crossbridges during activation for the control and thyrotoxic preparations (see text for discussion).

movement along arrows 2 and 3 (fig. 2) is also a characteristics of each type of myosin.

Thus the heat production associated with tension development can be analyzed in terms of "on" time and cycling rate (fig. 3). As a first approximation in quantifying the process of chemomechanical transduction consider the following model. Assume that the peak twitch is a function of the integrated rate at which the crossbridges cycle (f), average time each crossbridge is attached and in the tension producing configuration (τ) and the average stiffness of the crossbridge compliant element (S).

If the tension dependent heat is an index of the crossbridge cycling rate, and the strength of each myosin crossbridge is unity then the on time and cycling rates for the thyrotoxic preparation relative to control can be calculated. The thyrotoxic preparation develops force less efficiently than the control because of an increase in the cycling rate (f) and a decrease in the "on" time τ (fig. 3). Thus the efficiency of force development is inversely related to tension dependent heat or actin-activated myosin ATPase activity (1, 2). The ability of the heart to alter the structure of the myosin molecule synthesized in response to thyrotoxic stress appears to alter the rate limiting step of the actomyosin ATPase cycle (fig. 2, arrow 1) as well as the tension producing "on" time (fig. 2, arrows 2 and 3).

The combination of rapid myothermal measurements with high speed mechanical transient and enzyme kinetic analyses may provide additional data for testing the newer models of crossbridge behavior such as those proposed by *Eisenberg* and *Hill* (8), *Lymm* and *Taylor* (10), *Huxley* and *Simmons* (9), and *Podolsky* and *Nolan* (11).

Acknowledgement

L-thyroxine was kindly supplied by Flint Laboratories, Deefield, Illinois. The technical assistance of *Robert Goulette* was appreciated.

Zusammenfassung

Eine Herzvergrößerung beim Kaninchen als Folge von L-Thyroxin-Injektionen (täglich 0,2 mg/kg über 14 Tage) führt zu einer Steigerung der aktinaktivierten

Myosin-ATPase, der Verkürzungsgeschwindigkeit bei Nullast und der Geschwindigkeit der isometrischen Spannungsentwicklung. Durch Temperaturmessungen an rechtsventrikulären, isometrisch schlagenden Papillarmuskeln solcher Herzen wird der Beitrag des veränderten Myosins zum kontraktilen Wirkungsgrad bestimmt. Die spannungsabhängige Wärme pro Spannungseinheit ergibt sich aus schnellen myothermalen Messungen der Initialwärme, der spannungsunabhängigen Wärme und der isometrischen Kraft. Auf der Grundlage der spannungsabhängigen Wärme wird die Querbrückenkinetik *in vivo* bestimmt und untersucht, inwieweit Änderungen der Querbrückenkinetik zum Wirkungsgrad der Spannungsentwicklung beitragen. Im thyreotoxischen Herzen beträgt die maximal entwickelte Spannung 72% gegenüber den Kontrollen, während die spannungsabhängige Wärme pro Spannungseinheit 175% ausmacht. Diese *In-vivo*-Messungen stimmen mit Änderungen der *in vitro* gemessenen aktinaktivierten Myosin-ATPase überein. Eine Analyse dieser Daten anhand eines Modells, welches aus der Analyse von schneller Enzymkinetik und mechanischer Transienten entwickelt wurde, ergibt, daß der Querbrückenzyklus des thyreotoxisch-hypertrophierten Myosins im Vergleich zum normalen Myosin schneller abläuft und die Querbrücke für kürzere Zeit an das Aktin angeheftet ist. Diese Änderung des Zyklusablaufs könnte die Grundlage für eine inverse Beziehung zwischen der Myosin-ATPase-Aktivität und dem Wirkungsgrad der Spannungsentwicklung bilden.

References

1. *Banerjee, S. K., E. Morkin:* Actin-activated adenosine triphosphatase activity of native and N-ethylmaleimide-modified myosin from normal and thyrotoxic rabbits. Circulat. Res. **41**, 630–634 (1977).
2. *Alpert, N. R., R. Z. Litten, L. A. Mulieri:* Myothermal vs. enzymatic changes in thyrotoxic cardiac hypertrophy. The Physiologist **21**, 2 (1978).
3. *Mulieri, L. A., G. Luhr, J. Trefry, N. R. Alpert:* Metal film thermopiles for use with rabbit right ventricular papillary muscles. Amer. J. Physiol. **233** (5), C146–C156 (1977).
4. *Hamrell, B. B., N. R. Alpert:* The mechanical characteristics of hypertrophied rabbit cardiac muscle in the absence of congestive heart failure: the contractile and series elastic elements. Circulat. Res. **40**, 20–25 (1977).
5. *Shiverick, K. T., B. B. Hamrell, N. R. Alpert:* Structural and functional properties of myosin associated with compensatory cardiac hypertrophy in rabbit. J. Mol. Cell Cardiol. **8**, 837–851 (1976).
6. *Thomas, L. L., N. R. Alpert:* Functional integrity of SH_1 site in myosin from hypertrophied myocardium. Biochim. et Biophys. Acta **481**, 680–688 (1977).
7. *Alpert, N. R., L. A. Mulieri:* The partitioning of altered mechanics in hypertrophied heart muscle between the sarcoplasmic reticulum and the contractile apparatus by means of myothermal measurements. Basic Res. Cardiol. **72**, 153–159 (1977).
8. *Eisenberg, E., T. L. Hill:* A crossbridge model of muscle contraction. Prog. Biophys. Mol. Biol. **33**, 55–82 (1978).
9. *Huxley, A. F., R. M. Simmons:* Proposed mechanism of force generation in striated muscle. Nature **233**, 533–538 (1971).
10. *Lymm, R. W., E. W. Taylor:* Mechanism of adenosine triphosphate hydrolyses by actomyosin. Biochemistry **10**, 4617–4624 (1971).
11. *Podolsky, R. J., A. C. Nolan:* Muscle contraction transients, crossbridge kinetics and the Fenn effect. Cold Spring Harbor Symp. Quant. Biol. **37**, 661–668 (1972).

Authors' address:

Norman R. Alpert, Department of Physiology and Biophysics, University of Vermont College of Medicine, Given Medical Building, Burlington, Vermont 05405

Basic Res. Cardiol. **75**, 185–192 (1980)
© 1980 Dr. Dietrich Steinkopff Verlag, Darmstadt
ISSN 0300–8428

Paper, presented at the Erwin Riesch Symposium, Tübingen, April 3–7, 1979

Physiologisches Institut II, Universität Tübingen

Oxygen consumption and substrate uptake of the hypertrophied rat heart in situ*)

Sauerstoff- und Substratverbrauch des hypertrophierten Rattenherzens in situ

G. Kissling

With 3 figures and 1 table

Summary

A new heart preparation was developed which permits in situ measurements of myocardial oxygen consumption and substrate uptake in small animals. Using this new method the mechanical activity, as well as oxygen consumption and substrate uptake of the heart, was measured in Goldblatt rats with left ventricular hypertrophy of about 40%.
1. In agreement with former investigations on the hypertrophied rat heart, this model also shows that both the performance of the whole ventricle, as well as the contractile force per unit of cross-sectional area, is increased in the state of stable hypertrophy.
2. The absolute values of oxygen consumption and substrate uptake are increased in the hypertrophied hearts. However, oxygen consumption and substrate uptake as related to muscle mass and to wall stress were largely identical in hypertrophied and control hearts.
3. Hypertrophied hearts and controls utilize substrates according to their respective arterial blood concentration. Under our experimental conditions approximately 50% of the total energy in both groups is obtained from glucose, 30% from lactate, and 20% from fat. The relatively high consumption of lactate could be explained by the glucose uptake and lactate release of the erythrocytes.

An immense number of investigators have measured oxygen consumption and substrate uptake of the heart under various conditions. Cardiac energetics of the hypertrophied heart are of special interest, because alterations of cardiac energetics might contribute to the development of heart failure (3, 5). An often used model for investigating this topic in experimental cardiac hypertrophy is the hypertrophied rat heart. To our knowledge oxygen consumption and substrate uptake have only been measured in the rat in isolated preparations because the obtainmnet of in situ coronary-venous blood samples is made difficult by small animal size. However, the significance of measurements on isolated preparations is limited because any isolation of the heart leads to a deterioration of its contractile state.

---
*) Supported by the Deutsche Forschungsgemeinschaft.

Therefore, we have developed a new in situ heart preparation which includes elements of the Langendorff preparation as well as elements of the heart-lung preparation. Using this new method the mechanical activity, as well as the oxygen consumption and substrate uptake of the heart, was measured in Goldblatt rats 8 weeks after narrowing of one renal artery and in corresponding control animals.

Methods

Cardiac hypertrophy with an increase in left ventricular weight of about 40% was produced by coarctation of one renal artery (Goldblatt II). 8 weeks after coarctation the chest was opened under urethane anesthesia (1–1.4 g/kg body weight) and the animals were ventilated artificially. After opening the chest an electromagnetic flowprobe was placed around the trunk of the pulmonary artery. The left ventricle was pierced at the apex with a canula for pressure measurement and for withdrawal of arterial blood samples. The aortic pressure was measured using a second canula which was inserted into the ascending aorta immediately above the aortic valves. Subsequently, the aortic trunk, as well as the superior vena cava, were ligated, the latter directly in front of the right atrium. A third canula was ligated into the inferior vena cava for measuring central venous pressure and for withdrawing venous blood samples. Under these conditions the circulating was: left heart – coronary arteries – right heart – pulmonary circulation – left heart (fig. 1).

The circulating blood volume of this preparation was measured in 16 Goldblatt and control animals using Evans blue and was found to be 1.56 ml/100 g body weight in both groups. This value corresponds to 25% of the total blood volume of the animals.

The arterial pH was adjusted to 7.1–7.2 by ventilation with a 95% oxygen and 5% CO_2 gas mixture.

The following mechanical parameters were recorded: left ventricular pressure amplitude, left ventricular enddiastolic pressure, and the first derivative of left ventricular pressure; pulmonary flow; pressure in the aortic trunk; central venous pressure.

Ventricular wall stress and the maximum rate of stress development and of relaxation were calculated using the model of a thick-walled sphere (11).

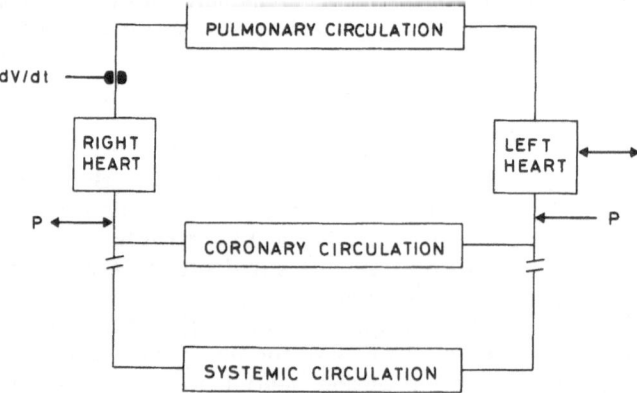

Fig. 1. Schematic diagram of the circulation after ligation of the aortic trunk and the venae cavae.

In our preparation steady-state values of the mechanical parameters were reached about 15 minutes after the ligation of the aortic trunk, and the hearts are able to work up to 3 hours under steady-state conditions. In these experiments, however, arterial and venous blood samples for the measurement of oxygen and substrate concentrations were taken after 30 minutes. After recording the diastolic pressure-volume relations, the animals were sacrificed and the heart weights and left ventricular weights were measured.

Oxygen consumption was measured using the arteriovenous oxygen difference (Lex O_2-Con) and pulmonary flow. Arterial hematocrit and arterial blood concentration of glucose, lactate, pyruvate and the arterial plasma concentration of esterized, nonesterized glycerine and of free fatty acids was measured before and 30 minutes after the ligation of the aortic trunk. Substrate uptake was calculated from the difference in concentrations before and after ligation and from the blood or plasma volume.

Results and Discussion

a) Mechanical parameters

In Goldblatt rats the developed pressure is significantly higher and the enddiastolic pressure significantly lower than in control animals, while the maximum rate of systolic pressure development and heart rate are identical in both groups. Systolic peak wall stress and the maximum rate of stress development and of relaxation are not statistically different in Goldblatt and control animals. In contrast, diastolic wall stress is lowered significantly in Goldblatt rats. Therefore it seems, that systolic wall stress is the regulatory parameter, i.e., the hypertrophied hearts have adjusted their preload such that the systolic wall stress remains constant under the enhanced pressure load.

However, it should be kept in mind that the contractile capability of the hypertrophied hearts is still increased. At a given enddiastolic pressure, systolic peak pressure, as well as the maximum rate of pressure development and of pressure fall, are significantly increased in Goldblatt rats. The calculated parameters of wall stress also point to an enhanced contractility of the hypertrophied hearts. At any given enddiastolic wall stress the peak wall stress and the maximum rate of stress development and of relaxation are significantly increased in Goldblatt rats.

Table 1.

	Experimental values (mM ATP)			Normalized values (mM ATP/g)		Per cent values %	
	Controls	Goldblatt	p	Controls	Gold-blatt	Controls	Gold-blatt
Glucose	0.908±0.108	1.301±0.113	<0.01	1.382	1.442	52	46.5
Lactate	0.484±0.034	0.941±0.154	<0.01	0.737	1.043	28	34
Pyruvate	0.015±0.008	0.010±0.003	ns	0.023	0.011	1	0.5
Triglycerides	0.294±0.088	0.528±0.192	ns	0.448	0.585	17	19
Free fatty acids	0.034±0.006	0.019±0.007	ns	0.052	0.021	2	1
Total	1.753	2.799		2.642	3.102		

These results are in agreement with former investigations of our group on the mechanical activity of the hypertrophied rat heart (9).

b) Oxygen consumption

Using pulmonary flow and the arteriovenous oxygen difference, the oxygen consumption was determined 30 minutes after ligation of the aortic trunk. Although the cardiac output in Goldblatt rats was diminished by 25%, the absolute value of oxygen consumption was increased by 48% due to an increased arteriovenous difference in oxygen concentration. However, oxygen consumption in relation to muscle mass and to wall stress parameters was not increased in the hypertrophied hearts. Figure 2 shows the dependence of oxygen consumption per minute and per g heart weight on the systolic peak wall stress (σ_{max}), the maximum rate of stress development ($d\sigma/dt_{max}$), the developed wall stress averaged over one minute ($\bar{\sigma}$), and the product of heart rate times wall stress over one minute ($\bar{\sigma} \cdot HR$). The closest correlations are between oxygen consumption and the maximum rate of stress development, on the one hand, and the product of heart rate times wall stress averaged over one minute, on the other hand.

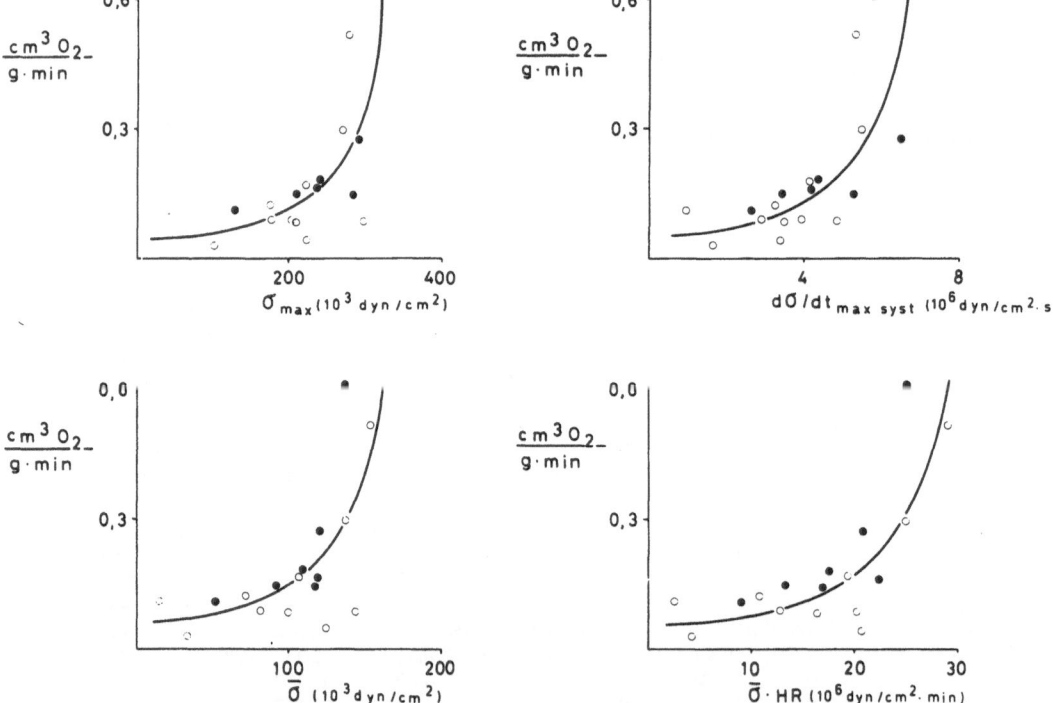

Fig. 2. Dependence of oxygen consumption per g heart weight and per minute on the systolic peak wall stress (σ_{max}), the maximum rate of stress development ($d\sigma/dt_{max\ syst}$), the developed wall stress averaged over one minute ($\bar{\sigma}$), and the product of heart rate times wall stress averaged over one minute ($\bar{\sigma} \cdot HR$). ○ Goldblatt rats, ● controls.

The average oxygen consumption of all control animals was 0.2173 ml O_2 per minute and per g heart weight at an average systolic peak pressure of 158 mmHg. At first sight this value corresponds very well with the results of *Gamble* et al. (4), who found an oxygen consumption of about 22 ml O_2 per minute and per 100 g left ventricular weight in the isolated, blood-perfused rat heart at comparable pressure values. However, the heart rates of their preparations were much higher (200–360 beats/min in comparison to ca. 160 beats/min in our experiments). Therefore, they found an oxygen consumption per beat and per 100 g left ventricular weight of 0.07 ml, whereas in our experiments the calculated O_2 consumption per beat and per 100 g heart weight was 0.146 ml.

Unfortunately *Gamble* and his coworkers have not measured the substrate uptake of the hearts. In our experiments oxygen consumption was measured after 30 minutes, during which the hearts worked almost isovolumetrically. At this moment the glucose concentration in the circulating blood was diminished to about 40% of its initial value. In other words, in this moment the proportion of fat on the energy supply of the heart must be relatively high. Therefore, the relatively high oxygen consumption of our preparations might be due to a low RQ value.

Oxygen consumption of the hypertrophied myocardium was investigated by *Gunning* and *Coleman* (6). In cat papillary muscles of right hypertrophied ventricles these authors measured an oxygen consumption of 1.17×10^{-3} µl O_2 per mg heart weight per gram developed tension and per contraction (control value: 0.56×10^{-3} µl O_2 per mg and per contraction). If our values obtained from rat myocardium are calculated in the same manner with the aid of a thick-walled sphere, an oxygen consumption results for the control animals of 0.55×10^{-3} µl O_2 per mg heart weight and per gram developed tension and per contraction. This value corresponds exactly with the results on normal cat papillary muscle. In our hypertrophied hearts, however, the calculated value is 0.46×10^{-3} µl O_2 per mg and per contraction, which is even somewhat lower than the control value.

The explanation of this discrepancy between the results of *Gunning* and *Coleman* and ours might be, that their experimental animals with hypertrophied right ventricles showed all signs of congestive heart failure with decreased isometric peak tension, decreased maximum rate of tension development, and decreased shortening velocity, whereas our Goldblatt rats showed no signs of cardiac failure with even enhanced peak wall stress and increased maximum rate of stress development. Therefore it seems that myocardial oxygen consumption increases only in the state of decompensatory hypertrophy.

c) Substrate uptake

If one examines the substrate uptake of the heart in situ, one must consider that not only the heart muscle, but also the erythrocytes take up substrate in the form of glucose. This fact may be of secondary importance in the total energy balance, because the glucose which is taken up from the erythrocytes is released by them in the form of lactate, which can also be utilized by the heart. However, it is important to take this fact into

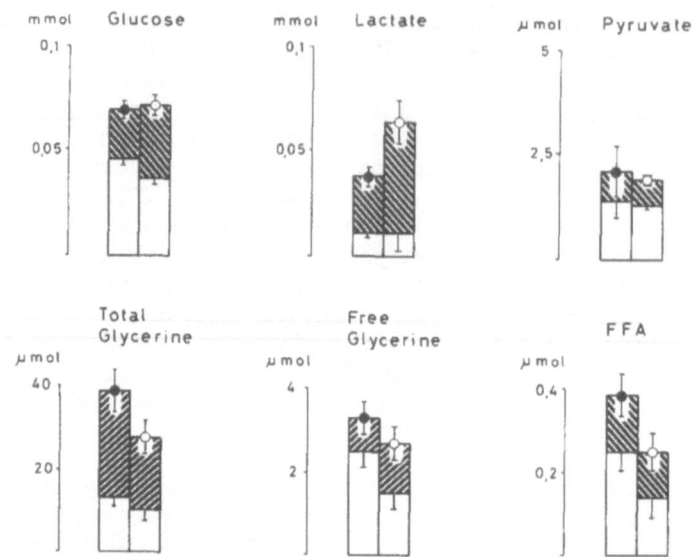

Fig. 3. Content of individual substrates in the blood at the beginning of the experiments (o Goldblatt rats, ● controls). For glucose, lactate, pyruvate, and free fatty acids, the hatched areas of the columns stand for the diminution of these substances due to myocardial uptake. The hatched areas of the total and free glycerine columns stand for the increase in these substances during the experimental period.

consideration when discussing cardiac consumption of individual substrates.

In vitro experiments on the glucose uptake and lactate formation of the erythrocytes in rat blood showed that the higher the hematocrit, the more glucose is taken up and the more lactate is released. On the basis of these measurements it was possible to take the metabolism of the erythrocytes into consideration. On average about 20% of the total consumed glucose was utilized by the erythrocytes; whereas in controls about 50% and in hypertrophied hearts about 30% of the lactate which was utilized by the myocardium originates from the metabolism of the erythrocytes.

Figure 3 shows the content of the individual substrates in the blood at the beginning of the experiments. In each case, the right columns refer to the values of Goldblatt animals. Although the experimental conditions as well as the circulating blood volume were identical in both groups, in the blood of the Goldblatt rats the content of lactate was significantly higher and the content of free fatty acids was significantly lower than in the controls. For glucose, lactate, pyruvate, and free fatty acids, the hatched areas of the columns stand for the diminution of these substances due to myocardial uptake. The hatched areas of the total and free glycerine columns, however, stand for the increase in these substances during the experimental period. The increase in free glycerine was assumed to be due to a splitting of triglycerides into glycerine and free fatty acids.

In Goldblatt rats glucose and lactate uptake are significantly greater than in the control animals, whereas the clearly enhanced splitting of triglycerides could not be proved statistically, due to greater scatter. The increased lactate uptke of the hypertrophied hearts is caused by an increased initial content of lactate in the blood. Pyruvate and free fatty acids are also consumed in proportion to their availability in the blood. The enhanced glucose uptake of the hypertrophied hearts, however, is not caused by a greater glucose content in the blood of the Goldblatt animals but rather by the fact, that the hypertrophied hearts extract more glucose than the controls.

The conditions for the increase of free glycerine are quite different. There is no relation between the amount of triglycerides in the blood and the formation of free glycerine. It is certainly true that the amount of triglycerides increases markedly after aortic ligation. However, the triglycerides are only cleaved to the extent that they are required by the heart. Under our experimental conditions the heart prefers to metabolize carbohydrates; thus, it only falls back on the esterized fatty acids when the carbohydrates are reduced. Therefore the formation of free glycerine depends on the initial amount of carbohydrates. If much carbohydrates are available in the blood, the heart consumes little fat and only if little carbohydrates are available, does the heart consume more fat.

Under the assumption that all substrates are totaly metabolized to CO_2 and water in the Krebs cycle, one can calculate the energy generated from the individual substrates in the form of ATP. The total heart energy consumption due to the individual substrates is presented in table 1. The hypertrophied hearts consume about 60% more substrate than the controls. The contribution of free fatty acids and pyruvate to the total energy is negligible. ATP consumption per g left ventricular weight is almost the same in both groups. In both groups approximately 50% of the total energy is obtained from glucose, 30% from lactate, and 20% from fat.

In contrast to our results the consensus view is that fatty acids are the most important cardiac substrate (5). Furthermore, in isolated rat heart preparations *Neely* et al. (10) showed that an increase in cardiac work is accompanied by an increased utilization of fatty acids, provided they are available in the blood. Therefore one should expect that in our preparation, in which the hearts work under high afterload, the main substrate should be fat.

On the other hand, it is well known that the heart utilizes the individual substrates according to their respective arterial concentration (2, 1). In our experimental animals the initial glucose and lactate concentration in the arterial blood was very high (14.4 mmol/l blood glucose and 7.1 mmol/l blood lactate in controls, and 14.2 mmol/l glucose and 11.9 mmol/l lactate in Goldblatt animals) and the initial FFA concentration was low (0.14 mval/l plasma in controls and 0.11 mval/l plasma in Goldblatt rats).

Furthermore, high lactate blood concentrations inhibit the cleaving of triglycerides (7). In agreement with these results, *Keul* et al. (8) measured only a 20.8% portion of fat in the energy supply of the heart in working human athletes with high blood levels of lactate. The relatively high portion of lactate in our experiments could be explained by the metabolism of the erythrocytes, which has been underestimated in the literature up to now. Our findings support the view that the heart utilizes substrates according to their respective arterial concentration.

Zusammenfassung

Es wurde ein neues Herzpräparat entwickelt, das auch an kleinen Tieren die Messung von Sauerstoff- und Substratverbrauch in situ ermöglicht. Mit dieser neuen Methode wurden sowohl die mechanische Aktivität als auch der Sauerstoff- und Substratverbrauch des Herzens an Goldblattratten mit einer linksventrikulären Hypertrophie von ca. 40% gemessen.

1. In Übereinstimmung mit früheren Untersuchungen am hypertrophierten Herzen wurde auch mit der neuen Methode im Stadium der stabilen Hypertrophie sowohl eine gesteigerte Leistungsfähigkeit des Gesamtventrikels als auch eine Erhöhung der querschnittsbezogenen Kraftentwicklung gefunden.

2. Der absolute Sauerstoff- und Substratverbrauch war bei den hypertrophierten Herzen erhöht. Bezieht man den gemessenen Sauerstoff- und Substratverbrauch jedoch auf die Muskelmasse und die entwickelte Wandspannung, dann ergeben sich für die hypertrophierten Herzen und die Kontrollen weitgehend übereinstimmende Werte.

3. Sowohl hypertrophierte Herzen als auch Kontrollen verbrauchen die einzelnen Substrate entsprechend ihrer jeweiligen Konzentration im arteriellen Blut. Unter unseren experimentellen Bedingungen wurden etwa 50% der gesamten Energie durch die Verbrennung von Glukose, 30% durch Laktat und 20% durch Fett bereitgestellt. Der relativ hohe Laktatverbrauch läßt sich durch die Glukoseaufnahme und Laktatproduktion der Erythrozyten erklären.

References

1. *Ballard, F. B., W. H. Danforth, S. Naegle, R. J. Bing:* Myocardial metabolism of fatty acids. J. Clin. Invest. **39**, 717–723 (1960).
2. *Bing, R. J.:* Myocardial metabolism. Circulation **12**, 635–647 (1955).
3. *Bing, R. J.:* Cardiac metabolism. Physiol. Rev. **45**, 171–213 (1965).
4. *Gamble, W. J., P. A. Conn, A. Edelji Kumar, R. Plenge, R. G. Monroe:* Myocardial oxygen consumption of blood perfused, isolated, supported rat heart. Amer. J. Physiol. **219**, 604–612 (1970).
5. *Gibbs, C. L.:* Cardiac energetics. Physiol. Rev. **58**, 174–254 (1978).
6. *Gunning, J. F., H. N. Coleman:* Myocardial oxygen consumption during experimental hypertrophy and congestive heart failure. J. Mol. Cell. Cardiol. **5**, 25–38 (1973).
7. *Hirche, Hj., H. D. Langohr:* Hemmung der Milchsäureaufnahme im Herzmuskel narkotisierter Hunde durch hohe arterielle Konzentration der freien Fettsäuren. Pflügers Arch. **293**, 208–214 (1967).
8. *Keul, J., E. Doll, H. Steim, U. Fleer, H. Reindell:* Über den Stoffwechsel des menschlichen Herzens. III. Der oxydative Stoffwechsel des menschlichen Herzens unter verschiedenen Arbeitsbedingungen. Pflügers Arch. **282**, 43–53 (1965).
9. *Kissling, G., T. Gassenmaier, M. F. Wendt-Gallitelli, R. Jacob:* Pressure-volume relations, elastic modulus, and contractile behaviour of the hypertrophied left ventricle of rats with Goldblatt II hypertension. Pflügers Arch. **369**, 213–221 (1977).
10. *Neely, J. R., K. M. Whitmer, S. Mochizuki:* Effects of mechanical activity and hormones on myocardial glucose and fatty acid utilization. Circulat. Res. **39**, Suppl. I 22–I 29 (1976).
11. *Sandler, H., H. T. Dodge:* Left ventricular tension and stress in man. Circulat. Res. **13**, 91–104 (1963).

Anschrift des Verfassers:

Dr. *G. Kissling,* Physiol. Institut II der Universität Tübingen, Gmelinstraße 5, 7400 Tübingen

Basic Res. Cardiol. **75**, 193–198 (1980)
© 1980 Dr. Dietrich Steinkopff Verlag, Darmstadt
ISSN 0300-8428

Paper, presented at the Erwin Riesch Symposium, Tübingen, April 3–7, 1979

*I.N.S.E.R.M. U2, Unité de Recherches de Pathologie Cardiovasculaire, Hôpital
Léon Bernard, 94450 Limeil-Brévannes*

Intracellular oxygen utilization in mechanically overloaded rat heart*)

Intrazelluläre Sauerstoff-Utilisation beim mechanisch überbelasteten Rattenherzen

J. Moravec

With 3 figures and 1 table

Summary

Bilateral hypertrophy of the heart was induced in rats by aorto-caval fistula. One
month after surgery, when the heart weight increased by about 60%, the hearts were
excised and perfused according to *Langendorff* with bicarbonate buffer containing
2.0 mM pyruvate (pH 7.4, 37 °C, 75 Torr). Steady-state reduction degree of respiratory components as well as the state of myoglobin O_2-saturation were monitored
throughout the experiment in the visible range by means of a rapid scanning
spectrophotometer. Double wavelength recordings of cytochrome aa_3 and myoglobin absorption changes were done during a short period of anoxia (N_2-equilibrated
solution) followed by reoxygenation of the preparation (O_2-equilibrated medium).
The time course of cytochrome aa_3 reoxidation was analysed with respect to
intracellular pO_2 changes as reflected by myoglobin saturation. The results of the
above experiments suggest that cytochrome aa_3 of overloaded hearts can be kept
fully oxidized at lower intracellular pO_2 (70 percent of Mb oxygenation) than in
control hearts (90 percent of Mb oxygenation). A prospective mechanism of the
observed phenomena as well as its impact on energy production of mechanically
overloaded myocardium are briefly discussed.

Recent advances in optical methods permitting an *in situ* monitoring of
mitochondrial function and tissue oxygenation (*Chance,* 1971; *Lübbers,*
1959) have allowed study of the state of energy production of intact organs
under a number of experimental conditions (*Chance,* 1978; *Rosenthal,*
1977; *Moravec,* 1978; *Jöbsis,* 1967; *Lübbers,* 1975). As concerns chronical
mechanical overloading of the myocardium, we still do not have enough
information about prospective alterations of mitochondrial energy production. Since in the heart muscle the latter is essentially aerobic, it
seemed to us to be worthy of interest to define conditions of oxygen
utilization by the mitochondria of normal and overloaded myocardium. In
the experiments described below, absorption changes related to myoglobin and cytochrome aa_3 were recorded simultaneously on the surface of
the left ventricle from rats with one-month lasting aorto-caval fistula and
the results compared with those obtained on hearts from control animals.

---

*) Supported by D.G.R.S.T. Contrat n° 74.7.0790.

Material and methods

Adult female Wistar rats were used throughout this study. The aorto-caval fistula was done under nembutal anesthesia (30 mg/kg) according to the technique introduced by *Hatt* et al. (this volume). The animals were sacrificed one month after the surgery and their hearts used for in vitro perfusion with Krebs-Henseleit bicarbonate buffer containing 2 mM pyruvate (37 °C, 100 cm H_2O, Langendorf preparation). The hearts were preperfused for 15 min with O_2-equilibrated solution ($pO_2 \simeq 600$ Torr) and then subjected to several short periods of anoxia ($pO_2 \simeq 60$ Torr) followed by reoxygenation. The hearts were allowed to recover completely between the two

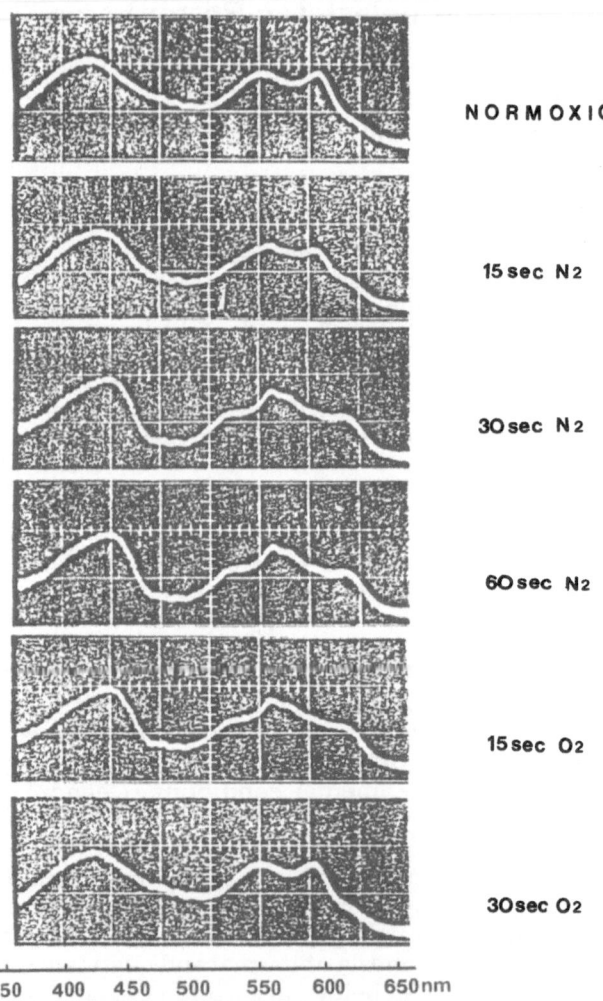

Fig. 1. Sequence of absorption spectra recorded during an anoxic cycle on the surface of the left ventricle of control heart. Note Mb deoxygenation at 540, at 580 nm and cytochrome aa$_3$ (606), cyt b (564) and cyt c (550) reduction. After the reoxygenation of the heart the initial redox conditions are reached in approximately 30 s. Calibration of the vertical axis: 0.250 OD/division.

anoxic cycles (H R, reoxidation of the component under study). Absorption changes related to myoglobin O_2 saturation and cytochrome aa_3 reduction degree were recorded by means of reflectance spectroscopy (*Chance*, 1971; *Lübbers*, 1959; *Jöbsis*, 1977). The rapid scanning spectroscope of Howaldtswerke Deutsche Werft AG, equipped with a double wavelength unit developed by *Brauser*, was used throughout this study (*Moravec*, 1978). More detailed description of the employed technique can be found in a preceding paper (*Moravec*, 1978).

Results and discussion

One month after the surgery, there was an 80% increase of the heart weight in most of the animals, most of this increment of the heart weight being related to cell hypertrophy (cf., *Hatt* et al.). Short anoxia led to both significant reduction of cytochrome aa_3 (cyt aa_3) and deoxygenation of myoglobin (Mb). During reoxygenation of the heart initial conditions were

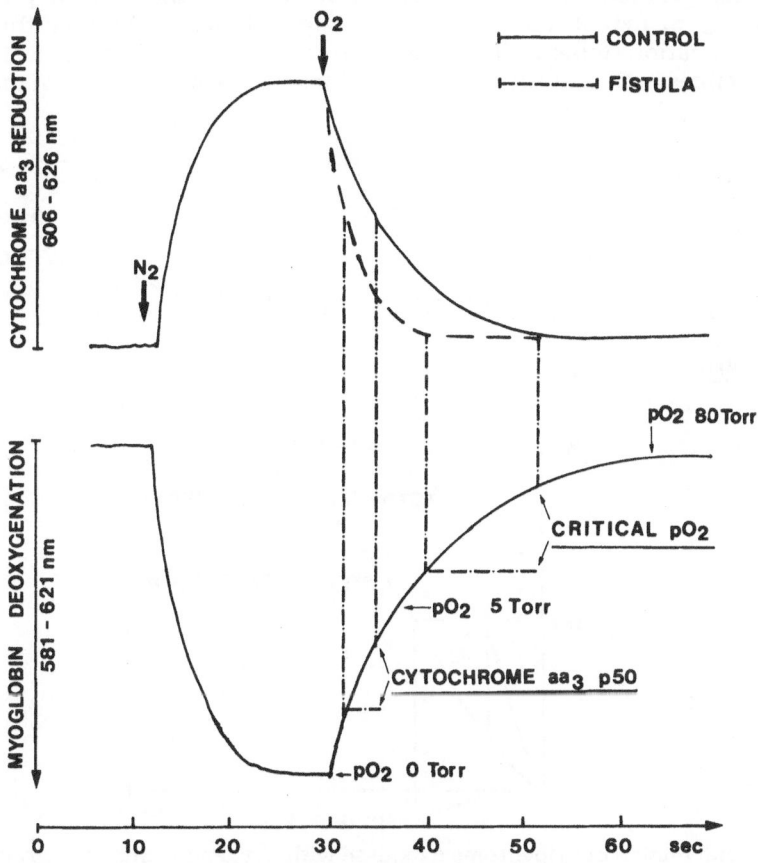

Fig. 2. Schematic representation of Mb and cyt aa_3 absorption changes during an anoxic transient. Note shortening of cyt aa_3 reoxidation in heart from the animal with aorto-caval fistula. No significant modification of time course of Mb reoxygenation could be detected. Cytochrome aa_3 p50 and the critical pO_2 seems to be shifted in overloaded heart.

Table 1. Effect of volume overload (1 month fistula) on cytochrome aa$_3$ and myoglobin recoveries from short anoxia.

	Cytochrome aa$_3$ (606–620 nm)		Myoglobin (581–621 nm)	
	dO.D. (dO.D.$_{N2}$–dO.D.$_{O2}$)	T (sec)	dO.D. (dO.D.$_{O2}$–dO.D.$_{N2}$)	T (sec)
Controls (n = 10)	0.070±0.010	21.75 ±2.02	0.910 ±0.020	41.66±5.40
1 Month ACF (n = 10)	0.065±0.010	13.20**±2.50	0.120*±0.010	41.25±8.20

* = p < 0.05, ** = p < 0.01

rapidly reestablished (fig. 1). Detailed analysis of a series of double
wavelength recordings have shown, however, that the speed of postanoxic
recovery of cytochrome aa$_3$ redox state is twice as high as that of Mb
reoxygenation (table 1). This observation seems to reflect the well-known
differences in O$_2$-saturation curves of these two compounds (*Chance* 1977).

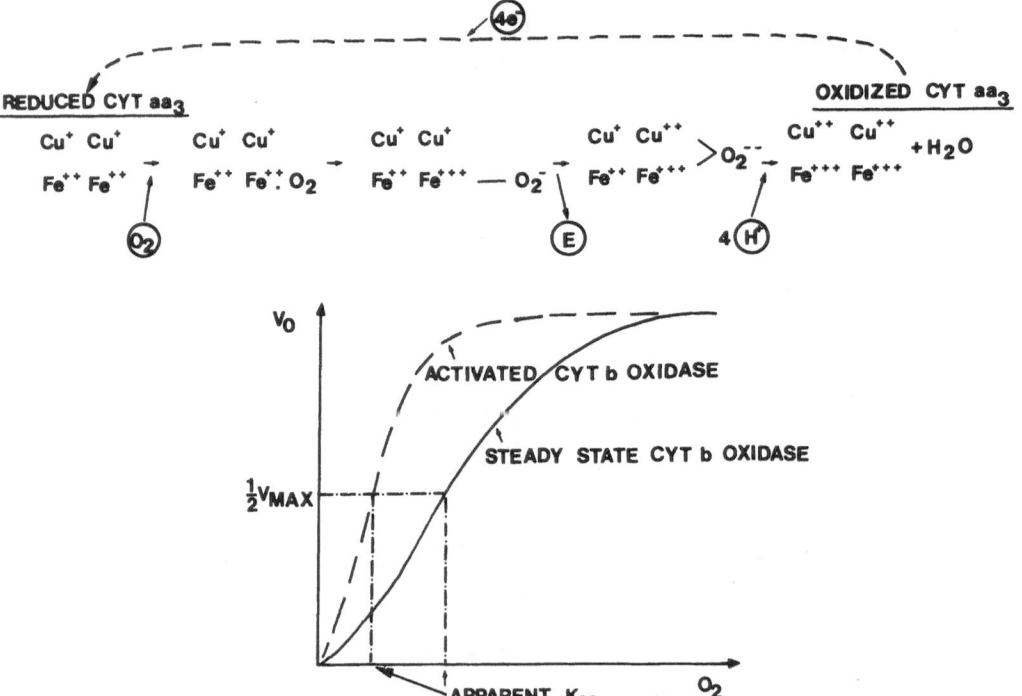

Fig. 3. Interaction of cytochrome c oxidase with oxygen (from *Antonini* et al.). Note
regulatory nature of cytochrome aa$_3$, resulting from the cooperation between Fe
and Cu subunits. At least four regulatory factors can be imagined: oxygen per se,
energy drain at coupling site III, local pH and substrate (reduced cyt c) availability.
The lower part of the figure shows that increased affinity for oxygen may result
from the activation of cytochrome c oxidase.

In volume overloaded hearts, we found an interesting modification of cyt aa_3 reoxidation: full oxidation of the respiratory chain was regularly obtained at considerably lower intracellular pO_2 extrapolated from simultaneously recorded Mb-O_2 saturation (fig. 2). This modification of "critical pO_2" was further suggested by a shortening of the time necessary for cytochrome aa_3 reoxidation during the period of reoxygenation of the preparation (table 1), while the time necessary for myoglobin reoxygenation was not changed. The above data might suggest that during the development of heart hypertrophy the affinity of cytochrome oxidase for dissolved oxygen has increased, which should be considered as an adaptive mechanism permitting the overloaded heart to maintain maximal respiratory rate even under conditions of decreased oxygenation. Among the factors capable of explaining the acceleration of cyt aa_3 reoxidation encountered in volume-overloaded rat hearts, the following ones seem most plausible: (1) existence of respiratory chain inhibition, (2) increased energy drain, (3) decreased apparent K_M (oxygen) of cytochrome oxidase (fig. 3). The work actually in progress in this laboratory should help to understand better the above-described phenomenon.

Zusammenfassung

Bei Ratten wurde eine beidseitige Hypertrophie des Herzens durch aortokavale Fistelbildung erzeugt. Einen Monat nach dem operativen Eingriff – nach einem Anstieg des Herzgewichts um etwa 60% – wurden die Herzen entnommen und nach *Langendorff* mit einer 2-mM-Pyruvat-Lösung (pH 7,4, 37 °C, 75 Torr, Zusatz eines Bikarbonatpuffers) durchströmt. Das Ausmaß der Abnahme der respiratorischen Komponenten und der Grad der Sauerstoffsättigung von Myoglobin wurden über die Gesamtdauer des Experiments mittels eines schnell registrierenden Spektrophotometers aufgezeichnet. Während einer kurzen Periode der Anoxie (N_2-equilibrierte Lösung) mit nachfolgender Reoxigenierung des Präparates wurden 2-Wellenlängen-Messungen von Cytochrom aa_3 und Absorptionsmessungen von Myoglobin durchgeführt. Der Zeitverlauf der Reoxigenierung von Cytochrom aa_3 wurde im Hinblick auf intrazelluläre Änderungen des pO_2 analysiert. Die Ergebnisse dieser Experimente lassen vermuten, daß das Cytochrom aa_3 des überbelasteten Herzens bei geringerem intrazellulärem pO_2 (70% der Mb-Oxigenierung) als bei Kontrollherzen (90% der Mb-Oxigenierung) voll oxidiert gehalten werden kann. Der vermutliche Mechanismus der beobachteten Phänomene und ihre Bedeutung für die Energieproduktion des mechanisch überbelasteten Herzens werden kurz diskutiert.

References

1. *Antonini, E., M. Brunori, A. Colosimo, C. Greenwood, M. T. Wilson:* Oxygen "pulsed" cytochrome oxidase: functional properties and catalytic relevance. Proc. Natl. Acad. Sci. (USA) **74**, 3128–3132 (1977).
2. *Chance, B., N. Graham:* A rapid scanning spectrophotometer. Rev. Sci. Instr. **42**, 941–958 (1971).
3. *Chance, B., J. B. Leigh:* Oxygen intermediates and mixed valence states of cytochrome oxidase. Proc. Natl. Acad. Sci. (USA) **74**, 4777–4780 (1977).
4. *Chance, B., C. Barlow, Y. Nakase, H. Takema, A. Meyevsky, R. Fischetti, N. Graham, J. Sorge:* Heterogeneity of oxygen delivery in normoxic and hypoxic states. Amer. J. Physiol. **4**, 809–820 (1978).

5. *Hatt, P. Y., K. Rakusan, P. Gastineau, M. Laplace, J. Moravec:* Aorto-caval fistula in the rat. An experimental model of heart volume overload. In press.
6. *Jöbsis, F. F., J. C. Duffield:* Oxidative and glycolytic recovery metabolism in muscle. J. Gen. Physiol. **50**, 1009–1029 (1967).
7. *Jöbsis, F. F., J. H. Keizer, J. C. Lamanna, M. Rosenthal:* Reflectance spectroscopy of cytochroma aa_3 in vivo. J. Appl. Physiol. **43**, 858–872 (1977).
8. *Lübbers, R. W., W. Niessel:* Rapid scanning spectrophotometer for rabbit heart perfused in vitro. Pflüg. Arch. Physiol. **268**, 281–295 (1959).
9. *Moravec, J., A. Corsin, P. Y. Hatt:* Dependence of myocardial redox systems on the concentration of exogenous substrate. In: Recent Advances in Studies on Cardiac Structure and Metabolism, vol. 10, *Roy, P. E., P. Harris* (Ed.) pp. 167–177 (Baltimore 1976).
10. *Moravec, J., G. Renault, P. Y. Hatt:* Alternations of mitochondrial function as detected in left ventricular myocardium of rats with acute aortic constriction. Basic. Res. Cardiol. **73**, 535–550 (1978).
11. *Petersen, L. C.:* On the mechanism of the cytochrome c oxidase reaction. Eur. J. Bioch. **85**, 339–344 (1978).
12. *Wodick, R., D. W. Lübbers:* Quantitative Analyse von Reflexionsspektren und anderen Spektren mit inhomogenen Lichtwegen an Mehrkomponentensystemen. Hoppe Seyler's Z. Physiol. Chem. **354**, 903–915 (1973).

Author's address:

Dr. *J. Moravec,* I.N.S.E.R.M. U2, Unité de Recherches de Pathologie cardiovasculaire, Hôpital Léon Bernard, 94450 Limeil-Brévannes (France)

Basic Res. Cardiol. **75,** 199–206 (1980)
© 1980 Dr. Dietrich Steinkopff Verlag, Darmstadt
ISSN 0300–8428

Paper, presented at the Erwin Riesch Symposium, Tübingen, April 3–7, 1979

*Abteilung für Experimentelle Chirurgie (Komm. Leiter: Prof. Dr. U. Mittmann) der
Chirurgischen Universitätsklinik Heidelberg und Kinderchirurgische Klinik der
Medizinischen Fakultät Mannheim der Universität Heidelberg
(Direktor: Prof. Dr. I. Joppich)*

Myocardial flow reserve in experimental cardiac hypertrophy*)

Die myokardiale Durchblutungsreserve bei experimenteller Herzhypertrophie

*U. Mittmann, U. B. Brückner, H. E. Keller, U. Kohler,
H. Vetter,* and *K.-L. Waag*

With 4 figures

Summary

The distribution of myocardial blood flow (MBF) was evaluated in pressure-induced LV hypertrophy of foxhounds. At the early stage of developing hypertrophy, i.e., 3 months after aortic banding (+ 53% LV weight) resting MBF and flow reserve were not significantly different from control hearts. One year after banding (+ 94% LV weight) myocardial flow reserve had clearly decreased.

Acute coronary stenosis of 60 and 70% cross-sectional area resulted in a moderate fall of flow reserve in controls and hearts with early hypertrophy. In hearts with extensive hypertrophy the drop of poststenotic MBF was considerably greater affecting preferentially the subendocardium.

The data suggest that myocardial blood flow was impaired before any signs of heart failure were observed. Furthermore a decrease of MBF may not be confined to forms of hypertrophy induced by renal and idiopathic hypertension.

Hypertrophic heart diseases may be associated with a decreased coronary blood flow (9). It is, however, not known whether the decrease of flow is confined to the late stages of hypertrophy. The term "progressive cardiosclerosis" used by *F. Z. Meerson* (7) may lead to the assumption that the decrease of myocardial blood flow (MBF) was merely a consequence of myocardial fibrosis stimulated by similar biochemical pathways which induce the hypertrophic growth of myocardial fibers. At least in patients with idiopathic hypertension, MBF appears to be impaired at an earlier stage of compensatory hypertrophy (10), the reason being either structural changes at the site of the small coronary arteries and arterioles ("coronary factor", 5) or a primary "myocardial factor" increasing coronary flow resistance or altering coronary autoregulation. ─

---

*) Supported by Deutsche Forschungsgemeinschaft, SFB 90, Heidelberg

So far, little is known about whether a coronary and/or myocardial factor may lead to an impaired myocardial perfusion in other forms of pressure-induced cardiac hypertrophy, e.g., aortic valvular stenosis, coarctation or massive aortic sclerosis without major coronary artery disease.

If myocardial hypertrophy (MH) per se were always associated with a decrease of MBF, any additional coronary stenosis would be likely to increase the risk of myocardial ischemia even though the coronary lesions were of minor extent.

Therefore the distribution of MBF was measured 3 months and 1 year after experimental induction of left ventricular hypertrophy in the dog. Additional moderate coronary stenosis was acutely induced in order to evaluate the potential risk of regional ischemia.

Methods

Myocardial hypertrophy was induced in 22 foxhounds by banding the ascending aorta immediately proximal to the brachiocephalic artery at the age of 4–10 weeks. The initial pressure gradient was 5–15 mm Hg.

In addition to a *control group* of 7 foxhounds (age 4–6 months) 13 dogs were restudied at an early stage of developing hypertrophy *(group I, "3 months MH")*. A second group of 4 dogs was studied 1 year after the banding procedure *(group II, "1 year MH")*.

All animals were premedicated with .6 mg/kg morphine sulphate and .15 mg/kg proprionyl-phenothiazine[1]). After induction of anesthesia (15 mg/kg pentobarbital) the animals were artificially ventilated with an N_2O/O_2 mixture (3:1). Light anesthesia was maintained by additional small doses of pentobarbital (3 mg/kg · hr). The thorax was opened in order to evaluate left ventricular (LV) function and O_2-consumption. These results will be reported elsewhere.

MBF was measured with the tracer microsphere method (8, 11). 5 different radioisotopes (J–125, Ce–141, Cr–51, Sr–85, Sc–46) were injected sequentially into the left atrium in the following experimental situations:

Estimation of
1. control (resting) blood flow
2. cardiac contractile reserve, infusion of 1 µg/kg · min norepinephrine
3. maximal coronary dilatation ("coronary flow reserve"), infusion of .4 mg/kg dipyridamole in 3 min
4. 60% stenosis of the left ant. desc. cor. artery (LAD) under maximal coronary dilatation
5. 70% LAD-stenosis under maximal coronary dilatation

Standardized coronary constriction was performed using a micrometer-type coronary constrictor described earlier in detail (3). LAD-flow changes were assessed with an electromagnetic flowprobe positioned immediately proximal to the constrictor. A fall of mean coronary perfusion pressure which normally occurs after injection of dipyridamole was prevented by means of a micrometer-type aortic constrictor.

At the end of the experiments the LAD was occluded and lissamine was injected i.a. distal to the point of occlusion in order to stain exclusively the myocardium supplied by the LAD. Afterwards the heart was excised and sectioned. Each specimen was subdivided into a subepicardial, midwall, and subendocardial sample. Blood flow in each sample was calculated as described earlier by *Wirth* et al. (11).

---

[1]) Combelen®

Results

Extent of hypertrophy

Based on the ratio of LV-weight (g)/body weight (kg) of 3.63 in the controls LV-weight had increased by 53% in group I (3 months MH). Mean aortic pressure gradient was 31 mm Hg.

In dogs of group II (1 year MH) LV-weight had increased by 94%. The aortic pressure gradient was 65 mm Hg.

5 dogs starting out with a slightly greater initial aortic pressure gradient at the time of the banding operation (10–15 mm Hg) died 111 ± 27 days later of LV failure. Their increase of LV weight amounted to 100%. However, none of the dogs included in the following data showed any "clinical" signs of cardiac failure, i.e. cardiac output < 75 ml/kg · min, LV enddiastolic pressure > 15 mm Hg, pleural effusion or ascites.

Myocardial blood flow, poststenotic area of the LV-free wall

Under resting conditions there was no major difference between mean MBF of control dogs or animals with MH. However, subendocardial flow of group II was 35 ml/100 g · min greater than in controls (fig. 1). No further statistical evaluation was attempted because of the small number of group II dogs studied (n = 4).

In the subepicardium (fig. 2) coronary flow reserve was nearly identical in controls and dogs with MH. Also the decrease of flow reserve after coronary stenosis of 60 and 70% was not different in all 3 groups.

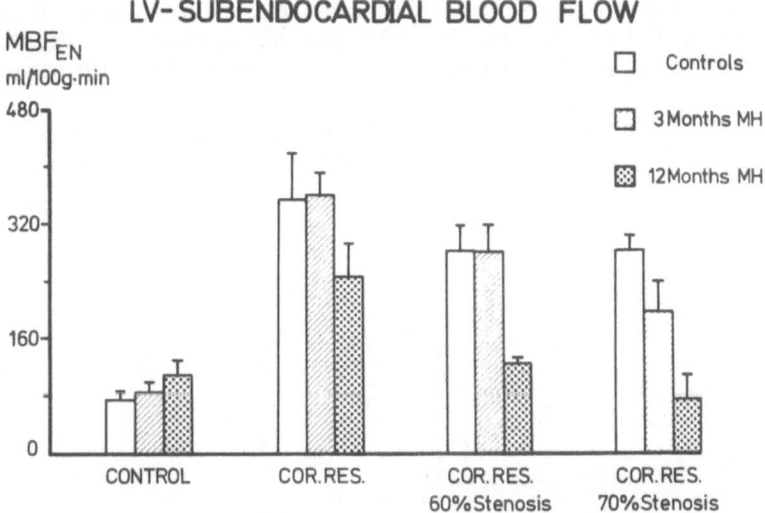

Fig. 1. Mean values (± SE) of subendocardial blood flow (MBF$_{EN}$) in the left ventricular free wall of control dogs and dogs with myocardial hypertrophy (MH). control = resting blood flow. cor. res. = coronary flow reserve, measured after i.v. injection of .4 mg/kg of dipyridamole. 60 and 70% acute stenosis of the left ant. desc. coronary artery. Note the substantial decline of subendocardial flow reserve in dogs with 12 months MH after induction of moderate coronary stenoses.

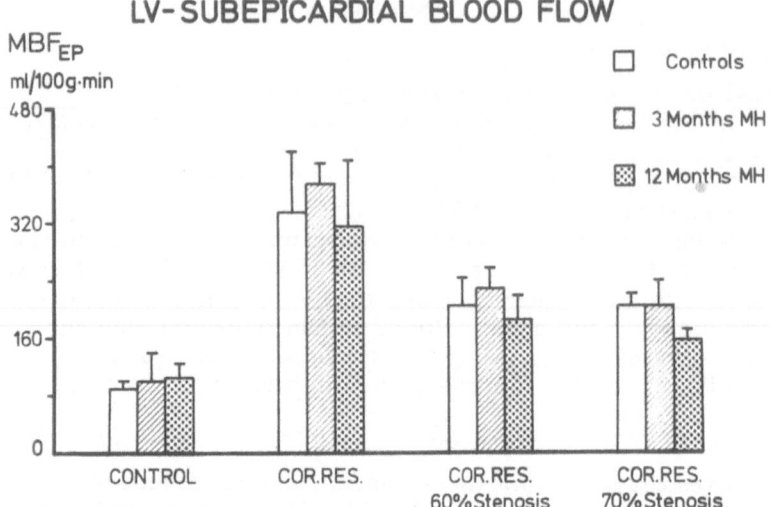

Fig. 2. Mean values (± SE) of subepicardial blood flow (MBF$_{EP}$) in the left ventricular free wall. For abbreviations see fig. 1. Subepicardial flow does not appear to be
significantly different when comparing control hearts and hearts with varying
degrees of myocardial hypertrophy (MH).

In contrast to the subepicardium flow reserve in the inner layers of the
heart (fig. 1) was clearly smaller in animals with a 1 year MH. Additional
60% LAD stenosis resulted in a further sharp decline of subendocardial
flow in group II hypertrophy. The 70% stenosis appears to indicate that
the decrease of subendocardial flow reserve is correlated with the extent

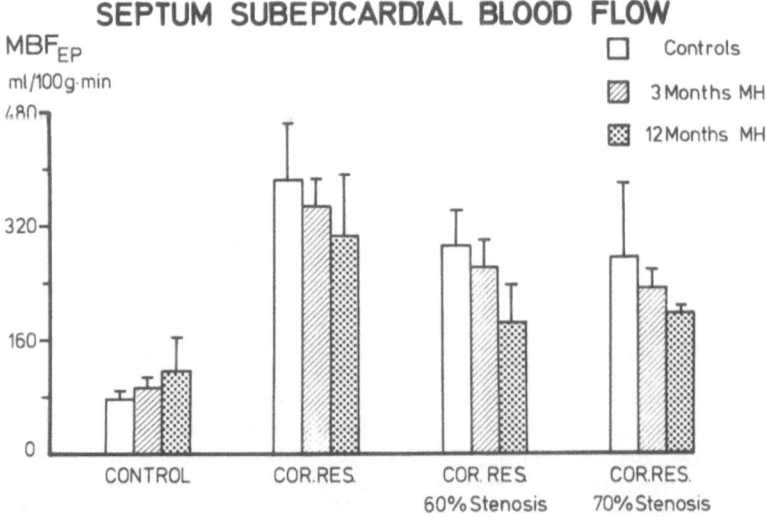

Fig. 3. Mean values (± SE) of myocardial blood flow in the part of the septum facing
the right ventricle ("subepicardial blood flow"). For abbreviations see fig. 1.

of MH. Subendocardial flow reserve decreased to 284 ± 20 ml/100 g · min in controls, to 195 ± 41 ml/100 g · min in group I dogs (p < .05 v.s. controls), and to 76 ± 33 ml/100 g · min in group II dogs.

After coronary dilatation and 70% LAD-stenosis the ratio of subendocardial/subepicardial flow was 1.39 in controls, .94 in group I and .48 in group II.

Myocardial blood flow, poststenotic area of the septum

Flow changes in the septum were comparable to those described in the LV free wall. Again there was no major difference between resting myocardial flow of controls and dogs with MH although MBF appeared to be slightly greater in animals with severe MH (figs. 3 and 4).

In the subepicardium (fig. 3) flow reserve of the hypertrophied hearts was slightly smaller than in controls. Additional moderate coronary stenosis, however, did not enlarge this difference.

As in the LV free wall, subendocardial flow reserve (fig. 4) of hearts with severe hypertrophy was clearly smaller than in controls and group I dogs. Moreover, the decrease of subendocardial flow reserve with 60 and 70% coronary stenosis was distinctly greater in MH group II as compared to controls and MH group I dogs.

MBF during infusion of catecholamines

1 μg/kg · min of norepinephrine was infused in 5 controls and 3 dogs of MH group II. The rise of subepicardial flow was practically identical in controls (212 ± 28 ml/100 g · min) and group II dogs (204 ± 30 ml/100 g ·

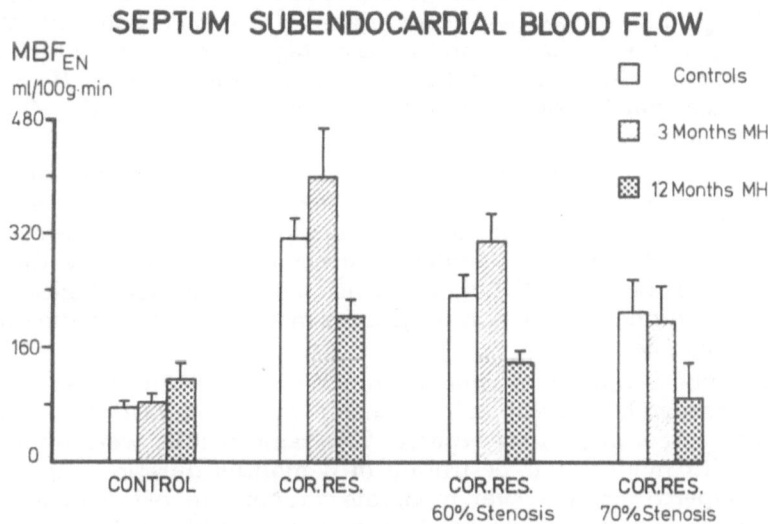

Fig. 4. Mean values (± SE) of subendocardial blood flow (MBF$_{EN}$) in the septum. For abbreviations see fig. 1. Subendocardial flow reserve is clearly smaller in dogs with 12 months myocardial hypertrophy (MH), particularly after induction of acute moderate coronary stenoses.

min). In contrast to the subepicardium flow to the inner layers of the heart increased to 252 ± 11 in controls and only to 177 ± 8 ml/100 g · min in group II animals.

Discussion

Evaluation of cardiac function and MBF in hypertrophied hearts is complicated by the fact that different experimental models used to induce an increase of cardiac wall thickness are likely to produce results which are difficult to compare. Experimental MH induced by renal hypertension appears to result in an underperfusion of the subendocardium (6). However, renal hypertension and essential hypertension can presumably result in primary structural changes of the coronary arteries (4, 5).

At the moment we cannot exclude that an altered renal function, e.g. a stimulation of the renin-angiotensin mechanism, may have played an additional role in our model of LV hypertrophy. Nevertheless, we will restrict the comparison of flow data to the results obtained in the same model of proximal aortic constriction. *Baird* et al. (1) observed a slight increase of resting MBF 280 days after proximal aortic constriction in dogs. Also *Holtz* et al. (2) reported a small and statistically not significant increase of resting flow 1 year after aortic banding in the dog.

As resting blood flow depends essentially upon the O_2 requirements at the time when the measurements are performed, the results will be particularly sensitive to the momentary contractile state of the heart, anesthesia etc. Therefore flow reserve is more likely to yield conclusive results as long as coronary perfusion pressures are comparable. *Holtz* et al. (2) described a significant decrease of flow reserve when the coronary arteries were maximally dilated with dipyridamole. Our own data indicate that flow reserve was unchanged in the early stages of developing MH. It was, however, clearly decreased in the 1 year hypertrophy group. It should be emphasized that the decrease of flow reserve was confined to the inner layers of the heart.

The fact that subendocardial flow increase after ventricular loading with norepinephrine was smaller than in controls supports the concept of a decreased flow reserve of the subendocardial muscle of severely hypertrophied hearts observed under pharmacological coronary dilatation. Apparently subendocardial underperfusion is no pharmacological artifact as long as coronary perfusion pressure is maintained during the injection of dipyridamole.

Induction of moderate coronary stenoses of 60 and 70% (cross-sectional area) in normal hearts results in no change of resting MBF (11) and a mild decrease of coronary flow reserve. The same results were obtained in hearts with moderate hypertrophy of 3 months duration (fig. 1–4). In severe hypertrophy, however, moderate coronary stenosis of no more than 60% results in a sharp decline of subendocardial blood flow to very low values. A sufficient compensatory increase of myocardial O_2 extraction would have been unlikely if maximal coronary dilatation had been stimulated by an actual increase of O_2 requirement instead of pharmacological coronary dilatation.

In summary, severe pressure-induced myocardial hypertrophy reduces coronary flow reserve before major signs of heart failure are observed. Additional moderate coronary stenosis results in a sharp decline of MBF jeopardizing preferentially the subendocardium, which presumably has the greatest O_2 requirement because of its larger wall tension.

A variety of factors may be responsible for the observed flow changes:
1. structural changes of the coronary vasculature,
2. decrease of myocardial contraction and particularly relaxation,
3. regional myocardial fibrosis,
4. metabolically induced derangement of coronary autoregulation.

Further experimental studies are being performed in order to evaluate the causes and the possible significance of the observed changes of MBF.

Zusammenfassung

Bei experimenteller LV-Druckhypertrophie (MH) wurde die myokardiale Durchblutungsverteilung gemessen. Im Frühstadium der MH, d. h. 3 Monate nach Stenosierung der Aorta asc. (LV-Gewicht + 53%), waren Ruhedurchblutung und Durchblutungsreserve nicht signifikant gegenüber einem Kontrollkollektiv verändert. Ein Jahr nach dem Eingriff (LV-Gewicht + 94%) war die Durchblutungsreserve jedoch erheblich eingeschränkt.

Akute Koronarstenosierung von 60 und 70% des Gefäßquerschnitts führte zu einer mäßigen Verminderung der Durchblutungsreserve der Kontrollherzen und der Herzen im Frühstadium der MH. Bei ausgeprägter MH dagegen war die poststenotische Durchblutungsreserve beträchtlich eingeschränkt, wobei die Herzinnenschichten besonders betroffen waren.

Offenbar ist die Myokarddurchblutung beeinträchtigt, bevor es zur manifesten Herzinsuffizienz kommt. Ferner ist zu vermuten, daß die Myokarddurchblutung nicht nur bei den Formen der MH vermindert ist, die durch renale oder essentielle Hypertonie zustande kommen.

References

1. *Baird, R. J., F. Dutka, M. Okumori, A. de la Rocha, M. M. Goldbach, T. J. Hill, D. C. MacGregor:* Surgical aspects of regional myocardial blood flow and myocardial pressure. J. Thorac. Cardiovasc. Surg. **69**, 17–29 (1975).
2. *Holtz, J., E. Bassenge, P. Bard, W. v. Restorff:* Regional myocardial blood flow at rest and during exercise in left ventricular hypertrophy. Pflügers Arch. Suppl. **359**, 18 (1975).
3. *Dietze, W., U. Mittmann, J. Schmier, R. H. Wirth:* Einfluß von Koronarstenose und Aortendruck auf Koronarfluß, Koronardruck und reaktive Hyperämie. Basic. Res. Cardiol. **71**, 309–318 (1976).
4. *James, Th.:* Small arteries of the heart. Circulation **56**, 2 (1977).
5. *Kathe, N.:* Die Veränderungen der Koronararterienzweige des Myocards bei Hypertonie. Beitr. path. Anat. **115**, 405 (1955).
6. *Kober, G.:* Regionale MBF im normalen und chronisch druckbelasteten linken Ventrikel. Z. Kreislaufforschg. **60**, 471 (1971).
7. *Meerson, F. Z.:* The Myocardium in hyperfunction, hypertrophy and heart failure. Circulat. Res. **24** and **25**, Suppl. II, 1–163 (1969).
8. *Rudolph, A. M., M. S. Heymann:* The circulation of the fetus in utero. Circulat. Res. **21**, 163–184 (1967).

9. *Strauer, B. E., M. Tauchert, H. W. Heis, K. Kochsiek, H. J. Bretschneider:* On the relations between coronary blood flow oxygen consumption und cardiac work in patients with and without angina pectoris. Int. Symp. Pisa, Minerva Medica, 465 (1972).

10. *Strauer, B. E.:* Personal communication.

11. *Wirth, R. H., U. B. Brückner, H. E. Keller, U. Mittmann:* Effects of moderate coronary stenosis on myocardial flow reserve in man and in the dog. Basic Res. Cardiol. (in press).

Für die Verfasser:

Prof. Dr. *U. Mittmann,* Abt. für Experimentelle Chirurgie der Chirurgischen Universitätsklinik Heidelberg, Im Neuenheimer Feld 347, 6900 Heidelberg

Basic Res. Cardiol. **75**, 207–213 (1980)
© 1980 Dr. Dietrich Steinkopff Verlag, Darmstadt
ISSN 0300–8428

Paper, presented at the Erwin Riesch Symposium, Tübingen, April 3–7, 1979

Physiologisches Institut der Universität München

Significance of the hexose monophosphate shunt in experimentally induced cardiac hypertrophy*)

Bedeutung des Hexosemonophosphat-Shunts während der Entwicklung einer experimentell induzierten Herzhypertrophie

H.-G. Zimmer, H. Ibel, and *E. Gerlach*

Whit 3 figures and 1 table

Summary
1. In three models of cardiac hypertrophy in rats (aortic constriction, application of a single dose of isoproterenol and daily injections of triiodothyronine) the biosynthesis of myocardial adenine nucleotides was enhanced.
2. In hypertrophying hearts due to aortic constriction and isoproterenol application, the activity of glucose-6-phosphate dehydrogenase and the available pool of 5-phosphoribosyl-1-pyrophosphate were increased indicating a stimulation of the hexose monophosphate shunt. In triiodothyronine-treated animals only the cardiac pool of 5-phosphoribosyl-1-pyrophosphate turned out to be elevated.
3. In all three models of cardiac hypertrophy, the enhancement of myocardial adenine nucleotide biosynthesis was exaggerated by ribose. It thus appears that the 5-phosphoribosyl-1-pyrophosphate pool is the limiting factor for the increase of adenine nucleotide biosynthesis under these conditions.
4. Long-term i.v. infusion of ribose (200 mg/kg/h) in isoproterenol-treated rats prevented the decrease of the cardiac ATP concentration induced by isoproterenol. However, the isoproterenol-induced stimulation of total cardiac protein synthesis was not altered, suggesting that the ATP decline may not be the trigger for stimulating protein synthesis in this model of myocardial hypertrophy.

Previous studies revealed that the biosynthesis of myocardial adenine nucleotides (AN) is enhanced during development of experimentally induced cardiac hypertrophy (1, 2). As far as the mechanism responsible for this enhancement is concerned, the available pool of 5-phosphoribosyl-1-pyrophosphate (PRPP) has been recognized as one of the most important factors involved (3, 4). PRPP is supplied via ribose-5-phosphate by the hexose monophosphate shunt. Since the hexose monophosphate shunt appears to be limiting for PRPP production, and thus for the biosynthesis of adenine nucleotides in the heart (3, 4), it was of interest to study this shunt in hypertrophying hearts in relation to changes in AN biosynthesis.

*) Supported by the Deutsche Forschungsgemeinschaft (Zi 199/1)

Methods

Cardiac hypertrophy was induced in rats by aortic constriction, by application of a single dose of isoproterenol (25 mg/kg) and by daily injections of 3,3',5-triiodo-L-thyronine (0.2 mg/kg). To evaluate the hexose monophosphate shunt, three different kinds of experimental approach were utilized:

1. The activity of glucose-6-phosphate dehydrogenase (EC 1.1.1.49), the first and rate-limiting enzyme of the hexose monophosphate shunt (5) was measured (6).
2. The available pool of cardiac 5-phosphoribosyl-1-pyrophosphate (PRPP), one of the endproducts of the hexose monophosphate shunt, was determined. For this purpose ^{14}C-adenine was i.v. administered in rats. PRPP is used in the reaction by which adenine is directly converted into AMP. Since AMP is in rapid equilibrium with ADP and ATP, the resulting radioactivity of the myocardial AN is an indirect measure of the available PRPP pool (2, 3).
3. The effect of i.v. applied ribose on the PRPP pool and on the biosynthesis of AN was studied. As previous investigations have shown, ribose bypasses the hexose monophosphate shunt in the heart and is rapidly converted via ribose-5-phosphate into PRPP (3). Rates of AN biosynthesis were calculated from the total radioactivity of myocardial AN due to the incorporation of i.v. injected 1–^{14}C-glycine and the mean specific activity of the precursor glycine (7). The concentrations of myocardial AN were determined according to the methods described by *Gerlach* et al. (8). Protein synthesis was assessed by measuring the incorporation of 1–^{14}C-glycine into total cardiac proteins (9).

Results

As is shown in figure 1, glucose-6-phosphate dehydrogenase activity was slightly elevated in hearts on the first day after aortic constriction, markedly enhanced on the second day and reached a maximum on the

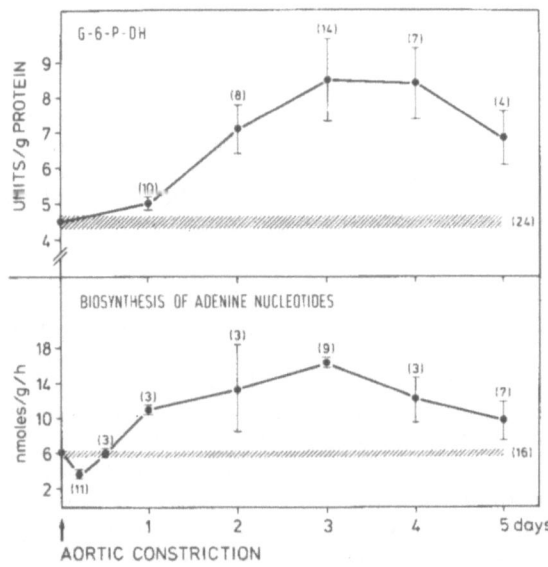

Fig. 1. Effect of aortic constriction on the activity of myocardial glucose-6-phosphate dehydrogenase (G-6-P-DH) and on the biosynthesis of cardiac adenine nucleotides. Mean values ± SEM, number of experiments in parentheses.

third day. Except for the initial decline, the changes in AN biosynthesis were almost parallel to those in the glucose-6-phosphate dehydrogenase activity. After application of isoproterenol (fig. 2), glucose-6-phosphate dehydrogenase activity did not change within the first 5 hours. An increase was found after 12 hours and a maximum was observed on the second day, whereas AN biosynthesis was maximally stimulated already within the first 12 hours. The enhancement found thereafter was maintained on a lower level. After daily injections of triiodothyronine (fig. 3), there were no alterations of glucose-6-phosphate dehydrogenase activity throughout the entire period of time studied, although AN biosynthesis did increase in a manner comparable to that observed in the other two models of cardiac hypertrophy.

In view of the different response of cardiac glucose-6-phosphate dehydrogenase activity in the three kinds of myocardial hypertrophy, it seemed of interest to examine whether the available pool of PRPP may also be affected differently. This, however, turned out not to be case. ^{14}C-Adenine incorporation into AN was increased to about the same extent in all three models indicating that the PRPP pool was elevated independently of the procedure by which hypertrophy was induced.

To find out whether the PRPP pool, although elevated in all three types of cardiac hypertrophy, may be a limiting factor for the enhancement of AN biosynthesis, studies with ribose were performed. Ribose bypasses the hexose monophosphate shunt and leads to an elevation of the PRPP pool and to an enhancement of AN biosynthesis in normal hearts (3). Ribose did exaggerate the increase of AN biosynthesis in all three models examined.

Further studies were performed on isoproterenol-stimulated hearts, in which ribose induced a marked exaggeration of the enhanced rate of AN

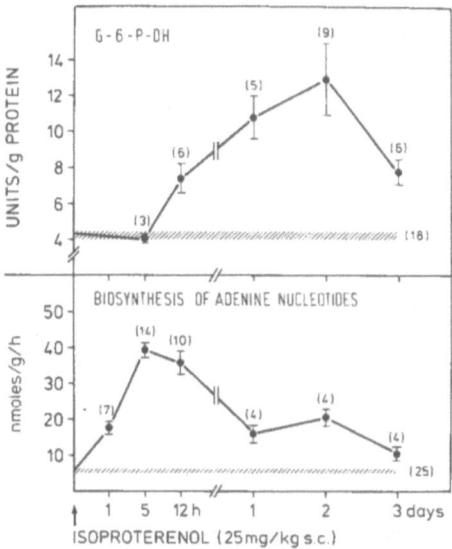

Fig. 2. Changes in glucose-6-phosphate dehydrogenase activity (G-6-P-DH) and in the biosynthesis of adenine nucleotides in rat hearts after a single injection of isoproterenol. Mean values ± SEM, number of experiments in parentheses.

biosynthesis (3). Since such an increased rate of AN biosynthesis could be expected to influence the well-known decrease of AN concentration (10), ribose was applied as constant i.v. infusion for 24 hours in unanesthetized, unrestrained rats (11), and the concentrations of AN were then deter-mined. As is evident from the data given in table 1, isoproterenol caused a decline of the cardiac ATP concentration. When ribose was constantly administerd, this decline did not occur. On the basis of this result, the hypothesis was tested according to which it is the ATP decline which may be the trigger for inducing the stimulation of cardiac protein synthesis occurring under these conditions (12). As can be seen from the data in table 1, cardiac protein synthesis was considerably increased 24 hours after application of isoproterenol. When ribose was i.v. infused for 24 hours, total cardiac protein synthesis turned out to be enhanced to about the same extent as after isoproterenol application alone despite the normalization of the ATP concentration.

Discussion

The three kinds of experimentally induced cardiac hypertrophy differ markedly with respect to the response of glucose-6-phosphate dehy-drogenase activity. It was found to be enhanced in parallel with the increase of AN biosynthesis after aortic constriction. After isoproterenol application, the increase of glucose-6-phosphate dehydrogenase activity appeared to correlate with the maintenance of the enhanced AN biosyn-thesis. In hypertrophying hearts due to daily administrations of triiodothyronine, however, glucose-6-phosphate dehydrogenase activity

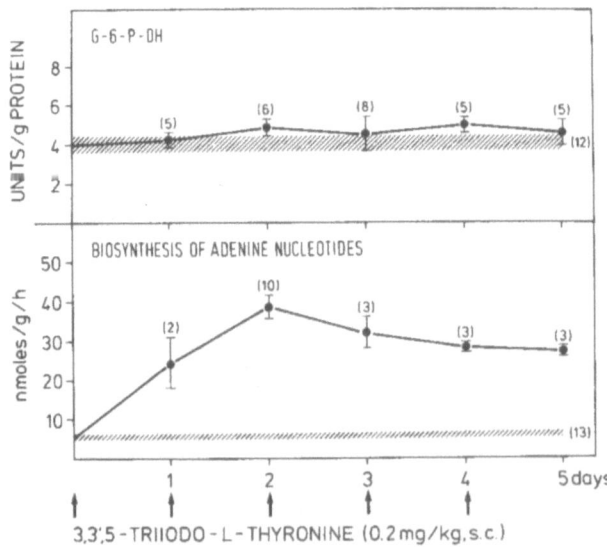

Fig. 3. Myocardial glucose-6-phosphate dehydrogenase activity (G-6-P-DH) and rates of adenine nucleotide biosynthesis in rat hearts under the influence of 3,3',5-triiodo-L-thyronine. Mean values ± SEM, number of experiments in parentheses.

was not altered at all. Despite these differences, the available pool of PRPP, one of the endproducts of the hexose monophosphate shunt, and the biosynthesis of AN were enhanced in all models of cardiac hypertrophy studied. It thus appears that the elevation of the myocardial PRPP pool is a major factor involved in the enhancement of AN biosynthesis which is common to all three models. However, different mechanisms may be involved in bringing about this elevation of the myocardial PRPP pool.

The essential role of the cardiac PRPP pool for the stimulation of AN biosynthesis is further supported by the results of our studies with ribose. Ribose induced a further increase of AN biosynthesis in hypertrophying hearts. Since ribose bypasses the hexose monophosphate shunt and leads to an elevation of the PRPP pool, these results suggest that the PRPP pool, although increased in all models, is a limiting factor for the enhancement of AN biosynthesis. At least in hypertrophying hearts due to aortic constriction and isoproterenol application, the available pool of PRPP seems to be limited by the hexose monophosphate shunt.

Another aspect of these studies concerns the possible trigger mechanism ascribed to the decrease in the ATP concentration in bringing about the stimulation of cardiac protein synthesis during development of hypertrophy (12). Constant i.v. infusion of ribose in isoproterenol-treated rats induced an increase in AN biosynthesis which was of such an extent (ca. 80 nmoles/g/h) that the concentrations of AN could be expected to be influenced. In fact, after 24 hours of continuous i.v. application of ribose, the well-known ATP decline induced by isoproterenol (4, 10) did not occur (table 1). Utilizing this experimental approach, the alleged trigger for stimulating cardiac protein synthesis (12) was removed. Thus, if the decrease of ATP would be an essential mechanism for the enhancement of protein synthesis, then the increase induced by isoproterenol should not occur anymore. However, despite the normal ATP concentration under the simultaneous treatment with isoproterenol and constant i.v. infusion of ribose, cardiac protein synthesis was increased to about the same extent as after isoproterenol application. These results, therefore, indicate that

Table 1. Concentrations of myocardial ATP and relative rates of total cardiac protein synthesis 24 hours after application of a single dose of isoproterenol (25 mg/kg) in rats which had received constant i.v. infusion of 0.9% NaCl and ribose (200 mg/kg/h), respectively. Mean values ± SEM, number of experiments in parentheses.

	ATP (μmoles/g)	Relative rates of protein synthesis expressed in per cent
Control	4.47 ± 0.08 (34)	100 ± 5.7 (4)
Isoproterenol + NaCl	3.17 ± 0.06 (9)	230 ± 16.9 (7)
Isoproterenol + Ribose	4.56 ± 0.29 (6)	226 ± 12.4 (9)

the decrease of the ATP concentration seems not to be the trigger for stimulating total cardiac protein synthesis at least in this model of experimentally induced cardiac hypertrophy.

Zusammenfassung

1. Die Biosynthese von myokardialen Adenin-Nukleotiden war während der Entwicklung einer experimentell induzierten Herzhypertrophie (Aortenkonstriktion, Applikation von Isoproterenol und tägliche Gaben von Trijodthyronin) gesteigert.
2. Die Aktivität der Glukose-6-phosphat-Dehydrogenase und die Verfügbarkeit von PRPP waren im Herzen nach Aortenkonstriktion und nach Isoproterenol-Gabe erhöht als Ausdruck einer Stimulation des Hexosemonophosphat-Shunts. Im Herzen von trijodthyroninbehandelten Ratten erwies sich nur der verfügbare PRPP-Pool als erhöht.
3. In allen drei Modellen der Herzhypertrophie wurde die Steigerung der Biosynthese von Adenin-Nukleotiden durch Ribose verstärkt. Dieser Befund läßt erkennen, daß die Verfügbarkeit von PRPP ein limitierender Faktor für die Steigerung der AN-Synthese im hypertrophierenden Herzen ist.
4. Durch Langzeit-Dauerinfusion von Ribose (200 mg/kg/h) wurde die isoproterenolinduzierte Verminderung der kardialen ATP-Konzentration verhindert. Dagegen blieb die isoproterenolbedingte Proteinsynthese-Steigerung unter diesen experimentellen Bedingungen unbeeinflußt. Der ATP-Abfall scheint demnach nicht der auslösende Mechanismus für die Stimulation der Protein-Synthese in diesem Modell der Herzhypertrophie zu sein.

References

1. *Zimmer, H.-G., C. Trendelenburg, E. Gerlach:* Acceleration of adenine nucleotide synthesis de novo during development of cardiac hypertrophy. J. Mol. Cell. Cardiol. **4**, 279–282 (1972).
2. *Zimmer, H.-G., E. Gerlach:* Changes of myocardial adenine nucleotide and protein synthesis during development of cardiac hypertrophy. Basic Res. Cardiol. **72**, 241–246 (1977).
3. *Zimmer, H.-G., E. Gerlach:* Stimulation of myocardial adenine nucleotide biosynthesis by pentoses and pentitols. Pflügers Arch. **376**, 223–227 (1978).
4. *Zimmer, H.-G., E. Gerlach:* Effect of beta adrenergic stimulation on myocardial adenine nucleotide metabolism. Circulat. Res. **35**, 536–543 (1974).
5. *Eggleston, L. V., H. A. Krebs:* Regulation of the pentose phosphate cycle. Biochem. J. **138**, 425–435 (1974).
6. *Glock, G. E., P. McLean:* Levels of enzymes of the direct oxidative pathway of carbohydrate metabolism in mammalian tissues and tumors. Biochem. J. **56**, 171–175 (1954).
7. *Zimmer, H.-G., C. Trendelenburg, H. Kammermeier, E. Gerlach:* De novo synthesis of myocardial adenine nucleotides in the rat: Acceleration during recovery from oxygen deficiency. Circulat. Res. **32**, 635–642 (1973).
8. *Gerlach, E., B. Deuticke, R. H. Dreisbach:* Zum Verhalten von Nucleotiden und ihren dephosphorylierten Abbauprodukten in der Niere bei Ischämie und kurzzeitiger Wiederdurchblutung. Pflügers Arch. **278**, 296–315 (1963).
9. *Zimmer, H.-G., G. Steinkopff, E. Gerlach:* Changes of protein synthesis in the hypertrophying rat heart. Pflügers Arch. **336**, 311–325 (1972).
10. *Fleckenstein, A.:* Specific inhibitors and promoters of Ca^{++} action. pp. 135–188. In: *Harris, P.* and *Opie, L.:* Calcium and the heart. Academic Press New York (1971).

11. *Zimmer, H.-G., H. Ibel:* Effects of isoproterenol and dopamine on the myocardial hexose monophosphate shunt. Experientia **35**, 510–511 (1979).
12. *Meerson, F. Z., V. D. Pomoinitsky:* The role of high-energy phosphate compounds in the development of cardiac hypertrophy. J. Mol. Cell. Cardiol. **4**, 571–597 (1972).

Authors' address:

Physiologisches Institut der Universität München, Pettenkoferstr. 12, 8000 München 2 (Germany)

Basic Res. Cardiol. **75,** 214–220 (1980)
© 1980 Dr. Dietrich Steinkopff Verlag, Darmstadt
ISSN 0300–8428

Paper, presented at the Erwin Riesch Symposium, Tübingen, April 3–7, 1979

Physiologisches Institut II, Universität Tübingen

The behavior of some enzymes of the hypertrophied and postnatally developing myocardium of the rat*)

Das Verhalten einiger Enzyme im Rattenmyokard bei Hypertrophie und während der postnatalen Entwicklung

U. Koehler and *I. Medugorac*

With 3 figures

Summary

The present study was undertaken in order to investigate the behavior of lactate dehydrogenase (LDH) and hexokinase (HK) in the mechanically overloaded and the postnatally developing left ventricle of the rat.

In Goldblatt rats (GBR) 2 to 4 months after operation total LDH activity was decreased by 7%, accompanied by an isoenzyme shift towards a higher M proportion. Swimming rats (SR) showed an 11% increase in LDH activity. HK activity was increased by 14% in GBR and unaltered in SR.

Histochemical investigations revealed no indication of heterogeneous alterations in various areas of the myocardium.

During postnatal development, a gradual increase of activity and H subunit proportion of LDH were observed. HK activity was increased after one week, but underwent a slow decrease thereafter. These changes are interpreted as processes of adaptation to the conditions of extrauterine life.

Enhanced mechanical load of striated muscle can lead to alterations of mechanical, morphological and biochemical parameters depending on the type, intensity and duration of the stress. The adaptation of cardiac muscle to mechanical overload leads to a more or less pronounced hypertrophy, the parameters of which vary with the character of the stimulus. Recent studies from our institute (1, 2, 3) reported on mechanical, morphological and biochemical alterations in heart muscle in the compensatory stage of hypertrophy induced by swimming-training and pressure overload.

Thus the intention of the present study was to complete this picture by investigating the behavior of some determinants of the left ventricular biochemistry of swimming rats and Goldblatt rats. Additionally, we wanted to be able to compare the compensatory stages of hypertrophy with postnatal adaptation of the left ventricle to the conditions of extrauterine life.

---

*) A part of this paper is taken from the unpublished doctoral thesis of *U. Koehler.*

Methods

Left ventricles of Goldblatt rats (GBR) 2 to 4 months after operation and of swimming rats (SR) were used for investigation. SR were subjected to swimming training 2 hours per day, 7 days a week for a period of 2 to 4 months. Nonoperated (CR_G) and sedentary animals (CR_S) of the same age served as controls for GBR and SR, respectively.

Tissue homogenization was performed according to (4). The homogenate was stirred with Triton-X-100 in order to free structure-bound hexokinase. Supernatant LDH activity was determined by measuring the rate of pyruvate reduction at 365 nm (5). LDH isoenzymes were separated electrophoretically using 5.5% PAA gels (6) and specifically dyed by utilizing the isoenzymes' capability of lactate oxidation (7). The relative quantities of LDH isoenzyme activities were obtained on the basis of densitometry of the stained bands carried out at 540 nm. The densitometer tracings were evaluated by planimetry.

Soluble HK activity was measured by coupling the HK reaction with the glucose-6-phosphate dehydrogenase reaction (8).

Supernatant protein concentration was determined according to *Lowry* et al. (9).

For histochemical investigation 14 µm thick cryostat sections were specifically stained for LDH (10), succinate dehydrogenase (SDH) (11), and acid- (pH 4.2) and alkali-stable (pH 10.4) myofibrillar ATPase (12).

Results and discussion

a) *Biochemical and histochemical investigations of the compensatory stage of hypertrophy (table 1)*

In GBR, LDH activity per gram wet weight was decreased by 7% as compared to controls ($p < 0.05$); HK activity per unit wet weight showed a 14% increase ($p < 0.01$); the concentration of soluble protein, a 12% decrease ($p < 0.001$). Thus the LDH/HK ratio in GBR was decreased by 15% as compared to control values ($p < 0.001$). The contribution of M subunits to total LDH activity in oxidizing lactate was increased from 28% to 32% (about 13%) ($p < 0.001$), cf. fig. 1a, b.

Table 1. Anatomical and biochemical changes in Goldblatt rats (GBR) and swimming rats (SR) as compared to respective control rats (CR_G and CR_S). LV = left ventricular weight, BW = body weight. Numbers of animals used are given in parentheses. Values are means ± SE; n.s. = $p > 0.05$.

Experimental group	LV/BW (mg/g)	LDH activity (IU/g wet wt.)	HK activity (IU/g wet wt.)	Soluble protein (mg/g wet wt.)
GBR	2.99 (19) ± 0.58	505 (20) ± 36	7.87 (19) ± 1.32	44.0 (20) ± 3.3
CR_G	1.90 (13) ± 0.20	543 (13) ± 42	6.92 (13) ± 0.38	50.1 (12) ± 3.7
GBR/CR_G	+ 57	− 7	+ 14	− 12
% change	$p < 0.001$	$p < 0.05$	$p < 0.01$	$p < 0.001$
SR	2.07 (14) ± 0.16	474 (14) ± 21	6.10 (15) ± 0.66	53.1 (12) ± 3.1
CR_S	1.84 (18) ± 0.15	429 (18) ± 36	6.11 (16) ± 0.52	51.8 (18) ± 4.5
SR/CR_S	+ 13	+ 11	± 0	+ 3
% change	$p < 0.001$	$p < 0.001$	n. s.	n. s.

The decreased LDH activity might indicate a lower capability of lactate utilization, whereas the increased soluble HK activity could indicate an enhanced capability of glucose decay. The ratio of these two pathways of energy supply to the myocyte seems to be altered towards a more pronounced capability of direct metabolization of glucose, which is expressed by the decreased LDH/HK ratio. Many authors have reported that hypoxic conditions are a stimulus for an isoenzyme shift towards a higher M proportion of LDH. Thus it is conceivable that such conditions occurred in the GBR hearts and contributed to the enhanced M proportion, which might then reflect an adaptation, and so a better resistance to hypoxic conditions. Furthermore, it has been reported that the activity of LDH isoenzymes rich in H subunits might be subjected to a more precise control than those rich in M subunits (13, 14); thus the quality of the regulation of the intracellular $NAD/NADH_2$ ratio could be affected by the isoenzyme shift and possibly also by the decrease of the LDH/HK ratio. Since this ratio seems to be of importance for the regulation of the macromolecular metabolism (15), it is conceivable that relations exist between the regulatory function of LDH and HK, on the one hand, and other morphological, biochemical and mechanical changes in hypertrophied myocardium, on the other hand.

In SR, LDH activity per unit wet weight was increased by 11% ($p < 0.001$). HK activity remained unchanged, as did the concentration of soluble protein, thus SR showed a 10% increase in the LDH/HK ratio as compared to control values ($p < 0.05$). Additional results also point to an enhanced M proportion in LDH of SR.

As the isoenzymes rich in H subunits are more markedly inhibited by high concentrations of lactate than are the M subunits, it is conceivable that the increase in LDH activity as well as the enhanced M proportion express an adaptation to the conditions of swimming in which increased amounts of lactate have to be metabolized by the heart. The increased LDH/HK ratio might indicate an increased provision of energy by lactate utilization during the swimming-period.

It is interesting that a comparison of these metabolic changes in both types of hypertrophy shows an analogy to the changes in mechanical

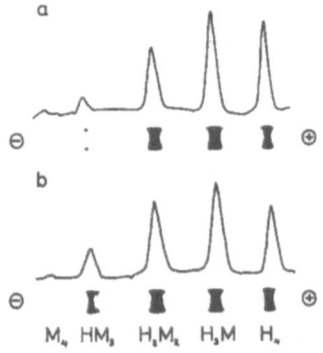

Fig. 1. Typical distribution of LDH isoenzymes in left ventricular myocardium of control rats (a) and Goldblatt rats (b).

properties and ATPase activity of contractile proteins (2). The maximum shortening velocity (Vmax) as well as the myofibrillar ATPase activity decrease parallel to the decrease of the LDH/HK ratio in GBR, whereas all of these parameters are increased in SR.

The histochemical detection of LDH did not show any apparent changes in intensity or distribution of staining in the cross sections of the left ventricles of GBR as compared to CR_G; neither did the sections for SDH as a mitochondrial enzyme. In the left ventricles of both GBR and CR_G the histochemical investigation of the acid- and alkali-stable myofibrillar ATPase in an acid (pH 4.2) or alkaline (pH 10.4) medium showed a homogeneous staining intensity over the entire cross section. No differences due to the different incubation media were observable. A comparison of SR with CR_S did not reveal any differences.

These findings show that overt regional changes in LDH, SDH, and the two types of ATPase do not occur in GBR, neither do they in SR. We may assume therefore that adaptive biochemical processes occur in all the cardiac muscle cells in a similar way, and not in single types of fibers, as is the case in skeletal muscle.

b) Changes in LDH and HK during postnatal development

Beginning from birth the pattern of isoenzymes is shifted impressively (fig. 2 a–d): the contribution of the M subunits to total LDH activity in

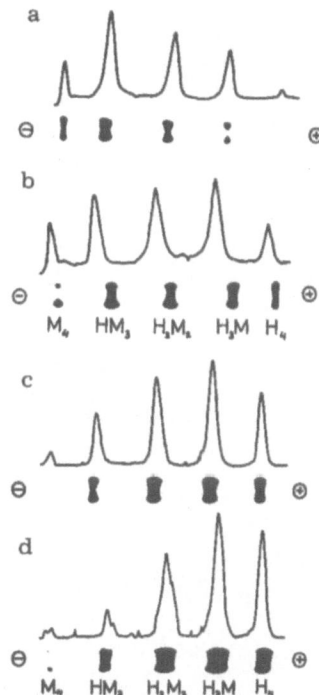

Fig. 2. Typical distribution of LDH isoenzymes in left ventricular myocardium of developing rats at the ages of 0 weeks (newborn rats) (a), 1 week (b), and 2 weeks (c), and adult rats (d).

oxidizing lactate is 60% at birth, 47% after one and 36% after two weeks, and then undergoes a slow decrease to the value of 28% in adult rats. Coincidentally, the activity of LDH per unit wet weight in reducing pyruvate shows an increase which decelerates gradually (fig. 3a). The HK activity per gram wet weight is increased after one week to a value about 13% above that at birth; subsequently, it decreases by degrees to about 13% below the value of the newborn rats (fig. 3a). The contribution of water to total ventricular wet weight decreases during the first four postnatal weeks from about 87% to 80%. This fact is partly responsible for the gain in LDH per unit wet weight reported here. Thus LDH activity per unit dry weight shows an initial decrease early after birth, and a continuous increase only thereafter (fig. 3b). Possibly this is due to processes of adaptation to extrauterine life. However, we calculated a continuous decrease in HK activity from the beginning of postnatal life, if related to dry weight (fig. 3b). Thus we found an increasing LDH/HK ratio. The changes in enzyme activities and the remarkable isoenzyme shift towards a predominance of those fractions which are said to work better under aerobic conditions (12, 13) made it conceivable that a progressive change takes place towards a more pronounced aerobic energy supply. This would also be supported by the well-known fact that postnatal tissue is less resistant to hypoxia than fetal tissue. Furthermore, the reported alterations might indicate the gradual formation of an increasingly effec-

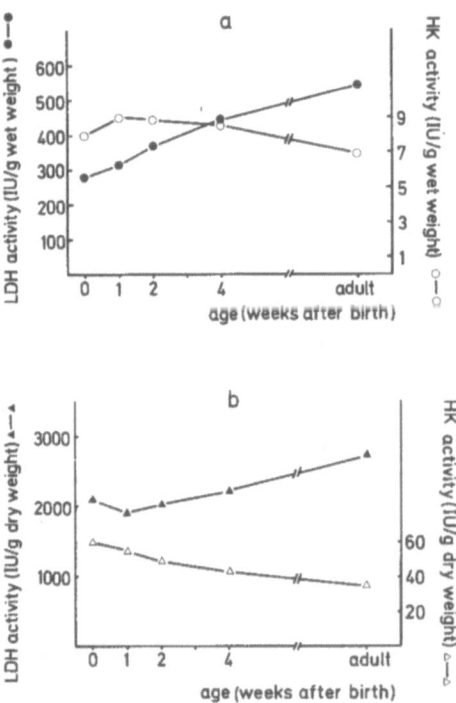

Fig. 3. Changes of enzyme activities in left ventricles of postnatally developing rats, related to wet (a) or dry (b) weight.

tive intracellular regulatory system for the NAD/NADH$_2$ ratio. The latter might be of great importance in cellular processes during postnatal development (cf. 15).

Zusammenfassung

Aktivitätsveränderungen der Lactatdehydrogenase (LDH) und der Hexokinase (HK) im linken Ventrikel der Ratte bei chronischer mechanischer Mehrbelastung und während der postnatalen Entwicklung waren Gegenstand der vorliegenden Untersuchung. Goldblattratten (GBR) zeigten 2 bis 4 Monte nach der Operation eine Abnahme der LDH-Aktivität um 7%, eine Zunahme des Anteils der M-Untereinheiten an der Gesamtaktivität um 13% sowie eine um 14% erhöhte HK-Aktivität. Schwimmratten (SR) hingegen wiesen nach 2- bis 4monatigem Training eine um 11% gesteigerte LDH-Aktivität auf, während die Aktivität der HK unverändert blieb. Histochemische Untersuchungen ergaben keinerlei Hinweise auf uneinheitliche Veränderungen in einzelnen Myokardarealen.

Im Verlaufe der postnatalen Entwicklung wurde ein Anstieg der LDH-Aktivität und des relativen Anteils der H-Untereinheiten an dieser festgestellt. Die HK-Aktivität stieg zunächst an, um anschließend wieder allmählich abzufallen. Diese Veränderungen werden als Ausdruck von Anpassungsvorgängen an die extrauterinen Lebensbedingungen interpretiert.

References

1. *Medugorac, I., R. Jacob:* Concentration and Adenosinetriphosphatase Activity of Left Ventricular Actomyosin in Goldblatt Rats during the Compensatory Stage of Hypertrophy. Hoppe-Seyler's Z. Physiol. Chem. **357**, 1495 (1976).
2. *Jacob, R., G. Ebrecht, A. Kämmereit, I. Medugorac, M. F. Wendt-Gallitelli:* Myocardial Function in Different Models of Cardiac Hypertrophy. Basic Res. Cardiol. **72**, 160 (1977).
3. *Medugorac, I.:* Characteristics of the Hypertrophied Left Ventricular Myocardium in Goldblatt Rats. Basic Res. Cardiol. **72**, 261 (1977).
4. *Bass, A., D. Brdiczka, P. Eyer, S. Hofer, D. Pette:* Metabolic Differentiation of Distinct Muscle Types at the Level of Enzymatic Organization. Eur. J. Biochem. **10**, 198 (1969).
5. *Boll, M. P.:* Untersuchungen zur Wechselwirkung zwischen der Lactatdehydrogenase und ihren Antikörpern. Diss. Bochum 1974.
6. *Dietz, A. A., T. Lubrano:* Separation and Quantitation of Lactic Dehydrogenase Isoenzymes by Disc Electrophoresis. Analyt. Biochem. **20**, 246 (1967).
7. *Schrauwen, J. A. M.:* Nachweis von Enzymen nach elektrophoretischer Trennung an Polyacrylamid-Säulchen. J. Chromatogr. **23**, 177 (1966).
8. *Falkenberg, F.:* Die Isoenzyme der Laktatdehydrogenase als Ursache für unspezifische Tetrazoliumsalz-Anfärbungen in Gelzymogrammen und die Isoenzyme der Hexokinase aus Schweinegeweben. Isolierung, biochemische und immunologische Charakterisierung. Diss. Bochum 1971.
9. *Lowry, O. H., N. J. Rosebrough, A. L. Farr, R. J. Randall:* Protein Measurement with the Folin Phenol Reagent. J. Biol. Chem. **193**, 265 (1951).
10. *Giebel, W.:* Die Hydrogenasen in der lateralen Cochleawand des Goldhamsters. Arch. Oto-Rhino-Laryng. **217**, 69 (1977).
11. *Arnold, M.:* Histochemie. pp. 156–157 (Berlin–Heidelberg–New York 1968).
12. *Müller, W.:* Temporal Progress of Muscle Adaptation to Endurance Training in Hind Limb Muscles of Young Rats. Cell. Tiss. Res. **156**, 61 (1974).
13. *Hultin, H. O.:* Effect of Environment on Kinetic Characteristics of Chicken Lactate Dehydrogenase Isoenzymes. pp. 69–85. In: Isozymes II, ed. *C. L. Markert* (New York 1975).

14. *Everse, J., N. O. Kaplan:* Mechanisms of Action and Biological Functions of Various Dehydrogenase Isozymes. pp. 28–34. In: Isozymes II, ed. *C. L. Markert* (New York 1975).
15. *Kun, E., A. C. Y. Chang, M. L. Sharma, A. M. Ferro, D. Nitecki:* Covalent Modification of Proteins by Metabolites of NAD$^+$. Proc. Natl. Acad. Sci. USA **73**, 3131 (1976).

Authors' address:

U. Koehler and Dr. *I. Medugorac,* Physiologisches Institut II der Universität Tübingen, Gmelinstr. 5, 7400 Tübingen

Basic Res. Cardiol. **75**, 221–222 (1980)
© 1980 Dr. Dietrich Steinkopff Verlag, Darmstadt
ISSN 0300–8428

Paper, presented at the Erwin Riesch Symposium, Tübingen, April 3–7, 1979

Medizinische Universitätsklinik, D-7400 Tübingen, Germany

Immunological parameters in patients with congestive cardiomyopathy

Immunologische Parameter bei Patienten mit kongestiver Kardiomyopathie

B. Maisch, P. A. Berg, and *K. Kochsiek*

Cardiomyopathies comprise those myocardial diseases that are not caused by coronary heart disease or mechanical overload. We studied 83 patients with cardiomyopathies, who were classified according to *Goodwin* (1970) (1):
1) 55 patients had congestive cardiomyopathy (COCM). 34 of them were of the primary, 21 of the secondary alcoholic type.
2) 28 patients had hypertrophic cardiomyopathy with or without obstruction (HOCM).

Since the etiology of COCM is unknown in most cases, we were interested in finding out if autoimmune reactions may play a role in the pathogenesis of the disease (2, 3). Autoimmune phenomena were studied by the detection of autoantibodies in the patients sera against several tissues, among them heart and skeletal muscle or vital rat cardiocytes.

Antibodies were either classified as heart-specific, such as antiinterfibrillary (IFA); as muscle-specific, such as antisarcolemmal (ASA) or antifibrillary (AFA); or as nonorgan-specific, such as antiendothelial (AEA), antimitochondrial (AMA), antinuclear (ANA) or smooth muscle antibodies (SMA). Among the 28 patients with HOCM heart-muscle-associated antibodies were detected rarely (IFA in 11%, ASA in 14%, AFA in 21%, 40 controls up to 5%). In patients with COCM, IFA of the IgG and IgM type were demonstrated in 35%, that is, three times as much as in HOCM with 11%. ASA and AFA were found in 20% each. In alcoholic myocardial disease antiinterfibrillary antibodies (IFA) with 24% were less frequent than in primary COCM. Nonorgan-specific autoantibodies against the endothelium of small vessels were found only in 10% to 11% of primary and secondary COCM. Two of three patients with COCM, who had a viral myocarditis in their history, showed ASA in association with nonorgan-specific AEA. This pattern of ASA and AEA can be attributed to viral myocarditis and is interpreted as a marker of the viral etiology of congestive cardiomyopathy.

Antinuclear antibodies (ANA) appeared in primary and secondary COCM with 36% and 38% respectively, that is four times as much as in controls. Three of the ANA-positive patients demonstrated anti-DNA antibodies but no SLE. In 6 patients with primary COCM (11%) a pattern of nonorgan-specific ANA with muscle-specific AFA without evidence of

ASA and AEA was present. This pattern observed in 11% of patients with primary COCM may be indicative of an autoimmune cardiomyopathy.

Among the muscle-associated antibodies only the antiinterfibrillary antibodies (IFA) showed myocardial specificity. ASA and AFA reacted with myocardial and skeletal tissue. For ASA and AFA either a common myocardial and skeletal antigen or a heterogenity of antisarcolemmal and antifibrillary antibodies must be postulated. In order to investigate the biological relevance of the antiheart antibodies we compared the immunofluorescent staining of dead rat cardiocytes with vital contracting rat cardiocytes. Only ASA reacted with conctracting muscle fibers, indicating that the sarcolemmal antigens are easily accessible at the surface of the membrane. These data also demonstrate that the membrane of the cardiocyte must be altered before antibodies against intracellular structures, such as antifibrillary, antiinterfibrillary or antinuclear antibodies, can penetrate.

The presence of heart-muscle-associated antibodies particularly of the IFA type can be associated with the severity of the heart disease according to the New York Heart Association (NYHA) classification. All patients with grade 4, severest form of cardiac insufficiency, 88% of patients with grade 3 and 49% with grade 2 revealed heart-muscle-associated antibodies. Only 30 % of patients with grade 1 had cardiac autoantibodies. These results are compatible with the finding that antibodies of the IFA-type were found in patients with a significantly ($2P < 0.05$) higher pulmonary wedge pressure of 19.8 ± 2.9 mm Hg when compared with patients without antibodies, whose pulmonary wedge pressure did not exceed 10.2 ± 3.1 mm Hg.

From our investigation of 55 patients with congestive and 28 patients with hypertrophic cardiomyopathy it can be concluded that:

1) In patients with HOCM no significant autoimmune phenomena could be demonstrated.
2) The pattern of muscle-specific ASA and nonorgan-specific AEA was found in 3 patients with COCM and may be indicative of the viral etiology of the cardiomyopathy.
3) Heart-specific antiinterfibrillary antibodies (IFA) occur in 35% of patients with COCM.
4) IFA indicate a COCM of high severity. We interpret their presence as an epiphenomenon of myocardial cell damage in progressive COCM.
5) ANA are present in 11% of patients with COCM; a pattern of muscle-specific AFA and nonorgan-specific ANA may indicate an autoimmune COCM.

References

1. *Goodwin, J. F.:* Congestive and hypertrophic cardiomyopathies. A decade of study. Lancet 1970/I, 733.
2. *Kirsner, A. B., Hess, E. V., Fowler, N. O.:* Immunologic findings in idiopathic cardiomyopathy: A prospective serial study. Amer. Heart J. 625–630 (1973).
3. *Sack, W., Sebening, H., Wachsmuth, E. D.:* Auto-Antikörper gegen Herzmuskelsarkolemm im Serum von Patienten mit primärer Cardiomyopathie. Klin. Wschr. **53**, 103–110 (1975).

Author's address:

Dr. *B. Maisch*, Medizinische Universitätsklinik, 7400 Tübingen

Basic Res. Cardiol. **75**, 223–233 (1980)
© 1980 Dr. Dietrich Steinkopff Verlag, Darmstadt
ISSN 0300–8428

Paper, presented at the Erwin Riesch Symposium, Tübingen, April 3–7, 1979

*The Laboratory of Pathophysiology of the Heart, Institute of General Pathology
and Pathophysiology, Academy of Medical Sciences, Moscow (USSR)*

On the mechanism of elevation of cardiac muscle functional capabilities in adaptation to exercise

Zum Mechanismus der Verbesserung der Leistungsfähigkeit des Herzens durch körperliches Training

F. Z. Meerson, V. I. Kapelko, and *C. Pfeiffer*)*

With 3 figures and 3 tables

Summary

The main parameters of contraction and relaxation of papillary muscle strips taken from the left ventricle of control and exercise-adapted rats were measured. The isotonic peak shortening velocity and contraction amplitude of thin strips under low loads in adapted animals were 1.5 times higher compared to the corresponding controls.

In thick strips an even greater difference in parameters of isotonic contraction was observed – 2.3 times more. This change, together with 1.5 times higher maximal load corresponding to maximal developed tension, suggested the increased resistance to hypoxia in myocardial cells during adaptation. These results have been interpreted as being due to the well-known increase in the myosin ATP-ase activity as well as the adaptive augmentation of the functional power of oxygen and substrates transport system in myocardial cells.

The relaxation velocity of the adapted cardiac muscle increased even more than the contractile parameters; the relaxation index was higher as compared to the controls. It was suggested that the adaptation caused an augmentation in the calcium pump functional power. The myocardial compliance and the positive inotropic response to high frequency of stimulation were also elevated in adapted cardiac muscle. In total, the results suggest that an elevation of maximal myocardial performance caused by the exercise adaptation may be due to a coordinative augmentation of the functional power of the three main systems of myocardial cells – the ionic transport system, myosin ATPase and the ATP resynthesis system.

It is well known that the maximal cardiac output and the cardiac work in trained subjects during maximal physical loads are 1.5–2 times higher as compared to untrained subjects (1, 2). This important achievement of adaptation is due not only to changes in neurohormonal regulation but also to stable structural changes developing in the cardiac muscle. In isolated hearts of rats adapted to exercise it was shown that the maximal work per unit of myocardial mass under optimal conditions are approxi-

---

*) Dr. *Pfeiffer* worked in Moscow during a Scientific Mission from Physiology Institute, Berlin, German Democratic Republic.

mately doubled as compared to untrained rat hearts (3–5). Nevertheless it was stated earlier that the tension developed by isolated papillary muscles (6) or the force developed per unit of left ventricular mass during the aorta clamping did not change after adaptation (7, 8) or only slightly increased (9, 10).

These results have led us to suggest that the adaptational changes developing in the cardiac muscle during training may be differently displayed in isotonic and isometric regimes of contractions. Thus the first aim of this work was the determination of the force-velocity curve for the myocardium of control and adapted animals.

The second aim was to evaluate the function of the relaxation system in myocardial cells of adapted animals. For this we measured the velocity of isotonic relaxation and determined its relation to contraction amplitude. This relation has been referred to earlier as "relaxation index" (11–13). It has been suggested that this index changes proportionally to the activity of the "calcium pump" of the sarcoplasmic reticulum. This pump mainly determines the velocity of myofibrillar relaxation as well as the quantity of Ca^{++} that has been retained in myofibrils and in this way can influence myocardial distensibility. For evaluation of the distensibility, the dependence of the muscle length on the resting load was determined.

The third aim was to evaluate the ionic transport mechanisms that regulate the quantity of activator Ca^{++} in the myoplasm. For this purpose we measured the rate and the magnitude of the positive inotropic effect caused by an increase in the frequency of contractions.

It is well known that the contraction and the relaxation of cardiac muscle, as well as the magnitude of a positive inotropic effect, are highly influenced by an adequate energy supply. The papillary muscle thickness is the critical factor that limits the oxygen diffusion to central areas and as a result – also limits muscle function (14, 15). To improve oxygen availability, we cut thin strips from papillary muscles and used strips of approximately equal thickness from both groups for comparison. The preliminary report of this work has recently been published (12).

Materials and methods

Adaptation to physical exercise

The male rats of initial weight of about 200 g were forced to swim in water at 32 °C 5 times a week for 7–11 weeks. The swimming time increased from 10 to 60 minutes a day for the first two weeks and then remained constant over 6 weeks. In the last 1–5 weeks the swimming time was diminished to 30 minutes. As a result of adaptation the left ventricular weight of 24 animals was $107 \pm 1.2\%$ compared to the value in control rats with the same body weight. 32 experiments were performed, of which 13 represented adapted animals and 19 controls.

Experimental equipment

Isolated papillary muscle strips taken from the left ventricle were placed in a glass chamber filled with oxygenated Krebs solution (Ca^{++} concentration = 1.2 mM) at 30 °C. The initial load was 0.25–0.5 g. The experimental design was previously described in detail (15). It was possible to vary the muscle load at fixed or released muscle length. Muscle shortening was detected with a sensitive capacitive transducer 51B21, the signal being amplified by a 51B02 Disa amplifier and registered on a Disa Universal Indicator by Cossor photocamera. The relaxation index was determined as a ratio between the relaxation velocity and the contractile amplitude.

Experimental procedure

Each experiment consisted of two parts. In the first part the force-velocity curve and the influence of strip extension on its length and isotonic contractile amplitude were determined. This part was performed at constant frequency of contractions – 20 per minute. The muscle extension was caused by progressive increments of resting loads from a minimal value of 50 mg up to a maximal value at which a definite diminution of the contractile amplitude was observed. Then the strip length corresponding to the optimum contractile amplitude was fixed and the force-velocity curve was determined by progressive increments in afterload. The extrapolation of this curve to abscissae allowed determination of the maximal isometric load corresponding to maximal developed tension.

In the second part of each experiment the inotropic effect of increased frequency of contractions was studied. There were three basic frequencies – 20, 60, and 120 per minute. At each basic level the stimulation frequency was abruptly increased twofold.

Results and discussion

The maximal contractile amplitude in control experiments was observed mainly at a load equal to 0.6 g/mm². Strips taken from adapted animals did not show such dependence; the contractile amplitude at loads of 0.2–0.6 g/mm² was roughly equal.

Table 1 represents data on contraction and relaxation parameters at equal loads – approximately 0.6 g/mm². Since these parameters in both

Table 1. The contraction and relaxation parameters of myocardial strips of controls and animals adapted to exercise (mean ± SE).

Indices	Control		Adaptation	
	thin strips (11)	thick strips (8)	thin strips (8)	thick strips (5)
Strip cross-sectional area (mm²)	0.57 ± 0.03	$0.95 \pm 0.05^{++}$	0.66 ± 0.04	$1.04 \pm 0.12^{++}$
Resting load (g/mm²)	0.67 ± 0.09	0.60 ± 0.09	0.57 ± 0.08	0.59 ± 0.20
Contractile amplitude (percent of muscle length)	9.0 ± 1.2	$5.8 \pm 0.6^{+}$	14.0 ± 2.0	13.1 ± 1.0
Contractile velocity (ML/sec)	1.20 ± 0.15	$0.76 \pm 0.09^{+}$	1.77 ± 0.22	1.74 ± 0.14
Time to contraction peak (msec)	117 ± 3	124 ± 4	125 ± 4	116 ± 6
Relaxation velocity (ML/sec)	1.44 ± 0.23	$0.80 \pm 0.10^{+}$	2.65 ± 0.55	2.14 ± 0.22
Relaxation index (sec⁻¹)	14.9 ± 0.9	13.6 ± 0.8	18.1 ± 1.2	16.2 ± 1.0

Figures in brackets denote number of experiments. Difference is significant at confidence level – [+] = $p < 0.05$, [++] = $p < 0.01$ as compared to corresponding thin strips.

groups were dependent on strip thickness, it was decided to divide each group into two subgroups with approximately equal muscle thickness within a single group. The thinner strips with estimated cross-sectional area of 0.57–0.66 mm² were called "thin strips", whereas the thicker strips with cross-sectional area of 0.95–1.04 mm² were called "thick strips". Data of table 1 and figure 1 revealed three main facts.

1. In control experiments the isotonic contractile amplitude and velocity of thick strips were 35–37% less as compared to thin strips, whereas in adapted animals this diminution of contractile function was not observed. This well-known functional depression in thicker muscles (14, 15) was more prominent at high afterloads (fig. 1A). In fact, the isotonic peak velocity of thick strips at a load of 0.6 g/mm² was only 36 percent less whereas the maximal load was more than 2 times less as compared to thin control strips. The observed phenomenon has been undoubtedly caused by a hypoxia of the central core of a muscle due to increased diffusion distance for oxygen.

The absence of this contractile diminution in adapted animal experiments (fig. 1B) seems to reflect increased capabilities of oxygen and pyruvate transport systems in cardiac muscle of adapted animals. In fact, the following observations were made in training animals: increase in myoglobin concentration (16), density of coronary capillaries (17, 18), as well as hexokinase and lactate dehydrogenase activities (16, 19).

The data suggest that under natural conditions oxygen and substrate transport represents a factor limiting cardiac function, while the exercise adaptation increased the critical value of this factor.

2. The velocity and amplitude of isotonic contractions at a light load were substantially higher in adapted animal experiments. The difference as compared to controls was 2.3 times for thick strips (p < 0.001) and + 55% for thin strips (p < 0.05). This difference became even greater when comparing the parameters at small load – 0,2 g/mm². As has been pointed

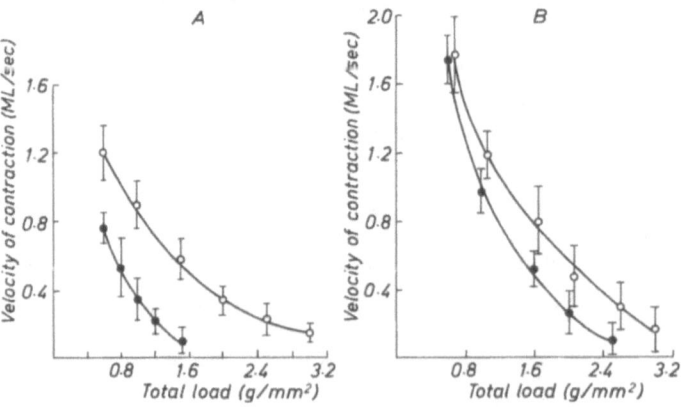

Fig. 1. The force-velocity curves of controls (A) and adapted animals (B) myocardial strips of different thickness – thin (open circles) and thick (closed circles). Abscissa – total load in g/mm², ordinate – velocity of contraction in muscle length per second (mean ± SE).

out earlier, the contractile parameters in control experiments were significantly less at this light load. Therefore the velocity and amplitude of the contraction of thin strips taken from adapted animals were two times higher compared to control values (table 2).

The adaptation-induced augmentation of the contractile velocity of thin strips under isotonic conditions with small loads seems not to be due to increased functional power of the energy supply because it is practically absent under nearly isometric conditions (fig. 1B) when, as it is known, the oxygen consumption is roughly 3 times higher (20). The more probable explanation may be based on the recently discovered fact that during adaptation myosin ATPase activity increases (21, 22). It is known that myosin ATPase activity is the main factor limiting the rate of turnover of actomyosin links and, finally, the velocity of contraction (23, 24). But this advantage was not revealed in the isometric regime.

This finding can be explained by assuming that the role of myosin ATPase activity in isometric contraction is not so large as in isotonic contraction. In fact, active sites of actin and myosin protofibrils can be in opposition to each other for a rather long time during isometric contraction when shortening is minimal or absent. The force developed is determined chiefly by the quantity of actomyosin bonds which depends on myofibrillar content in a cell. It was shown that calculation of developed tension per unit of area occupied by myofibrils in skeletal muscle cells gives a value which is quite compatible with the corresponding value for cardiac muscle (25). Another reason to support the discussed idea comes from studies on animals with different states of thyroid activity. Hypo- or hyperthyroidism is definitely followed by corresponding changes in myosin ATPase activities and maximal isotonic velocity of contraction, while maximal developed tension remains quite stable (26–28).

A different situation sometimes arose under a higher and more intensive regime of exercise over a prolonged time. This led to a 15–20% increase in left ventricular weight. Although maximal isotonic velocity of contraction against a light load was also somewhat higher in adaptation, a relatively greater increase in maximal tension developed by whole papillary muscles of trained rats was reported (29, 30). The observed changes were similar to our findings on thick strips. Whether the above-mentioned

Table 2. The contractile parameters of myocardial strips at small load (0.2 g/mm^2).

	Thin strips		Thick strips	
	control (9)	adaptation (8)	control (5)	adaptation (4)
Contractile amplitude (percent of muscle length)	6.9 ± 1.4	$13.8 \pm 2.3^+$	4.2 ± 1.1	$12.5 \pm 2.8^+$
Contractile velocity (muscle length/sec)	1.1 ± 0.17	$2.1 \pm 0.32^+$	0.7 ± 0.18	$1.9 \pm 0.18^{++}$

Difference is significant as compared to controls at confidence level of $^+ = p < 0.05$, $^{++} = p < 0.01$.

changes were caused by adaptation due to increased functional power of
energy supply, or were the result of a concomitant increase in myofibrillar
content, such as that observed in greyhounds (31), is a question which
requires further investigation.

3. Myocardial strips taken from adapted animal hearts differed from
controls by higher relaxation velocity. The difference was even more than
the difference in the contractile velocity and amplitude. The relaxation
index was higher in adapted animal experiments by about 20% ($p < 0.05$)
(table 1). The difference was observed at any tested frequency of contractions in the range from 60 to 300 per minute (fig. 2).

This fact was reported earlier (12); it correlates very well with the
observation of a lesser diastolic defect, that is, less incomplete diastolic
relaxation of the isolated heart of adapted animals upon sudden increase
in stimulation frequency (5). These data suggest that the training increases
the functional power of the relaxation system of myocardial cells. Quite
recently this postulate was confirmed by a direct study of calcium binding
velocity on cardiac sarcoplasmic reticulum fragments (32). It was found
that the fragments from the cardiac muscle of adapted animals exhibited
17–40% higher initial velocity of calcium accumulation as compared to
controls. This value closely coincides with the observed increase in the
relaxation index by 20%. The good correlation between the physiological
and biochemical indices of the relaxation process has also been observed
in cardiac compensatory hypertrophy, which is characterized by a pro-
foundly decreased functional power of the cardiac relaxation system (12,
15, 33, 34). Elevated left ventricular dP/dt during relaxation is the most
consistent finding in trained rats (4, 35).

The relaxation index determined under cardiac catheterization in vivo
was 30% higher in adapted animals as compared to controls (35). This
change was followed by a 17% increase in the diastolic pause duration at
equal heart rate.

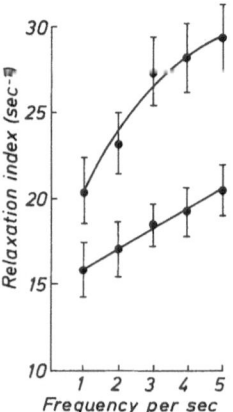

Fig. 2. Effect of increasing frequency of contractions on the relaxation index
represented by the ratio (in sec^{-1}) between the relaxation velocity and isotonic
contractile amplitude for myocardial strips of controls (lower curve) and adapted
(upper curve) animals (mean ± SE).

The adaptation-induced increase in the functional power of the cardiac relaxation system may exert profound effects on other aspects of cardiac performance. First, the more powerful calcium pump can extract more calcium ions from myofibrils and in this way can cause their more complete relaxation and increase the compliance of the cardiac muscle. Second, the more powerful calcium pump can facilitate cardiac function at high contraction frequencies. The higher relaxation index has been shown to combine with a greater positive inotropic effect (11, 13). Both suggestions were tested in this investigation.

The compliance of myocardial strips measured by the degree of their extension in response to increasing resting loads was found to be quite the same in thick and thin strips. But adapted animal strips showed higher compliance (fig. 3) at equal resting tension. The difference becomes statistically significant at a resting tension of 0.3 g/mm^2 and higher. For an extension of myocardial strips by 10% of initial length in adapted animal experiments it was necessary to apply a load of 0.55 ± 0.07 g/mm^2, whereas in the control experiments 0.90 ± 0.09 g/mm^2, that is, 1.5 times higher load was required. Increased compliance of the myocardium exerted by training seems to contribute to augmentation of the ventricular diastolic volume in training subjects.

An increase in stimulation frequency usually exerts a negative inotropic effect on rat ventricular muscle (36–39). In recent years it was found that a diminution of Ca^{++} concentration in the perfusate (38) or an improvement of energy supply (37, 39) can generally restore a positive inotropic effect of higher frequency in mammalian myocardium. In our experiments the Ca^{++} concentration was lowered and the possibility of inadequate oxygenation was diminished by the use of rather thin strips. Under these conditions the control myocardial strips showed no change in the contractile amplitude when the stimulation frequency was increased

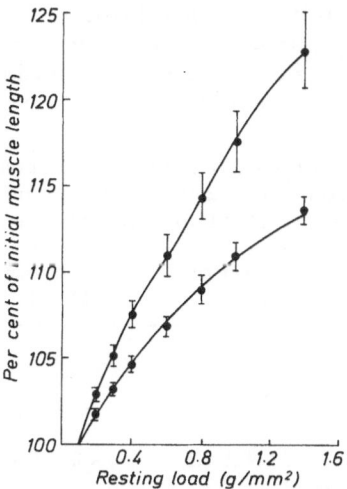

Fig. 3. The relation between the resting loads and the degree of extension of myocardial strips of control (lower curve) and adapted (upper curve) animals. Strip length at minimal load 0.1 g/mm^2 was taken as a reference point.

from 60 to 120 per minute, but they showed a 20-percent increase of amplitude when the stimulation frequency increased from 120 to 240 per minute. The adapted myocardial strips showed the definite positive inotropic effect ($+ 14 \pm 2$ %) which was significantly different from the control ($p < 0.05$) at increments of stimulation frequency from 60 to 120 per minute. The difference became higher at increments of stimulation frequency from 120 to 240 per minute (table 3). In adaptation experiments both the degree of the positive inotropic effect, and the rate of its development and disappearance, were significantly higher as compared to control values. Thus, the exercise adaptation leads to the increment of inotropic response to high stimulation frequency which combines with the higher relaxation index (fig. 2).

The higher functional power of the calcium pump in myocardial cells of adapted animals can possibly exert an effect on the ATP resynthesizing process. The higher the quantity of Ca^{++} ions accumulating into the sarcoplasmic reticulum is, the less is the quantity of Ca^{++} taken by mitochondria. It is known that mitochondrial Ca^{++} uptake is linked to electron transport and competes with ATP resynthesis (40). It follows that a lesser mitochondrial Ca^{++} uptake at high frequencies of contraction that is probable in adaptation should lead to some increase in the degree of the oxygenation-phosphorylation coupling and to an increase in cardiac efficiency. In fact, such a change was observed under oxygen deficit conditions (3), but was not so prominent at better conditions (4).

The suggested change would promote an increase in the functional power of the aerobic ATP resynthesis during intensive function. At maximal load on the heart caused by an aorta clamping, it was shown recently that the ATP concentration in the myocardium of the trained animals decreased much less than in control animals, whereas the contractile function intensity in adapted animals was significantly higher (41). From these results one can suggest that the exercise adaptation increases the functional capacity of aerobic ATP synthesis.

On the whole, the results suggest that an increase in maximal functional capabilities of the heart caused by adaptation to physical exercise seems to be due to coordinative increment of the functional power of three

Table 3. The degree and rate of positive inotropic effect caused by sudden increase in stimulation frequency from 120 to 240 per minute and rate of disappearance of this effect at inverse fall of frequency (mean $\pm$ SE).

	Control (8)	Adaptation (11)	Difference in percent	
Degree of positive inotropic effect (percent of initial amplitude)	20 ± 6	61 ± 10	$+ 41$	$p < 0.01$
Time to half inotropic effect (sec)	7.4 ± 0.5	4.8 ± 0.4	$- 35$	$p < 0.01$
Time to moment at which half of positive effect disappeared (sec)	8.5 ± 0.8	6.0 ± 0.5	$- 30$	$p < 0.02$

main myocardial cell systems – the ionic transport system, myosine ATP-ase and the ATP resynthesis system.

Zusammenfassung

An Papillarmuskelstreifen vom linken Ventrikel trainingsadaptierter Ratten wurden die wesentlichen Parameter der Kontraktion und Erschlaffung gemessen. Wurden dünne Muskelstreifen benutzt, so war die maximale Verkürzungsge-schwindigkeit und Kontraktionsamplitude unter geringer Last bei adaptierten Tieren um 1,5mal höher als bei entsprechenden Kontrollen. Bei dicken Streifen wurde noch eine größere Differenz (bis zum 2,3fachen der Kontrollen) gemessen. Diese Änderung, zusammen mit einer 1,5mal höheren Last, welche der maximalen Spannungsentwicklung entspricht, läßt bei Herzmuskelzellen während der Adap-tation eine gesteigerte Resistenz gegenüber Hypoxie vermuten. Die Ergebnisse werden als Folge der wohlbekannten Steigerung der Myosin-ATPase-Aktivität und einer adaptiv gesteigerten Leistungsfähigkeit des Sauerstoff- und Substrat-Trans-portsystems der Myokardzelle interpretiert.

Die Erschlaffungsgeschwindigkeit des adaptierten Herzmuskels war höher als die der Kontrollen; der Relaxationsindex stieg sogar mehr an als die Parameter der Kontraktion. Als Ursache wird eine adaptive Leistungssteigerung der Ca^{++}-Pumpe angenommen. Auch die Dehnbarkeit des Myokards und die positiv inotrope Ant-wort auf hochfrequente Reizung waren beim adaptierten Herzmuskel erhöht.

Insgesamt legen die Ergebnisse nahe, daß eine Steigerung der maximalen Leistungsfähigkeit des Myokards als Folge einer Anpassung an körperliches Trai-ning auf eine koordinative Steigerung der funktionellen Leistung dreier Systeme in der Myokardzelle bezogen werden kann, nämlich des Ionentransports, der Myosin-ATPase und des ATP-synthetisierenden Systems.

References

1. *Astrand, P. O., T. Cuddy, B. Saltin, J. Stenberg:* Cardiac output during submaxi-mal and maximal work. J. Appl. Physiol. **19**, 268–274 (1964).
2. *Komadel, L., E. Barta, M. Kokavetz:* Physiological augmentation of the heart (Bratislava 1968).
3. *Penpargkul, S., J. Scheuer:* The effect of physical training upon the mechanical and metabolic performance of the rat heart. J. Clin. Invest. **49**, 1859–1868 (1970).
4. *Bersohn, M. M., J. Scheuer:* Effects of physical training on end-diastolic volume and myocardial performance of isolated rat hearts. Circulat. Res. **40**, 510–516 (1977).
5. *Meerson, F. Z., V. I. Kapelko, S. I. Shaginova:* Contractile function of the myocardium in adaptation to physical load (Russ.) Cardiologia (Mos.) **13**, 5–18 (1973).
6. *Amsterdam, E. A., J. Wickmann-Coffelt, G. Choquet, T. Kamiyama, J. Lenz, R. Zelis, D. T. Mason:* Response of the rat heart to strenuous exercise: physical, biochemical and functional correlates (abstr.). Clin. Res. **20**, 361 (1972).
7. *Krames, B., D. W. Northup:* Isometric tension development in the hyper-trophied heart. Fed. Proc. **23**, 359 (1964).
8. *Meerson, F. Z., L. S. Rozanova:* Force and velocity of myocardial contraction in cardiac hypertrophy produced by experimental lesion and training. (Rus.) Pat. Fiziol. Exp. Ther. (Mos.) **11**, 18–22 (1967).
9. *Codini, M. A., T. Lipintsoi, J. Scheuer:* Cardiac responses to moderate training in rats. J. Appl. Physiol. Respirat. Environ. Exercise Physiol. **42**, 262–266 (1977).
10. *Steil, E., M. Hansis, A. Hepp, I. Kissling, R. Jacob:* Cardiac hypertrophy due to physical exercise – an example of hypertrophy without decrease of contractility: unreliability of conventional estimation of contractility by simple parameters.

In: Recent Advances in Studies on Cardiac Structure and Metabolism (ed. *A. Fleckenstein, N. S. Dhalla*) University Park, **5**, 491–496 (1975).

11. *Meerson, F. Z., V. I. Kapelko:* Role of the connection between the force of contraction and the velocity of relaxation of the myocardium in the adaptation of the heart to increasing loads. (Rus.) Cardiologia (Mos.) **13**, 19–30 (1973).

12. *Meerson, F. Z., V. I. Kapelko:* Contraction and relaxation of the myocardium in compensatory hypertrophy and the state of physical training. Proceed. Second USSR-USA symposium on Myocardial Metabolism, Sochi, 249–271 (1975).

13. *Meerson, F. Z., V. I. Kapelko:* The significance of the interrelationship between the intensity of the contractile state and the velocity of relaxation in adapting cardiac muscle to function at high work loads. J. Mol. Cell. Cardiol. **7**, 793–806 (1975).

14. *Henderson, A. H., R. J. Craig, R. Gorlin, E. H. Sonnenblick:* Free fatty acids and myocardial function in perfused rat hearts. Cardiov. Res. **4**, 466–472 (1970).

15. *Meerson, F. Z., V. I. Kapelko:* The contractile function of the myocardium in two types of heart adaptation to increased load. Cardiology **57**, 183–199 (1972).

16. *Troshanova, E. S.:* Effect of experimental training on biochemical indices of cardiac muscle (Rus.). Bull. Exp. Biol. Med. **32**, 287–293 (1951).

17. *Tepperman, J., D. Pearlman:* Effects of exercise and anemia in coronary arteries of small animals as revealed by the corrosion-cast technique. Circulat. Res. **9**, 576–584 (1961).

18. *Stevenson, J. A. F., V. Fekeli, P. Rechnitzer, J. R. Beaton:* Effect of exercise on coronary tree size in the rat. Circulat. Res. **15**, 265–269 (1964).

19. *Walpurger, G., H. Anger:* Die enzymatische Organisation des Energiestoffwechsels im Rattenherzen nach Schwimm- und Lauftraining. Z. Kreislaufforschg. **59**, 438–449 (1970).

20. *Coleman, H. N.:* Effect of alterations in shortening and external work on oxygen consumption of cat papillary muscle. Amer. J. Physiol. **214**, 100–106 (1968).

21. *Wilkerson, J. E., E. Evonuk:* Changes in cardiac and skeletal muscle myosin ATP-ase activities after exercise. J. Appl. Physiol. **30**, 328–330 (1971).

22. *Bhan, A. K., J. Scheuer:* Effects of physical training on cardiac actomyosin adenosine triphosphatase activity. Amer. J. Physiol. **223**, 1486–1490 (1972).

23. *Barany, M.:* ATP-ase activity of myosin correlated with speed of muscle shortening. J. gen. Physiol. **50**, 197–216 (1967).

24. *Katz, A. M.:* Relationships between mechanical and chemical phenomena in the myocardium. In: Cardiac hypertrophy, ed. *N. Alpert,* Acad. Press 85–88 (1971).

25. *Sonnenblick, E. H., W. W. Parmley, R. S. Buccino, J. F. Spann:* Maximum force development in cardiac muscle. Nature (Engl.) **219**, 1056–1050 (1960).

26. *Yazaki, Y., M. S. Raben:* Effect of thyroid state on the enzymatic characteristics of cardiac myosin. A difference in behaviour of rat and rabbit cardiac myosin. Circulat. Res. **36**, 208–215 (1975).

27. *Strauer, B. E., W. Schulze:* Experimental hypothyroidism: depression of myocardial contractile function and hemodynamics and their reversibility by substitution with thyroid hormones. Basic Res. Cardiol. **71**, 624–644 (1976).

28. *Skelton, C. L., J. Y. Su, P. E. Pool:* Influence of hyperthyroidism on glycerol-extracted cardiac muscle from rabbits. Cardiov. Res. **10**, 380–384 (1976).

29. *Kämmereit, A., I. Medugorac, E. Steil, R. Jacob:* Mechanics of the isolated ventricular myocardium of rats conditioned by physical training. Basic Res. Cardiol. **70**, 495–507 (1975).

30. *Mole, P. A.:* Increased contractile potential of papillary muscles from exercise-trained rat hearts. Amer. J. Physiol.: Heart a Circul. Physiol. **3**, H 421–H 425 (1978).

31. *Carew, T. E., J. W. Covell:* Left ventricular function in exercise-induced hypertrophy in dogs. Amer. J. Cardiol. **42**, 82–88 (1978).

32. *Penpargkul, S., D. I. Repke, A. M. Katz, J. Scheuer:* Effect of physical training on calcium transport by rat cardiac sarcoplasmic reticulum. Circul. Res. **40**, 134–138 (1977).

33. *Meerson, F. Z., V. I. Kapelko, A. A. Nourmatov:* Physiological evaluation of the capacity of the diastole mechanism. Acta cardiol. **26**, 547–567 (1971).

34. *Sordahl, L. A., W. B. McCollum, W. G. Wood, A. Schwartz:* Mitochondria and sarcoplasmic reticulum function in cardiac hypertrophy and failure. Amer. J. Physiol. **224**, 497–502 (1973).

35. *Kapelko, V. I., L. M. Giber:* Response of the heart to functional load in control and trained rats. (Rus.) Sechenov's Physiol. J. USSR **63**, 597–599 (1977).

36. *Henderson, A. H., D. L. Brutsaert, W. W. Parmley, E. H. Sonnenblick:* Myocardial mechanics in papillary muscles of the rat and cat. Amer. J. Physiol. **217**, 1273–1279 (1969).

37. *Kapelko, V. I.:* Effect of thickness of isolated papillary muscles on strength of contraction at different frequencies (Rus.) Bull. Exp. Biol. Med. **70**, 1352–1354 (1970).

38. *Forester, G. V., G. W. Mainwood:* Interval dependent inotropic effects in the rat myocardium and the effect of calcium. Pflüg. Arch. **352**, 189–196 (1974).

39. *Henry, P. D.:* Positive staircase effect in the rat heart. Amer. J. Physiol. **228**, 360–364 (1975).

40. *Lehninger, A. L.:* Mitochondria and calcium ion transport. Biochem. J. **119**, 129–139 (1970).

41. *Meerson, F. Z., L. Golubeva:* Effect of preliminary adaptation to basic factors of environment on the ATP concentration and the phosphorylation potential in the myocardium at acute overload of the heart. (Rus.) Doklady Acad. Sci. USSR **210**, 989–992 (1973).

Authors' address:

Prof. Dr. *F. Z. Meerson,* Institute of General Pathology and Pathophysiology, Academy of Medical Sciences, Moscow (USSR)

Basic Res. Cardiol. **75**, 234–243 (1980)
© 1980 Dr. Dietrich Steinkopff Verlag, Darmstadt
ISSN 0300–8428

Paper, presented at the Erwin Riesch Symposium, Tübingen, April 3–7, 1979

Department of Medicine, University of Munich, Klinikum Großhadern

Systolic stress, coronary hemodynamics and metabolic reserve in experimental and clinical cardiac hypertrophy*)

Wandspannung, koronare Hämodynamik und metabolische Reserve bei experimenteller und klinischer Herzhypertrophie

B. E. Strauer and *S. B. Bürger*

With 5 figures and 2 tables

Summary

The degree of LV hypertrophy may be determined by the relationships between mass-to-volume ratio and systolic wall stress. Systolic wall stress correlates directly with the MVO_2 and inversely with LV function. In chronic hypertrophic heart disease (a) normal stress, (b) low stress and (c) high stress hypertrophy may occur. Low stress hypertrophy has normal LV function and normal or decreased MVO_2, whereas high stress hypertrophy mostly has depressed function and an increased MVO_2. The MVO_2 is directly correlated to LV mass. This relationship is influenced by the variable degree of LV mass, by the mass-to-volume ratio and by inotropic interventions. Systolic stress reserve, the ratio of maximum to instantaneous systolic wall stress, averages 4.5. Similar reserves are present for the coronary (4.9) and for the metabolic reserve (4.6). It is concluded that systolic wall stress represents one of the major determinants of LV performance and of myocardial oxygen consumption.

Left ventricular functional reserve and working capacity depend on the heart's ability to appropriately increase (a) myocardial oxygen consumption and (b) coronary blood flow secondary to changes in (c) myocardial performance. Consequently, close relationships between these three variables ought to be expected for the normal, hypertrophied and dilated ventricular myocardium. This study was therefore aimed at investigating:
1. the appropriateness or degree of left ventricular (LV) hypertrophy in chronic hypertrophic heart disease,
2. the relationships between systolic wall stress, mass-to-volume ratio and ventricular function,
3. the influence of LV geometry on myocardial oxygen consumption and coronary blood flow, and
4. the quantification of three reserve capacities of the heart, i.e., the systolic stress reserve, the metabolic reserve and the coronary reserve.

---

*) Supported by the Deutsche Forschungsgemeinschaft

Materials and methods

Studies were carried out in a total of 301 patients with normal LV function and with various diseases of the heart. Methodological details have been published previously (1–5, 7, 8, 11–14). Quantitative ventriculography was performed in all patients. Wall stress was calculated frame by frame from ventriculograms until the peak value (maximum) of circumferential systolic wall stress was obtained (9, 11–13). LV mass and LV mass-to-volume ratio were determined from enddiastolic chamber dimensions. Coronary blood flow was determined by the argon method with gas chromatographic analysis of argon in the arterial and coronary sinus blood (1, 2, 11–14).

In a second study, LV function and LV geometry were determined in 52 normotensive and in 64 spontaneously hypertensive rats (SHR, strain Okamoto-Aoki) in situ (3). The age of rats varied 15–70 weeks for both groups. Details of methods have been described elsewhere (3). LV pressures and LV wall dynamics were analyzed (a) for control conditions (auxotonic), (b) for isometric contractions (aortic clamping) and (c) under the influence of pharmacological interventions: norepinephrine (2–5 µg/kg · min), isoprenaline (2–5 µg/kg · min) and propranolol (2–10 mg/kg).

Results

I. Stress and function

LV size as determined by the enddiastolic volume showed an inverse relationship with LV function as evidenced by the LV ejection fraction (fig. 1). Similar relationships were present between the enddiastolic vol-

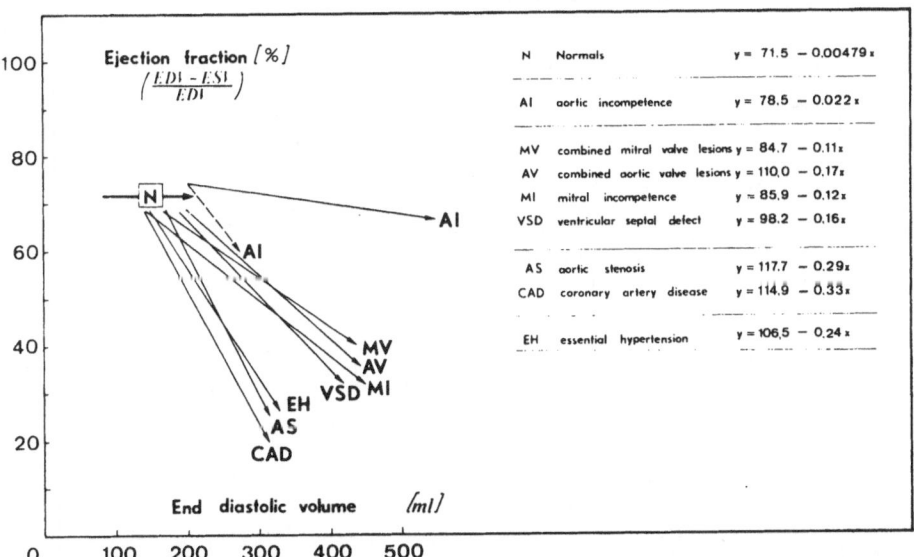

Fig. 1. Relationship between the enddiastolic volume and the left ventricular ejection fraction in normals as well as in various diseases of the human heart (n = 400) (11). Linear correlation between both variables was assumed. Note the quite different course of regression lines in (a) pure volume overload, (b) combined valvular and septal defects and (c) pressure overload as well as in coronary artery disease.

ume and time or velocity-related auxotonic ejection phase parameters (MNSER: mean normalized systolic ejection rate, V_{CF}: mean circumferential fiber shortening (11). With increase in enddiastolic volume the ejection fraction decreased for all patient groups. However, steepness of this characteristic was quite different: lowest decrease in LV function with increase in enddiastolic volume was present for volume-overloaded aortic incompetence, whereas largest decrease was found for chronic pressure overload due to aortic stenosis and essential hypertension as well as for coronary artery disease. This means that considerable decrease in LV function occurs at an only small LV enlargement in chronic pressure overload and in coronary artery disease, whereas in chronic volume overload even large increase in LV size may have normal LV function. The different course of these characteristics most probably may be related to different contractile state and/or to different loading conditions of the left ventricle. At an equal enddiastolic volume an increase in contractility increases shortening and hence the LV ejection fraction. Likewise therapeutic reduction of afterload may enhance LV function. The opposite effects should be expected with negatively inotropic interventions, with an increase in afterload and with abnormal increase or decrease in LV preload. Thus, it seems probable that the different course of this relationship in chronic volume and pressure overload reflects different LV performance (11). From the diagnostic point of view, these relationships may help to evaluate LV function from the heart size of chest X-rays, provided the reason for LV hypertrophy is known (11) (e.g., pressure overload, volume overload, coronary artery disease).

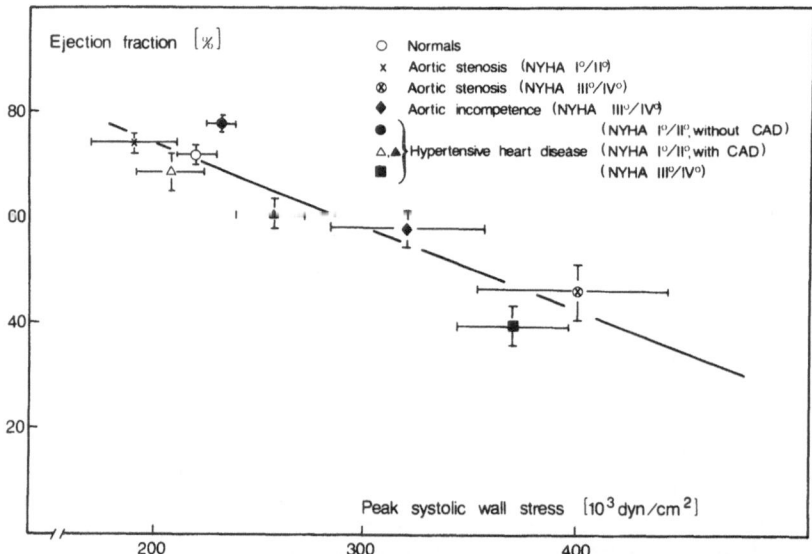

Fig. 2. Relationship between peak systolic circumferential wall stress of the left ventricle and the LV ejection fraction. Note the inverse behavior of both variables indicating decrease in LV function with increase in LV afterload (systolic wall stress).

Except for changes in contractility, the altered LV loading conditions may decrease LV function with increase in heart size. At comparable systolic pressure and mass an increase in enddiastolic volume leads to an increase in systolic wall stress. Accordingly, the relationship between wall stress and function has been determined for a large number of patients with chronic pressure and volume overload (fig. 2). With increase in systolic wall stress the ejection fraction markedly decreased. Doubling of stress led to reduction in the LV ejection fraction by approximately 50 per cent. Since systolic wall stress results from systolic pressure and mass-to-volume ratio, it equals the afterload which is imposed to the left ventricular wall. It therefore may be concluded that heart size, i.e. enddiastolic volume, and systolic wall stress are important determinants of left ventricular performance (14).

II. Myocardial oxygen consumption

Myocardial oxygen consumption which was determined in a total of 251 patients was lowest in the normotensive patients with coronary vasculitis, it was normal in concentric and clinically compensated LV hypertrophy, and it was largest in dilated hearts with aortic valve disease (table 1). There was no correlation between the oxygen consumption and ventricular function parameters, as cardiac index, isovolumic contractility indices and ejection phase parameters.

Total LV oxygen consumption was linearly related to total LV muscle mass in the normals and in chronic LV overload (14). At comparable LV mass an increased oxygen consumption occurred in high stress hypertro-

Table 1. Tabular representation of left ventricular (LV) ejection fraction, LV mass, LV mass-to-volume ratio, peak systolic circumferential wall stress (T_{syst}), myocardial oxygen consumption per weight unit (MVO_2) and total oxygen consumption (LVO_2). CAD = coronary artery disease, SVD = small vessel disease (coronary and systemic immune vasculitis at normal coronary arteriogram), AS = aortic stenosis, AI = aortic incompetence, HOC = hypertrophic obstructive cardiomyopathy, EH = essential hypertension, MI = mitral incompetence, MV = combined mitral valve lesions.

	N=	EJECTION FRACTION [%]	LV MASS [GM/M^2]	LV MASS TO VOLUME RATIO [GM/ML]	T_{SYST} [10^3 DYN/CM^2]	$M\dot{V}O_2$ [$ML/MIN \cdot 100$ G]	$L\dot{V}O_2$ [ML/MIN]
NORMALS	12	72 ± 2	92 ± 6	1.21 ± 0.12	220 ± 9	7.98 ± 0.52	13.3 ± 2.1
CAD	36	52 ± 11	145 ± 22ˣ	1.12 ± 0.16	236 ± 18	7.9 ± 0.39	20.6 ± 3.2
SVD	8	69 ± 8	84 ± 14	1.18 ± 0.21	206 ± 22	6.4 ± 0.6ˣ	9.7 ± 0.91ˣ
AS*	6	74 ± 4	145 ± 10ˣˣ	2.1 ± 0.31	192 ± 23	8.1 ± 0.8	21.1 ± 2.3ˣˣ
AS**	9	46 ± 11	190 ± 17•	1.01 ± 0.11	396 ± 95ˣˣ	14.9 ± 1.6•	51.0 ± 6.9•
AI	12	58 ± 7	174 ± 22•	1.12 ± 0.13	329 ± 36ˣ	14.2 ± 1.4•	45.4 ± 4.7•
HOC	12	78 ± 6	~228	~3.78	142 ± 52	8.6 ± 1.21	35.3 ± 3.6
EH	92	62 ± 6	152 ± 12•	1.52 ± 0.33	266 ± 18ˣˣ	10.7 ± 0.38•	29.3 ± 4.1•
MI	20	63 ± 9	132 ± 11ˣ	1.19 ± 0.09	267 ± 11ˣ	9.82 ± 0.21ˣˣ	21.6 ± 0.92
MV	44	62 ± 12	149 ± 9ˣˣ	1.20 ± 0.10	248 ± 32ˣ	9.22 ± 0.99ˣ	24.9 ± 2.9ˣ

AS* : CLINICALLY COMPENSATED (NYHA I°/ II°), CONCENTRIC HYPERTROPHY
AS**: CLINICALLY DECOMPENSATED (NYHA III°/ IV°), LV DILATATION

ˣ p <0.05   ˣˣ p <0.01   • p < 0.001

phy due to compensated aortic stenosis and aortic incompetence, whereas decreased oxygen consumption was found for coronary artery disease with aneurysm and for coronary vasculitis. In other words: there was significant relationship between the LV mass and the oxygen consumption in the normals and in clinically compensated hypertrophy, and there was lower or greater oxygen consumption relative to muscle mass when stress or myocardial viability were affected (table 1).

The mass-to-volume ratio was inversely related to the myocardial oxygen consumption per mass unit (table 1). At isobaric conditions largest mass-to-volume ratio and lowest oxygen consumption was found in hypertrophic obstructive cardiomyopathy, whereas in decompensated aortic stenosis and aortic incompetence lowest mass-to-volume ratio was associated with largest myocardial oxygen consumption. Normotensive patients with normal LV function or with coronary artery disease were shifted to lower oxygen consumption at comparable mass-to-volume ratio.

Since the mass-to-volume ratio, at equal systolic pressure, represents the major determinant of systolic wall stress, correlation was performed between stress (x) and oxygen consumption (y). A significant relationship was found between both variables (y = 3.28 ± 0.028 x, r = 0.78) (9, 10). Patients with decompensated aortic valve disease were within the upper range, and the normotensive normals were within the lower range of this

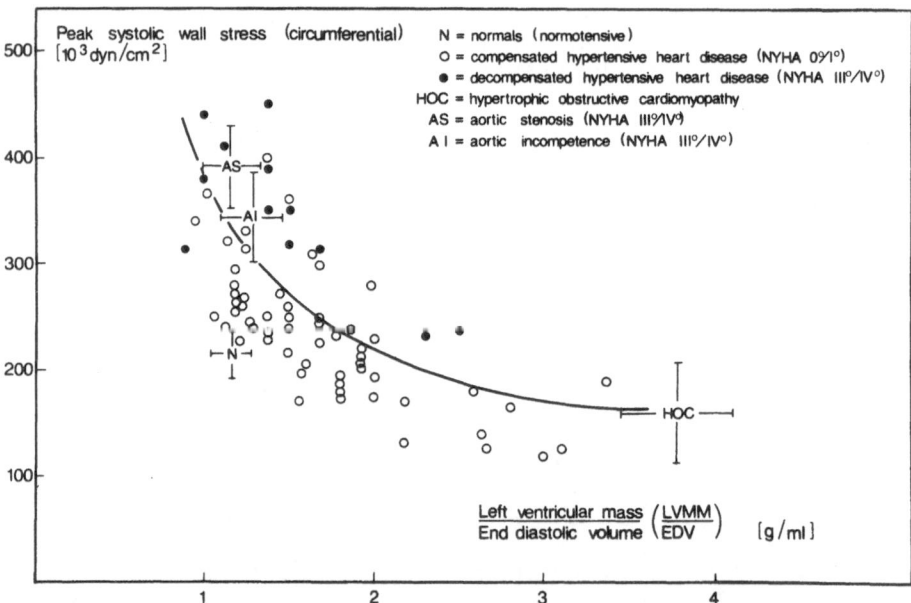

Fig. 3. Relationship between the LV mass-to-volume ratio and peak systolic circumferential wall stress. The curve represents mean values of patients with hypertensive (hypertrophic) heart disease (n = 92). Unilinear relationship was present for all patient groups investigated. Patient groups with nonhypertensive (= normotensive) hypertrophic heart disease are characterized by an isobaric curve, which is shifted to lower stress at comparable LVMM/EDV ratio, or to higher LVMM/EDV ratio at comparable wall stress respectively (see fig. 4).

relationship. Extrapolation to zero stress resulted in an intercept of 3.28 ml/min × 100 g. This value, though somewhat higher, corresponds quite well with the oxygen consumption of the empty beating heart. Steepness of this regression indicates an increase in the myocardial oxygen consumption by 2.8 ml/min × 100 g per an increase in systolic stress by 100 (10^3 dyn/cm^2) for the normals as well as for coronary artery disease and hypertrophic heart disease.

III. Appropriateness of LV hypertrophy

In patient groups with hypertrophic heart disease an inverse relationship existed between the mass-to-volume ratio and peak systolic wall stress (fig. 3). The largest mass-to-volume ratio was found in hypertrophic obstructive cardiomyopathy, and lowest values were present in decompensated pressure and volume overload. Concentric LV hypertrophy due to essential hypertension and aortic stenosis was within this correlation, whereas normotensives were shifted to lower systolic stress at equal mass-to-volume ratio, that is, to a lower isobaric relationship.

With regard to this characteristic, at least 3 types of LV hypertrophy may be separated in chronic hypertrophic heart disease:
1. appropriate hypertrophy which keeps systolic wall stress normal even at extreme pressure load, as a result of an appropriate increase in the mass-to-volume ratio parallel to pressure load,
2. inappropriate, i.e., low-stress hypertrophy, which is associated with marked increase in LV mass out of proportion to intraventricular volume (e.g. HOC), and

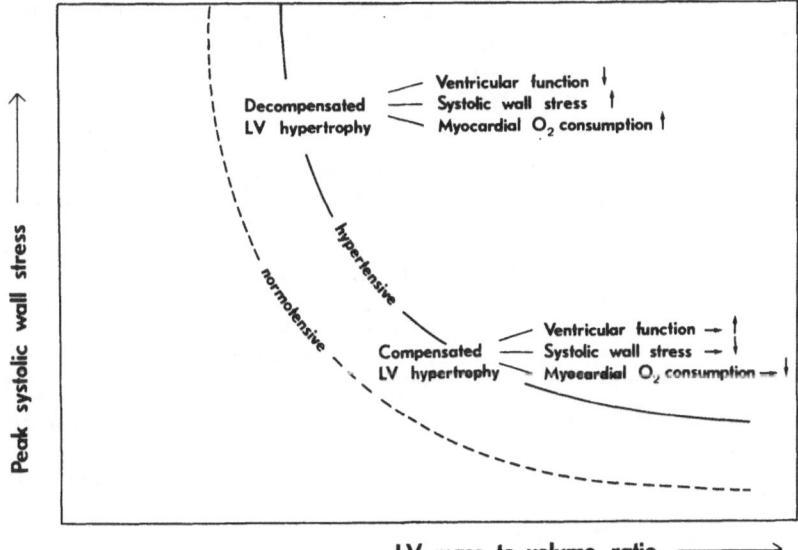

Fig. 4. Diagrammatic representation of the relationship between the LV mass-to-volume ratio (abscissa) and peak systolic circumferential wall stress (ordinate) at hypertensive and normotensive isobarics for different degrees (appropriateness) of LV hypertrophy (compensated, decompensated).

3. inappropriate, i.e., high-stress hypertrophy, which is characterized by excess dilatation out of proportion to ventricular mass development (e.g., decompensated volume and pressure overload). Thus, at least 2 forms of inappropriate hypertrophy may occur in chronic hypertrophic heart disease.

From the metabolic point of view, high-stress hypertrophy has increased oxygen consumption per unit mass with an impairment of LV function (fig. 4). In contrast, low-stress hypertrophy may have normal or even decreased oxygen consumption per LV mass unit with normal LV function. This may help to explain, for example, the existence of normal, decreased or increased oxygen consumption per unit LV mass in chronic pressure or volume overload: despite large pressure load, the oxygen consumption may be normal or even decreased in aortic stenosis as long as heart size and systolic wall stress are normal or decreased respectively. On the other hand, the same pressure load may have high oxygen consumption, when LV dilatation occurs and when systolic wall stress increases.

IV. Cardiac reserves

Lowest wall stress, which was found in compensated essential hypertension, averaged 100 ± 12 and largest stress was 450 ± 46 (10^3 dyn/cm^2) for decompensated hypertensive heart disease (table 2). The ratio of the maximum and minimum stress was 4.5. Similar range, i.e., 4.9, was present for the coronary reserve. Furthermore, quantitatively similar values were also obtained for the metabolic reserve, i.e., for the ratio of maximum and minimum oxygen consumption in compensated and decompensated pressure overload (4.6). It is obvious from these findings, that the human heart has a maximum 4.5 range in chronically increasing its systolic wall stress. This will lead to a similar increase in myocardial oxygen needs, which almost exclusively have to be covered by an adequate increase in

Table 2. Stress reserve, metabolic reserve and coronary vascular reserve (= coronary reserve) of the human heart based on the assessment of minimum and maximum systolic wall stress (T_{syst}), myocardial oxygen consumption (MVO_2) and coronary blood flow of the left ventricle (V_{cor}). Note the quantitatively similar values for all of the three reserves.

		MINIMUM	MAXIMUM	$\dfrac{\text{MAXIMUM}}{\text{MINIMUM}}$		
T_{SYST}	[10^3 DYN/CM^2] [*]	100 ± 12	450 ± 46	4,5	=	STRESS RESERVE
MVO_2	[ML/MIN · 100 G] [**]	$5,2 \pm 0,3$	$24 \pm 2,9$	4,6	=	METABOLIC RESERVE
V_{COR}	[ML/MIN · 100 G] [***]	79 ± 12	392 ± 26	4,9	=	CORONARY RESERVE

[*] ESSENTIAL HYPERTENSION. [**] CHRONIC VALVULAR AND HYPERTENSIVE PRESSURE OVERLOAD.

[***] NORMALS (BEFORE AND AFTER DIPYRIDAMOLE : 0,5 MG/KG)

coronary flow (1). It may be likely to assume that the quantitative similarity of stress and metabolic and coronary reserves may have its clinical significance in the close relationship of these 3 reserves to each other, even if factors other than wall stress may influence myocardial oxygen consumption in hypertrophic heart disease.

With regard to this concept, low initial wall stress would be associated with large stress reserve, whereas the latter would be reduced at high initial stress. With an increased wall stress, both, the myocardial oxygen consumption and coronary blood flow would also be increased, thus limiting the corresponding metabolic and coronary reserves. Consequently, the evaluation of one of these reserves, i.e., of the stress, the metabolic or the coronary reserve, would be appropriate in evaluating a correlate for the heart's working capacity.

In studies on isolated human ventricular myocardium, which was obtained during prosthetic mitral valve replacements from patients with LV hypertrophy due to mitral valve disease, the maximum tension development at L_{max} averaged 5–6 g/mm^2. This would approximately correspond to wall stress values of about 500–600 (10^3 dyn/cm^2) (fig. 5). Assuming similar maximum wall stress, the stress reserve could be defined as the ratio of maximum to initial wall stress (12). By inotropic interventions an alteration in systolic stress reserve could be obtained, since maximum systolic wall stress (T_{max}) is reduced (negative inotropism) or increased (positive inotropism). Likewise, shifts of the isobaric curves

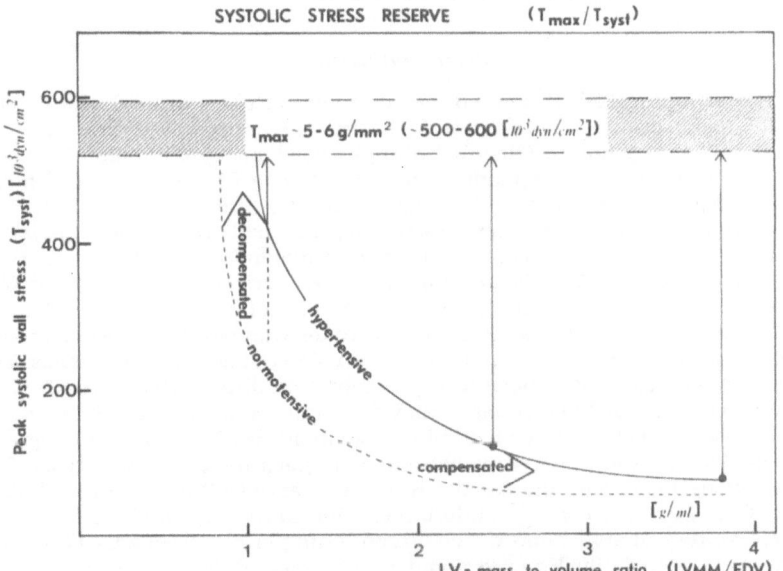

Fig. 5. Relationship between the LVMM/EDV ratio and peak systolic circumferential wall stress. The hatched region represents the maximum stress which may be developed by the intact ventricle. The value of 500–600 (10^3 dyn/cm^2) is estimated from experiments in hypertrophied, isolated human ventricular myocardium as well as on experiments in normotensive (nonhypertrophic) and on hypertensive (hypertrophic) rats.

at different systolic pressure would probably lead to an increase (lowering of systolic pressure) or decrease (systolic pressure rise) of systolic stress reserve (fig. 5).

In order to confirm this clinical concept of systolic stress reserve, the mass-to-volume ratio and systolic wall stress were analyzed in 52 normotensive and 64 hypertrophied spontaneously hypertensive rats (SHR) in situ (3). Systolic stress reserve (aortic clamping) was 2.5-fold for both the normotensive rats and the concentrically hypertrophied SHR. 60–70 week-old, decompensating SHR had higher initial stress values and lower stress reserve. Stress reserve could be altered by 20–40 percent under inotropic interventions to lower and greater values respectively: propranolol reduced maximum systolic wall stress dose-dependently by 20–40 percent, while maximum systolic wall stress was increased by norepinephrine or isoprenaline by 20–25 percent. Higher doses of norepinephrine (more than 10 μg per kg per min) resulted in no further increase in stress reserve, because initial systolic wall stress increased markedly by an increase in systolic pressure, while maximum systolic wall stress showed no further increase thus resulting in a decrease in stress reserve. Maximum systolic wall stress after rapid volume load (40 ml/kg × min until reaching peak cardiac output) and aortic clamping was approximately 500×10^3 dyn/cm^2 in normotensive rats and in compensated SHR, thus approximately corresponding to the maximum tension development of isolated ventricular myocardium. Stress reserve under these conditions was 3.1-fold in both normotensive rats and in compensated SHR.

Zusammenfassung

Der Hypertrophiegrad wird von der Beziehung zwischen Masse–Volumen–Relation und Wandspannung determiniert. Es besteht eine direkte Beziehung zwischen systolischer Wandspannung (Nachbelastung) und dem myokardialen Sauerstoffverbrauch. Systolische Wandspannung und Funktionsgrößen des linken Ventrikels (Auswurffraktion, zeitnormierte Auswurfparameter) sind invers korreliert. Am chronisch hypertrophierten Herzen lassen sich prinzipiell drei Hypertrophieformen voneinander abgrenzen: (a) Hypertrophie mit normaler Wandspannung, (b) Hypertrophie mit erniedrigter Wandspannung und (c) Hypertrophie mit erhöhter Wandspannung. Bei niedriger Wandspannung sind Ventrikelfunktion und myokardialer Sauerstoffverbrauch normal, während bei erhöhter Wandspannung Abnahmen der Ventrikelfunktion und Zunahmen des myokardialen Sauerstoffverbrauches auftreten. Bei vergleichbarer Wandspannung besteht eine direkte Beziehung zwischen der linksventrikulären Muskelmasse und dem linksventrikulären Sauerstoffverbrauch. Diese Beziehung ist vom Funktionszustand des Myokards abhängig. Die systolische Wandspannungsreserve beträgt am hypertrophierten Herzen 4,5. Quantitativ ähnliche Reserven sind für die Koronarreserve (4,9) und die metabolische Reserve (4,6) nachweisbar. Veränderungen der koronaren und metabolischen Reserven werden überwiegend durch Veränderungen der Mechanik (Wandspannungsreserve) beeinflußt. Es wird somit geschlossen, daß die systolische Wandspannung (Nachbelastung) eine der wesentlichen Determinanten der Ventrikelfunktion und des myokardialen Energiebedarfes repräsentiert.

References

1. *Bretschneider, H. J., L. Cott, G. Hilgert, R. Probst, G. Rau:* Gaschromatographische Trennung und Analyse von Argon als Basis einer neuen Fremdgas-

methode zur Durchblutungsmessung von Organen. Verh. dtsch. Ges. Kreislaufforschg. **32**, 267 (1966).

2. *Bretschneider, H. J., G. Hellige:* Pathophysiologie der Ventrikelkontraktion – Kontraktilität, Suffizienzgrad und Arbeitsökonomie des Herzens. Verh. dtsch. Ges. Kreislaufforschg. **42**, 14 (1976).

3. *Bürger, S. B., A. Meinardus, B. E. Strauer:* Hypertrophiegrad und Dynamik des linken Ventrikels bei der spontanen essentiellen Hypertonie der Ratte. Klin. Wschr. **56**, 207 (1978).

4. *Kochsiek, K., H. W. Heiss, M. Tauchert, B. E. Strauer:* Koronarreserve und Sauerstoffverbrauch bei hypertrophischer obstruktiver Cardiomyopathie. Verh. dtsch. Ges. inn. Med. **77**, 880 (1971).

5. *Kochsiek, K., M. Tauchert, L. Cott, J. Neubaur:* Die Koronarreserve bei Patienten mit Aortenvitien. Verh. dtsch. Ges. inn. Med. **76**, 214 (1970).

6. *Linzbach, A. J.:* Heart failure from the point of view of quantitative anatomy. Amer. J. Cardiol. **5**, 370 (1960).

7. *Strauer, B. E., I. Brune, H. Schenk, D. Knoll, E. Perings:* Lupus cardiomyopathy: Cardiac mechanics, hemodynamics, and coronary blood flow in uncomplicated systemic lupus erythematosus. Amer. Heart J. **92**, 715 (1976).

8. *Strauer, B. E., A. Scherpe:* Ventricular function in coronary hemodynamics after intravenous nitroglycerin in coronary artery disease. Amer. Heart J. **95**, 210 (1978).

9. *Strauer, B. E., S. B. Bürger:* Dynamic geometry of the left ventricle in essential hypertension. Circulation **56**, (Suppl. II) III–451 (1977).

10. *Strauer, B. E., K. H. Heitlinger, S. B. Bürger:* Coronary hemodynamics and myocardial oxygen consumption in essential hypertension. Circulation **56** (Suppl. II) III–818 (1977).

11. *Strauer, B. E.:* Änderungen der Kontraktilität bei Druck- und Volumenbelastungen des Herzens. Verh. dtsch. Ges. Kreislaufforschg. **42**, 69 (1976).

12. *Strauer, B. E.:* Das Hochdruckherz. (Berlin–Heidelberg–New York 1979).

13. *Strauer, B. E., K. Beer, K. Heitlinger, B. Höfling:* Left ventricular systolic wall stress as a primary determinant of myocardial oxygen consumption: Comparative studies in patients with normal left ventricular function, with pressure and volume overload and with coronary heart disease. Basic Res. Cardiol. **72**, 306 (1977).

14. *Strauer, B. E.:* Myocardial O_2 consumption in chronic heart disease: The role of wall stress, hypertrophy and coronary reserve. Amer. J. Cardiol. **44**, 730 (1979).

Authors' address:

Prof. Dr. *B. E. Strauer,* Department of Medicine, University of Munich, Klinikum Großhadern, Marchioninistraße 15, D-8000 München 70

Basic Res. Cardiol. **75**, 244–252 (1980)
© 1980 Dr. Dietrich Steinkopff Verlag Darmstadt
ISSN 0300-8428

Paper, presented at the Erwin Riesch Symposium, Tübingen, April 3–7, 1979

Physiologisches Institut II, Universität Tübingen

Contracture type and fibrosis type of decreased myocardial distensibility. Different changes in elasticity of myocardium in hypoxia and hypertrophy*)

Kontraktur- und Fibrosetyp bei verminderter myokardialer Dehnbarkeit. Unterschiedliche Veränderungen der Elastizität des Myokards bei Hypoxie und Hypertrophie

Ch. Holubarsch

With 4 figures and 2 tables

Summary

Resting length-tension relationships were measured in rat trabecular muscle strips under control (O_2) and contracture (N_2) conditions as well as in preparations of Goldblatt II (8-week stage) and control rats. For the evaluation of the diastolic elastic properties, diastolic stress at l_{max}, stress-strain relationships, the relation between tangent modulus $\dfrac{\Delta\sigma}{\Delta\varepsilon}$ and stress σ, and the function ln stress $\sigma = f$ (strain ε) were calculated and plotted. It was shown that the hypoxic contracture corresponds to the calcium-caffeine contracture – an experimental contracture model already investigated earlier. In contrast to these contracture-induced alterations, Goldblatt II hypertrophied myocardium corresponded to the fibrosis type. This type was already analyzed in an experimental model of myocardium-tendon tandem preparation. Additional investigations of hydroxyproline concentration of the same biological material showed in contrast to other studies that the collagen content may already be increased in this early stage of hypertrophy. Thus, altered distensibility of Goldblatt myocardium is certainly primarily due to increased connective tissue content.

Diastolic pressure-volume relationships can be changed either by acute interventions, such as hypoxia, or by chronic heart diseases, such as pressure-induced hypertrophy. In the latter case, alterations in chamber geometry and wall thickness have to be distinguished from those in diastolic elastic properties of the myocardial tissue itself. In order to recognize such changes of myocardial elasticity, resting length-tension relationships of nonhypertrophied muscle strip preparations were measured under control and hypoxic conditions, and hypertrophied myocardium of Goldblatt II rats was also investigated.

---

*) Supported by the Deutsche Forschungsgemeinschaft

These results were compared with those of earlier studies of experimental models of contracture and fibrosis. Using heart muscle strips, two experimental models of alterations of diastolic myocardial elasticity were analyzed by means of stress-strain relationships and the relation between tangent elastic modulus $\frac{\Delta\sigma}{\Delta\varepsilon}$ and stress σ (9; 10). Firstly, a shift of the stress-strain relationship was observed in the contracture-type (induced by the application of 10 mM caffeine and 7.5 mM calcium) without any significant alteration of the slope of the linear $\frac{\Delta\sigma}{\Delta\varepsilon} = f(\sigma)$ function. Secondly, in the experimental fibrosis model (i.e., a tandem preparation of healthy myocardium and a tendonous tissue strip), both the stress-strain relationship and the slope of the $\frac{\Delta\sigma}{\Delta\varepsilon} = f(\sigma)$ function were significantly shifted.

In this study, we intended to examine whether changes of myocardial distensibility of hypoxic and hypertrophied myocardium can be recognized and attributed to one or the other of the above types.

Methods

Experimental procedures and model preparations

Myocardial trabeculae were taken from the left ventricle of Wistar rats having a body weight between 160 and 240 g. The animals were anesthetized with urethane (2.5 g/kg body weight). Both ends of the muscle strips were fixed to small steel hooks by means of ligatures, and the preparations were arranged in a muscle bath perfused with tyrode solution (NaCl 130.5, NaH_2PO_4 0.83, $NaHCO_3$ 20.0, KCl 4.9, glucose 23.7 mM, bubbled with 95 % O_2 and 5 % CO_2, 32 °C). The myocardial muscle strips were stimulated using a frequency of 0.2 Hz, and contracted isometrically. After a recovery period of one hour, length-tension relationships were recorded by stepwise releases of 0.1 mm every 30 sec from l_{max} (i.e., the muscle length at which developed tension is maximum). This procedure was repeated three times in each muscle preparation.

Contracture was induced by the administration of 7.5 mM calcium and 10 mM caffeine (9). In these muscles, diastolic stress at l_{max} doubles 20 to 40 min after the pharmacological intervention.

Under these contracture conditions, length-tension relationships were also recorded in the same manner described above.

A simple fibrosis model was created by arranging a strip preparation of healthy myocardium in series with a strip of tendon from the M. digitorum II or Achilles tendon, both preparations with almost the same cross-sectional area. After recording 4 length-tension relationships, the single portions of the tandem preparation were decoupled, and length-tension curves were recorded separately from both the tendonous and the myocardial strips.

Hypoxic and hypertrophied myocardium

In order to produce hypoxic contracture, heart rate was increased to 1.0 Hz, and tyrode solution was bubbled with 95 % N_2 and 5 % CO_2. Thus an average increase of resting tension was observed at l_{max} of about 40%. Length-tension relationships were recorded again as described above.

Arterial hypertension was induced in Wistar rats (body weight 150 g) by narrowing the left renal artery using silver clips (Goldblatt II). When blood pressure was measured by the tail cuff method under ether narcosis, values of 180 mm Hg were exceeded. The increase of left ventricular muscle mass was relatively small when absolute mass values were compared, but high (85 %) when ventricular mass values were related to body weight. 8 weeks after renal artery coarctation, length-tension relationships were measured from myocardial muscle strips of control and hypertrophied left ventricles. In order to avoid possible errors due to different sizes of muscle strip preparations, 8 pairs of preparations were chosen with almost the same dimensions from control and hypertrophied hearts, respectively, as shown in table 1.

Evaluation of passive elastic properties

In order to keep distortion of the length-tension data by plastic and viscoelastic effects to a minimum, tension values were taken from 0.1 mm releases 30 sec after stress relaxation. (1) Stress σ was calculated (F/A) and related to strain ε, which was evaluated by $(l-l_0)/l_0$. The muscle length at zero stress is l_0, which was measured after registration of the third length-tension relationship in each experiment. (2) The tangent elastic modulus $\frac{\Delta\sigma}{\Delta\varepsilon}$ was also calculated for each measured point of the length-tension relationship, and related to stress σ (σ = b(σ – c)) (19).

The slope b was determined by means of linear regression analysis. (3) The natural logarithm of stress σ (ln σ) was calculated and plotted as a function of strain ε. As already shown by *Little* (16) and *Kitabatake* (15), a linear function was observed in the range of 0.10 < ε < 0.35.

For details of investigations of hydroxyproline concentration see (17).

Results

In earlier studies, it was shown that the application of 10 mM caffeine and 7.5 mM calcium induces a shift of stress-strain relationships in myocardial muscle strips of rats and cats (9). In contrast to this shift, figure 1 shows schematically the unaltered relation between the tangent elastic modulus and stress σ, whereas the ln σ = f (strain σ) function shows a clear parallel shift without any change of the slope of the linear function.

In figure 2, the summarized results from 8 muscle strip preparations under control and hypoxic contracture conditions are illustrated. Although the plots of the averaged stress-strain relationships differ clearly under both conditions and stress σ at l_{max} was increased significantly by

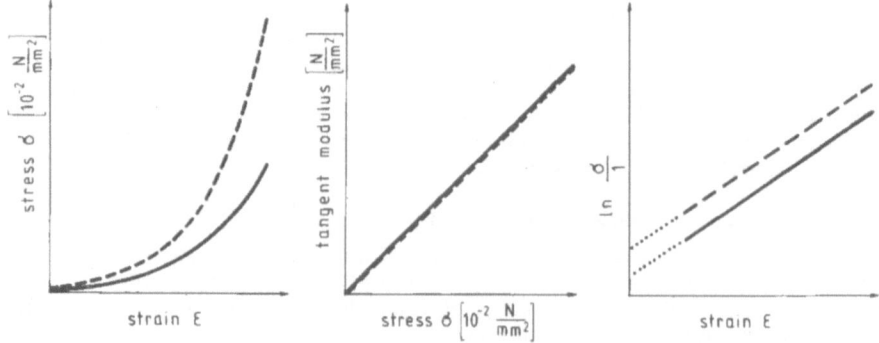

Fig. 1. Stress-strain relationships (left), tangent modulus versus stress σ (middle), and ln σ versus strain ε (right) under control (—) and calcium-caffeine contracture conditions (– – – –). Schematic plots according to *Holubarsch* and *Jacob* (9).

Table 1.

	Controls	Goldblatt II
Muscle length	5.94 ± 1.24 mm	6.00 ± 1.36 mm
Cross-sectional area	0.62 ± 0.13 mm^2	0.59 ± 0.15 mm^2
Developed tension at l_{max} (stimulation frequency 0.2 Hz)	$6.18 \pm 0.91 \cdot 10^{-2}$ N/mm^2	$8.55 \pm 1.25 \cdot 10^{-2}$ N/mm^2

40 %, the relation between the tangent elastic modulus and stress is not significantly altered as already shown in the calcium caffeine contracture. In the right diagram of figure 2, the plot of ln stress σ against strain ε results in a parallel shift of the linear function.

In order to simulate myocardial fibrosis, myocardial muscle strips were arranged in series with strips of tendon (10). The stress-strain relationships of these tandem experiments are schematically shown in figure 3. In contrast to the contracture experiments, both the slope of the tangent modulus – based on stress σ – as well as the slope of the ln stress σ = f (strain ε) function are significantly altered when compared to normal myocardium.

Resting length-tension relationships of myocardium were measured in 12 Goldblatt und 12 control rats 8 weeks after coarctation of the left renal artery. 8 pairs of muscle strips were chosen for evaluation of stress-strain relationships (see methods). Diastolic stress values measured at l_{max} were 80 % higher in hypertrophied than in control myocardium. It is evident from figure 4 that the shift of stress-strain relationships is accompanied by a significant increase of the slope $\dfrac{\Delta \sigma}{\Delta \varepsilon} = f (\sigma)$ and the ln σ = f (ε) functions.

Because of the similarity of the results of the fibrosis model and Goldblatt myocardium, a fibrosis in the Goldblatt myocardium was assumed as the cause of diminished distensibility. In order to check this assumption,

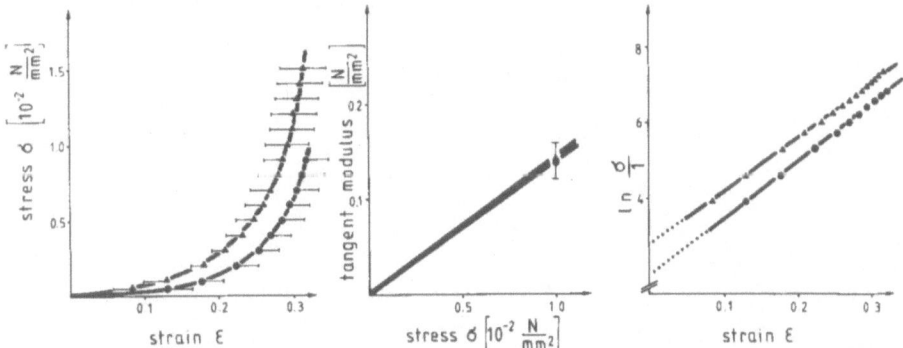

Fig. 2. Stress-strain relationships (left), tangent modulus versus stress σ (middle), and ln σ versus strain ε (right) under control (- ● - ● -) and hypoxic contracture (▲-▲-▲-▲-) conditions. Stress and strain values obtained from 8 experiments. Horizontal and vertical bars represent standard deviation.

Table 2. Hydroxyproline concentrations.

Control hearts	Goldblatt hearts (8 weeks after coarctation)	
2.36 ± 0.22 µg/mg dry weight	2.92 ± 0.15 µg/mg dry weight	
n = 8	n = 8	(p < 0.001)

hydroxyproline concentrations were evaluated from the left ventricular wall of the same Goldblatt and control rat hearts (17). As table 2 shows, hydroxyproline concentration is significantly higher in Goldblatt than in control myocardium in this investigated specimen.

Discussion

There is general agreement about the effect of caffeine on skeletal and heart muscle resulting in twitch potentiation and contracture development (literature see (9)). The effect of this drug on SR functioning as the structural mediator of sarcoplasmic calcium levels – is such that the calcium uptake by the SR is diminished or slowed. This effect leads to an increased sarcoplasmic calcium level during diastole and development of contracture tension.

In contrast to the caffeine-calcium contracture, myocardial metabolism is substantially changed under conditions of hypoxia. The resulting reduction of ATP has been described manifoldly in hypoxic as well as in ischemic contracture (7; 8; 13; 14; 20). Three possible basic mechanisms have to be discussed to explain hypoxic contracture. (1) ATP deficiency is so severe that rigor complexes are generated. (2) ATP deficiency impairs calcium uptake by the SR resulting in increased sarcoplasmic calcium levels, i.e., hypoxic contracture is comparable with the caffeine calcium contracture (12). (3) Decrease of sarcoplasmic ATP levels and Mg^{2+} concentrations can change the pCa-tension relationship of the contractile proteins and therefore increase actual diastolic stress without any change of the sarcoplasmic calcium concentration in diastole (6; 21). But two

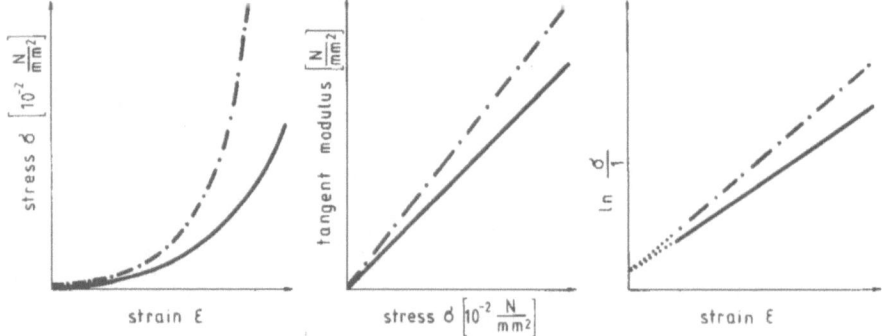

Fig. 3. Stress-strain relationships (left), tangent modulus versus stress σ (middle) and ln σ versus strain ε (right) of normal myocardium (———) and tendon-myocardium tandem preparation (27 % tendonous portion at l_{max}, – · – · – · –). Schematic plots according to *Holubarsch* and *Jacob* (10).

assumptions have to be made for this third explanation: In the physiological situation, the sarcoplasmic calcium concentration should have a value in the range of pCa = 7, i.e., in the vicinity of the inferior part of the unaltered activation curve. Furthermore, the alteration of the intracellular pH should have a smaller effect on the activation curve than Mg^{2+} and ATP alterations, because the decreasing pH antagonizes the effects of Mg^{2+} and ATP diminutions on the activation curve, at least in the case of ischemic contracture.

Irregardless of the true cause of hypoxic contracture, the results indicate a formal similarity between hypoxic and calcium-caffeine contractures. In both conditions, stress-strain relationships are altered without significant changes of the slope b of the tangent elastic modulus plotted as a function of stress. Thus, each increase of $\dfrac{\Delta\sigma}{\Delta\varepsilon}$ is accompanied by a proportional increase of diastolic stress. Mathematical analysis reveals that the stress-strain relationship under contracture conditions can be considered as an affinitive transformation of the original resting stress-strain relationship.

Three methods are used in the literature for detecting alterations of diastolic elastic properties of hypertrophied myocardium. (1) The biochemical method is the evaluation of hydroxyproline. With this method, *Bartošová* et al. (2) found an increase of collagen tissue in the following models of hypertrophy: repeated isoprenaline injections, experimental aortic stenosis, long-term adaption to simulated altitude and long-term adaption to physical stress. With the same method *Buccino* et al. (5) also demonstrated an increase in collagen tissue in pulmonary artery stenosis. (2) Resting tension at l_{max} can indicate alterations of diastolic elastic properties of myocardium. *Bing* et al. (3) showed that resting tension at l_{max} is increased parallel with a significant increase of hydroxyproline concentration in hearts exposed to aortic arch constriction. On the other hand, *Spann* et al. (22) did not find any significant change of resting

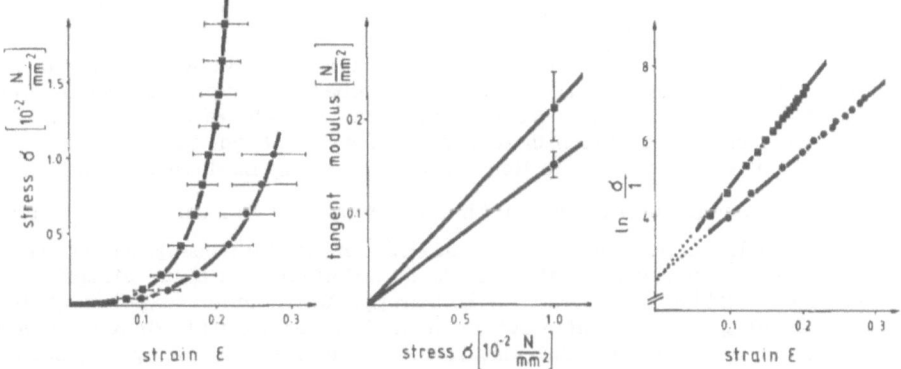

Fig. 4. Stress-strain relationships (left), tangent modulus versus stress σ (middle) and ln σ versus strain ε (right) of normal control myocardium (- ● - ● - ● -) and Goldblatt hypertrophied myocardium of the 8-week stage (- ■ - ■ - ■ -). Values were averaged from 8 experiments. Horizontal and vertical bars represent standard deviation.

tension in myocardium hypertrophied due to pulmonary artery constriction. (3) The evaluation of stress-strain relationships and tangent elastic modulus of resting myocardium is a further method. *Alpert* et al. (1) showed a significant increase in the slope of the elastic modulus versus stress for resting myocardium hypertrophied due to pulmonary artery stenosis.

Other factors, such as an increase in the ratio of contractile proteins to unit muscle mass or functional subcontracture (18), may also influence the resting hypertrophied myocardium. Therefore the purpose of this study was to compare resting tension values, stress-strain relationships, tangent elastic modulus based on stress and hydroxyproline concentrations. The results show that in the Goldblatt myocardium all parameters can be increased significantly as early as 8 weeks after renal artery coarctation. This also applies to the hydroxyproline concentration in contrast to another specimen investigated earlier (11). These results correspond excellently to our findings in the tandem fibrosis model. One must exercise caution, however, in comparing the presented model with hypertrophied myocardium, because tissues are arranged in series in the tandem preparation, whereas muscle and fibrous tissues can be arranged in series, and/or parallel with the contractile proteins in hypertrophied myocardium.

It is obvious that the increment of collagen tissue in Goldblatt hearts is not only due to the pressure overload as in other models of hypertrophy. The main source of the increase of collagen tissue has to be attributed to the alterations of coronary blood vessels, as already described by our group for the 24-week stage of Goldblatt hearts (23). This study and one paper of this issue (4), however, show that vasculopathy can occur in Goldblatt rats as early as 8 weeks after operation.

Acknowledgement

I wish to thank Dr. *I. Medugorac* for the determination of hydroxyproline concentrations.

Zusammenfassung

Ruhe-Dehnungs-Beziehungen wurden an Hand von 8 Rattentrabekeln unter Kontroll- (O_2) und Kontrakturbedingungen (N_2) ebenso wie von Präparaten von 8 Goldblatt-Herzen der Ratte (8-Wochen-Stadium) ermittelt. Zur Beurteilung der diastolischen elastischen Eigenschaften wurde die diastolische Spannung bei l_{max}, „stress-strain"-Beziehungen, die Relation zwischen tangentiellem Elastizitätsmodul $\frac{\Delta\sigma}{\Delta\varepsilon}$ und „stress" σ sowie die Funktion ln „stress" $\sigma = f$ (strain ε) errechnet und dargestellt. – Es zeigte sich, daß die hypoxische Kontraktur bezüglich der elastischen Eigenschaften vollständig der Calcium-Coffein-Kontraktur entspricht – einem bereits früher von unserer Arbeitsgruppe untersuchten experimentellen Modell. Demgegenüber konnten auf der Grundlage der Elastizitätsberechnungen die Veränderungen bei der Goldblatt-Hypertrophie dem Fibrosetyp zugeordnet werden; auch dieser Typ der Elastizitätsänderung war in vorausgegangenen Experimenten an Tandempräparaten, bestehend aus Sehne und Myokard, bereits analysiert worden. Zusätzliche Hydroxyprolin-Bestimmungen an demselben Experimentiergut zeigten im Gegensatz zu früheren Befunden, daß der Kollagengehalt bereits im 8-Wochen-Stadium der Goldblatt-Hypertrophie gesteigert sein kann, und waren mit den mechanischen Parametern voll vereinbar.

References

1. *Alpert, N. R., B. B. Hamrell, W. Halpern:* Mechanical and biochemical correlates of cardiac hypertrophy. Circulat. Res. **34/35** II, 71–82 (1974).
2. *Bartošová, D., M. Chmapil, B. Korecký, O. Poupa, K. Rakušan, Z. Turek, M. Vízek:* The growth of the muscular and collagenous parts of the rat heart in various forms of cardiomegaly. J. Physiol. **200**, 285–295 (1969).
3. *Bing, O. H. L., S. Matsushita, B. L. Fanburg, H. J. Levine:* Mechanical properties of rat cardiac muscle during experimental hypertrophy. Circulat. Res. **28**, 234–245 (1971).
4. *Borchard, F.:* Catecholamine contents and morphology of the adrenergic nerves in experimental hypertrophy. Basic Res. Cardiol. **75**, 118–125 (1980).
5. *Buccino, R. A., E. Harris, J. F. Spann, E.H. Sonnenblick:* Response of myocardial connective tissue to development of experimental hypertrophy. Amer. J. Physiol. **216 (2)**, 425–428 (1969).
6. *Cummings, J. R.:* Electrolyte changes in heart tissue and coronary arterial and venous plasma following coronary occlusion. Circulat. Res. **8**, 865–870 (1960).
7. *Greene, H. L., M. L. Weisfeldt:* Determinants of hypoxic and posthypoxic myocardial contracture. Amer. J. Physiol. **232 (5)**, H 256–H 533 (1977).
8. *Hearse, D. J., P. B. Gorlick, S. M. Humphrey:* Ischemic contracture of the myocardium: Mechanisms and prevention. Amer. J. Cardiol. **39**, 986–993 (1977).
9. *Holubarsch, Ch., R. Jacob:* Evaluation of elasticity by means of length-tension relationships in a model of isolated ventricular myocardium from rat and cat papillary muscle under conditions of contracture. Basic Res. Cardiol. **73**, 442–458 (1978).
10. *Holubarsch, Ch., R. Jacob:* Evaluation of elastic properties of myocardium. Experimental models of fibrosis and contracture in heart muscle strips. Z. Kardiol. **68**, 123–127 (1979).
11. *Jacob, R., E. Ebrecht. A. Kämmereit, I. Medugorac, M. F. Wendt-Gallitelli:* Myocardial function in different models of cardiac hypertrophy. An attempt at correlating mechanical, biochemical, and morphological parameters. Basic Res. Cardiol. **72**, 160–167 (1977).
12. *Jacob, R., Ch. Holubarsch, H. Moser, B. Brenner:* Quantification of changes in myocardial elasticity under hypoxia. Experiments on whole heart preparations and isolated muscle strips. Clin. Cardiol. (in press).
13. *Jarmakani, J. M., T. Nagatomo, G. A. Langer:* The effect of calcium and high-energy phosphate compounds on myocardial contracture in the newborn and adult rabbit. J. Mol. Cell. Cardiol. **10**, 1017–1029 (1978).
14. *Jarmakani, J. M., T. Nagatomo, M. Nakazawa, G. A. Langer:* Effect of hypoxia on myocardial high-energy phosphates in the neonatal mammalian heart. Amer. J. Physiol. **235 (5)**, H 475–H 481 (1978).
15. *Kitabatake, A., H. Suga:* Diastolic stress-strain relation of nonexcised blood-perfused canine papillary muscle. Amer. J. Physiol. **234 (4)**, H 416–H 420 (1978).
16. *Little, R. C.:* The effect of acute hypoxia on the viscoelastic properties of the myocardium. Amer. Heart J. **92**, 609–614 (1976).
17. *Medugorac, I., R. Jacob:* Concentration and adenosinetriphosphatase activity of left ventricular actomyosin in Goldblatt rats during the compensatory stage of hypertrophy. Hoppe-Seyler's Z. Physiol. Chem. **357**, 1495–1503 (1976).
18. *Meerson, F. Z.:* Insufficiency of hypertrophied heart. Basic Res. Cardiol. **71**, 343–354 (1976).
19. *Mirsky, I., W. W. Parmley:* Assessment of passive elastic stiffness for isolated heart muscle and the intact heart. Circulat. Res. **33**, 233–243 (1973).
20. *Rich, T. L., A. J. Brady:* Potassium contracture and utilization of high-energy phosphates in rabbit hearts. Amer. J. Physiol. **226 (1)**, 105–113 (1974).

21. *Rupp, H.:* Modulation of Ca^{2+}-induced tension generation by myofilaments. – An analysis of the effect of magnesium adenosine triphosphate, magnesium, pH and sarcomere length. Basic Res. Cardiol. (in press)
22. *Spann, J. F., R. A. Buccino, E. H. Sonnenblick, E. Braunwald:* Contractile state of muscle obtained from cats with experimentally produced ventricular hypertrophy and heart failure. Circulat. Res. **21**, 341–354 (1967).
23. *Wendt-Gallitelli, M. F., G. Ebrecht, R. Jacob:* Morphological alterations and their functional interpretation in the hypertrophied myocardium of Goldblatt hypertensive rats. J. Mol. Cell. Cardiol. **11**, 275–287 (1979).

Author's address:

Dr. *Ch. Holubarsch,* Physiologisches Institut II, Universität Tübingen, Gmelin-straße 5, D-7400 Tübingen

Basic Res. Cardiol. **75,** 253–261 (1980)
© 1980 Dr. Dietrich Steinkopff Verlag, Darmstadt
ISSN 0300–8428

Paper, presented at the Erwin Riesch Symposium, Tübingen, April 3–7, 1979

Physiologisches Institut II, Universität Tübingen

Elastic and contractile properties of the myocardium in experimental cardiac hypertrophy of the rat Methodological and pathophysiological considerations*)

Elastische und kontraktile Eigenschaften des Rattenmyokards bei experimenteller Herzhypertrophie Methodenkritische und pathophysiologische Gesichtspunkte

R. Jacob, B. Brenner, G. Ebrecht, Ch. Holubarsch,
and *I. Medugorac*

With 2 figures

Summary

Two essential parameters of myocardial mechanics, the diastolic stress-strain relationship and the maximum unloaded shortening velocity have been analysed in the pressure-hypertrophied myocardium of Goldblatt rats and compared with the alterations appearing in other models of hypertrophy (spontaneous hypertension, aortic stenosis, swimming training).

An augmentation of collagen content is apparently the decisive reason for a decrease in myocardial distensibility in Goldblatt rats – primarily due to hypertensive vasculopathy. In the early stages of this model, however, the significance of other factors such as a hypertrophy of inner membranes or even (unlikely) diastolic residual activation cannot be definitely excluded. In the other models the alteration in distensibility is slight or nonsignificant in the investigated stages. The study suggests that a substantial decrease in myocardial distensibility is not an inherent feature of the hypertrophy process.

The maximum unloaded shortening velocity is reduced in all models of pressure-induced hypertrophy, in contrast to hypertrophy due to swimming training. This reduction can be demonstrated also under optimal electromechanical coupling conditions in native preparations as well as in thin, nonfibrotic, glycerinated myocardial fibres. When an inner load or shortening-induced inactivation is taken into account by extrapolating the length-velocity curves at different Ca^{++} concentrations, then a Ca^{++}-independent, initial maximum velocity can be demonstrated at the starting length of the respective quick releases. This method also yields a Ca^{++}-independent reduction of V_{max} in the pressure-hypertrophied myocardium.

Hemodynamic overload of the heart leads to structural and functional alterations at the subcellular, cellular and whole heart levels. Both the

---

*) Supported by the Deutsche Forschungsgemeinschaft

properties of the myocardium in diastole, and myocardial contractile capability can be affected. The present study deals with two particularly prominent and functionally relevant alterations in the mechanics of the hypertrophied myocardium: 1) a decrease in diastolic myocardial distensibility which occurs in some models of experimental hypertrophy (6; 8; 9; 11) and 2) a reduction in maximum unloaded shortening velocity which has been demonstrable even in early stages of all the forms of experimental pressure hypertrophy investigated by our group up to now (8, 9).

An essential question is whether a reduction in distensibility is an inherent property of hypertrophied myocardium or merely occurs in late stages or in certain models as a result of increased connective tissue content. With regard to maximum unloaded shortening velocity, a basic problem of hypertrophy research is clarification of whether a decrease in this parameter under chronic pressure load should be attributed to alterations in processes of electromechanical coupling or the contractile apparatus itself. A further cause of altered shortening velocity could be a change in parallel elasticity. Shortening velocity is dependent upon the actual load and thus upon the parallel elastic structures which bear a variable proportion of the total load. Moreover, both distensibility and shortening velocity can be influenced by the formation of noncontractile material arranged in series with functioning sarcomeres. Thus, there are several aspects linking both of these alterations.

The present study is based on investigations performed primarily on Goldblatt rats with unilateral renal artery coarctation and also includes observations from hypertrophied hearts of rats with spontaneous hypertension, experimental aortic stenosis or chronic swimming training. Methodological problems are necessarily discussed in addition to correlative considerations and pathophysiological implications.

Methods

Left ventricular hypertrophy was induced in young male Wistar rats by unilateral renal artery constriction (Goldblatt II). Left ventricular mass was increased by 30% to 55% as compared with controls of the same age.

A portion of the experiments were also performed using other models of cardiac hypertrophy. A group of rats was subjected to coarctation of the ascending aorta directly distal to the aortic valve which produced a left ventricular hypertrophy of 10% to 30% compared to age-matched controls. Investigations on spontaneously hypertensive rats were performed on 10-month-old animals with 150–170 mm Hg systolic blood pressure (tail cuff method under ether anesthesia) and approximately 50% left ventricular hypertrophy. Further comparisons were made using swim-trained rats after an 8-week training period resulting in a moderate increase in left ventricular mass (8–15%) (10).

The experiments were carried out on trabecular preparations from the rear wall of the left ventricle. The muscle strips were fixed in a measuring apparatus described by *Gülch* (2). A temperature-controlled (32 °C) tyrode solution was used for perfusion (concentration in mM: glucose 25, NaCl 130.5, KCl 4.9, $CaCl_2$ 2.2, NaH_2PO_4 0.8, $NaHCO_3$ 30.0). The solution was constantly bubbled with 95% O_2 and 5% Co_2 (pH = 7.4).

In order to record diastolic length-tension relationships, the muscle strip was released by 0.1 mm every 30 s beginning at l_{max}, i.e., the muscle length at which developed tension is maximum. In this manner three length-tension relationships were measured in each preparation and transformed into stress-strain relationships (stress $\sigma = \dfrac{F}{A}$; strain $\varepsilon = \dfrac{l-l_o}{l_o}$). The tangent modulus was also calculated using $\dfrac{\Delta\sigma}{\Delta\varepsilon}$ from various points of the stress-strain relationship. (For further methodological details see 5, 6.)

The active isometric length-tension relations were recorded under steady state conditions and the force-velocity relations were determined from afterload contractions as well as from isometric and isotonic quick release experiments (for methodological details see 2, 3, 9, 10).

Furthermore, trabecular preparations were glycerinated for at least 30 minutes. The average diameter and length of all preparations were 0.30 ± 0.03 mm and 2.0 ± 0.4 mm, respectively. At the beginning of each experiment the preparation was prestretched to the sarcomere length of 2.15 µm (average of 50 sarcomeres over the whole length of the preparation); this procedure was carried out in relaxing solution and under microscopical observation. Quick release experiments were performed at 6.5 °C using activation solutions with defined Ca^{++} concentrations and an ATP regenerating system. The shortening velocity was plotted as a function of momentary length (1).

The hydroxyproline concentration was measured in samples of 10 to 50 mg of dry tissue.

A myofibrillar preparation was made from each single left ventricle. Each preparation was checked for purity using SDS-polyacrylamide (10%) gel electrophoresis. Myofibrillar ATPase activity was determined by measuring the liberation of inorganic phosphate in a final volume of 2 ml (at 35 °C and a pH of 7.6). (For further methodical details of biochemical analysis see 13 and references therein.)

Results and discussion

Distensibility of the hypertrophied myocardium

The question of whether chronic alterations in the enddiastolic ventricular pressure-volume relationship can be explained exclusively geometrically, that is, by an increase in wall thickness or by growth-induced increase of the ventricular radius, has been discussed in the literature for a long time. In addition to morphological alterations in tissue texture and composition, a functional component of changed distensibility has also been postulated by some authors (for literature see 9, 10). An incomplete relaxation occurring with increasing stimulation frequency is regarded as an early sign of an impaired function of the hypertrophied myocardium; the cause has been sought in reduced relaxation velocity due to impaired function of the sarcoplasmic reticulum. The same cause, however, has been postulated for changes in the resting tension curve (14).

With regard to incomplete relaxation, the qualification must be made that this phenomenon cannot always be attributed to reduced relaxation velocity. Thus, by the 8-week stage, the myocardium of Goldblatt rats shows a tendency towards an increase in diastolic tension under relatively moderate stimulation frequencies. In this case, however, the incomplete relaxation is primarily the result of prolonged systolic activation due to prolongation of the action potential (4).

Using stress-strain values of a normal resting tension curve, two compartments can be distinguished if one plots the tangent modulus (E) as a function of stress (σ) or the logarithm of stress ($\ln\sigma$) as a function of strain (ε), i.e., relative lengthening (8). The steeper compartment is most likely due to involvement of connective tissue structures. The following considerations will exclusively deal with the left portion of the resting-tension curve.

Preparatory investigations suggest differentiation of distinct types of decreased distensibiliy (5, 6, 7). On the basis of experimental models we refer to the first type as the "fibrosis type". It is characterized by a steeper slope of the relation between the tangent elastic modulus (E) and stress (σ) below l_{max} as well. The second type is referred to as the "contracture type" which is observed, for example, in a caffeine-Ca^{++} contracture or in hypoxic contracture. In this case of residual diastolic coupling the tangent elastic modulus increases proportionally to stress, and thus the E-σ curve under contracture cannot be separated from the control curve. When the logarithm of stress is plotted against strain, a parallel shift occurs.

Figure 1 shows the resting tension curve and the relation between elastic modulus and stress in different models of experimental hypertrophy. A decrease in myocardial distensibility is most distinct in Goldblatt

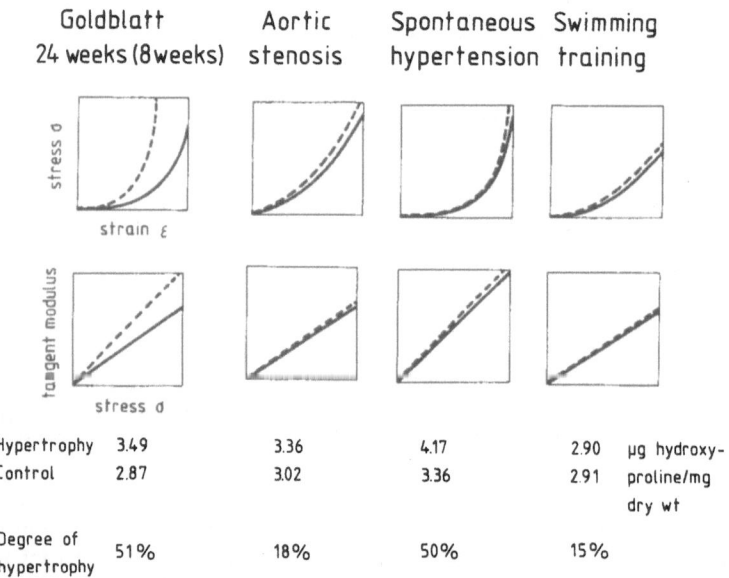

	Goldblatt 24 weeks (8weeks)	Aortic stenosis	Spontaneous hypertension	Swimming training	
Hypertrophy	3.49	3.36	4.17	2.90	µg hydroxy-
Control	2.87	3.02	3.36	2.91	proline/mg dry wt
Degree of hypertrophy	51%	18%	50%	15%	

Fig. 1. Stress-strain relations, tangent modulus-stress relations and hydroxyproline concentrations in various models of cardiac hypertrophy. The individual graphs and data are based on the mean values of myocardium from 10 hypertrophied ventricles and 10 age-matched controls. Hydroxyproline concentration was determined in the corresponding left ventricles (S.D. ca. 10% of the mean values). *Goldblatt hypertension:* In the earlier stages diastolic distensibility can be unchanged or already decreased. – *Aortic stenosis:* 7 weeks after operation. – *Spontaneous hypertension:* The animals were 40 weeks old. Controls were provided by normal Sprague-Dawley rats of the same age (SuT:SDT strain, Süddeutsche Versuchstierfarm, Tuttlingen). – *Swimming training:* 2 hours daily, for 10 weeks.

rats after 24 weeks. In this stage all investigated groups of Goldblatt rats revealed a considerable steepening of the tangent modulus-stress relation. Frequently, a significant shift of the original stress-strain curve toward higher stress values is recognizable as early as the 6–8 week stage. The change in slope of the tangent modulus-stress relation, however, is occasionally less clear at the earlier stages. – A slight tendency toward decreasing distensibility is also suggested in experimental stenosis, 4–6 weeks after operation. In spontaneously hypertensive rats the plot of the tangent modulus-stress relationship is relatively steep, but only insignificantly different from the respective controls. In swimming rats, on the other hand, one could expect at most a possible increase in distensibility according to the literature (see 10). In our material, however, no significant alterations are present and in no case do we find a flattening of the stress-strain relation. Thus, according to our investigations, the increased diastolic volume of the athletic heart can be exclusively attributed to muscle fibre growth and cannot be the result of decreased myocardial tone as proposed by some other authors (for literature see 10).

The altered myocardial distensibility of Goldblatt rats in the 24-week stage clearly conforms to the "fibrosis type". In this group there was an increase in the hydroxyproline concentration of 22% which is probably due primarily to hypertensive vasculopathy. The respective changes in myocardial hydroxyproline concentration in rats with experimental aortic stenosis and swimming rats are reflected in comparable slight decrease or constancy of distensibility in these groups. Two points require further clarification, however: 1) Remarkably, the distinct difference in hydroxyproline concentration between the spontaneously hypertensive rats and their controls only leads to an insignificant decrease in distensibility. 2) As mentioned above, in earlier stages of Goldblatt hypertrophy a decrease in distensibility was occasionally found which did not show a pronounced increase in hydroxyproline concentration and could not be clearly attributed to either type.

Several causes could explain these discrepancies. In the case of spontaneously hypertensive rats the corresponding controls already had a high collagen content and a steeper plot of the elastic modulus-stress relation. It should be considered that not only the content, but also the arrangement of connective tissue – diffuse formation on the one hand, localized scars on the other hand – should be of significance. The methodological problems could be of greater importance for both points, however, because in these experiments the hydroxyproline concentration has only been determined in the respective whole ventricle and not in the individual muscle strip preparation.

If, on the other hand, an increased resting tension in early stages of Goldblatt hypertension were due, or partially due, to an impaired function of the sarcoplasmic reticulum, i.e., an increased myoplasmic Ca^{++} concentration in diastole, then this increase should be reducable by experimental reduction of the Ca^{++} concentration, at least in the range of moderate preload. Investigations designed to cause a reduction of sarcoplasmic Ca^{++} concentration are underway. Up to now it can be stated that simple removal of Ca^{++} from the bath solution did not influence the resting tension curve of control or Goldblatt left ventricular myocardium.

The addition of 3 mM EGTA with the intention of obtaining a further reduction in the myoplasmic Ca^{++} concentration was likewise unsuccessful, although the systolic action was completely suppressed.

In conclusion: A substantial increase in diastolic myocardial stiffness is obviously not an inherent feature of the hypertrophy process. Although there are serious indications that the connective tissue content is the decisive cause of reduced diastolic distensibility of Goldblatt myocardium, the potential significance of other changes is still unanswered, for example, a hypertrophy of the inner membranes. A conceivable diastolic residual activity of cross bridges causing a contracturelike reduction in distensibility is improbable, but cannot be definitively ruled out in the early stages of Goldblatt hypertension. This question requires further investigations involving more sophisticated methodological approaches.

Unloaded shortening velocity

In contrast to the slightly increased value of the swimming rats, maximum shortening velocity under external zero load, as determined on the basis of isometric or isotonic quick release experiments or by analysis of afterloaded contractions, was already reduced by 25–30% in early stages of pressure-induced hypertrophy. Goldblatt rats revealed a further continuous decrease of the apparent V_{max} over the first 6-month period. A slight, age-dependent reduction was also seen in the controls (8, 9).

The unloaded shortening velocity at external zero load ("apparent V_{max}") is significantly dependent on the Ca^{++} concentration (3). In earlier investigations on the native hypertrophied myocardium we attempted to define the contribution of the contractile system alone to the alterations in V_{max} by optimizing the electromechanical coupling conditions (8). However, the significance of these investigations was limited primarily because control of the Ca^{++} concentration in the external medium did not permit precise definition of the myoplasmic Ca^{++} concentration.

In glycerinated preparations, however, the degree of activation can be exactly controlled. Furthermore, the influence of parallel elasticity should be diminished by destruction of the surface membrane and the inner membranes.

The apparent value of V_{max} was also shown to be Ca^{++}-dependent in glycerinated muscle fibres. If, however, an internal load or a length dependent inactivation is taken into account by extrapolating the length-velocity relations (corresponding to different Ca^{++} concentrations) to the starting length of the respective quick releases, then serious indications result for a Ca^{++}-independent V_{max} as shown in normal myocardium (1).

In view of these considerations we used thin glycerinated fibre preparations in reexamining the question of whether the unloaded shortening velocity in the pressure-hypertrophied myocardium is reduced independently of the conditions of electromechanical coupling. Fibrosis was ruled out in each preparation by light microscopic examination. In an early stage of Goldblatt hypertension, the value of V_{max} evaluated by extrapolation to the starting length of the respective quick release was decreased by ca. 30% as compared with age-matched controls (fig. 2). The apparent V_{max} at a Ca^{++} concentration which ensures full activation of the contractile

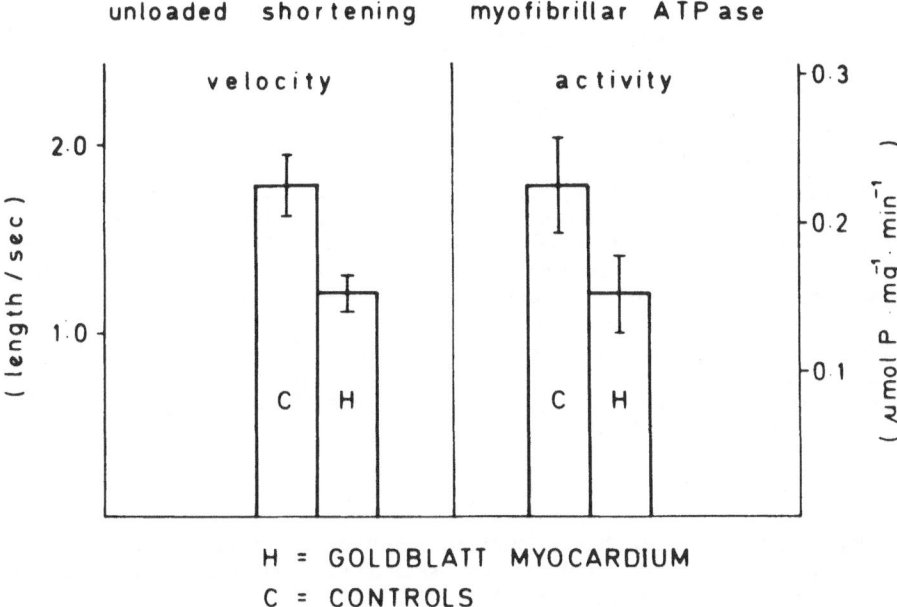

unloaded shortening   myofibrillar ATPase

Fig. 2. Maximum unloaded shortening velocity and myofibrillar ATPase activity of hypertrophic myocardium of Goldblatt rats (6-week stage) and age-matched controls (mean ± S.D.; C: n = 8; H: n = 8).
The (extrapolated) value of maximum shortening velocity at the starting length of the respective quick release was estimated in glycerinated fibers by extrapolating the length-velocity relations at different Ca^{++} concentrations.
Myofibrillar ATPase activity was determined in the corresponding ventricles.

system was also significantly different in hypertrophied myocardium of Goldblatt rats and controls. Myofibrillar ATPase activity was reduced by a comparable degree.

In conclusion: The results definitely show that maximum unloaded shortening velocity of the pressure-hypertrophied myocardium is reduced independently of processes of electromechanical coupling. The formal correlation of our data is compatible with the concept of an inner relationship between maximum unloaded shortening velocity and enzyme activity of the contractile proteins (12).

Zusammenfassung

Zwei wesentliche Parameter der myokardialen Mechanik, die Elastizität des erschlafften Herzmuskels sowie die Maximalgeschwindigkeit der lastfreien Verkürzung, wurden beim druckhypertrophierten Myokard von Goldblatt-Ratten analysiert und mit den Veränderungen bei anderen Hypertrophiemodellen (Ratten mit spontaner Hypertension, Aortenstenose und nach chronischem Schwimmtraining) verglichen.

Für die Dehnbarkeitsabnahme des Myokards bei Goldblatt-Ratten ist offensichtlich die Vermehrung des Kollagengehalts entscheidend, vorwiegend als Folge einer hypertensiven Vaskulopathie. In den Frühstadien dieses Hyper-

260   Basic Research in Cardiology, Vol. 75, No. 1 (1980)

trophiemodells kann jedoch ein Einfluß anderer Faktoren noch nicht ausgeschlossen werden, z. B. einer Hypertrophie innerer Membranen oder eine – wenn auch unwahrscheinliche – diastolische Restankopplung des kontraktilen Systems. Bei den anderen Modellen ist die Änderung der Dehnbarkeit in den untersuchten Stadien geringfügig oder nicht signifikant. Die Ergebnisse der Studie lassen vermuten, daß eine wesentliche Dehnbarkeitsabnahme nicht zum Wesen des Hypertrophieprozesses selbst gehört.

Die Maximalgeschwindigkeit der lastfreien Verkürzung ist bei allen Modellen der Druckhypertrophie vermindert, im Gegensatz zum Modell der Schwimmratten. Diese Abnahme läßt sich beim nativen Myokard und bei dünnen, nichtfibrosierten glycerinisierten Muskelfasern auch unter optimalen elektromechanischen Kopplungsbedingungen zeigen. Wird eine innere Last berücksichtigt, indem man die Längen-Geschwindigkeits-Beziehungen unter unterschiedlichen Ca^{++}-Konzentrationen extrapoliert, so ergibt sich bei der Ausgangslänge der „quick releases" eine Ca^{++}-unabhängige lastfreie, initiale Verkürzungsgeschwindigkeit. Aufgrund dieses Verfahrens läßt sich eine Ca^{++}-unabhängige Minderung von V_{max} beim druckhypertrophierten Myokard nachweisen.

References

1. *Brenner, B., R. Jacob:* Calcium activation and maximum unloaded shortening velocity. Investigations on glycerinated skeletal and heart muscle preparations. Basic Res. Cardiol. **75**, 40–46 (1980).
2. *Gülch, R. W.:* A critical analysis of myocardial force-velocity relations obtained from damped quick-release experiments. Basic Res. Cardiol. **69**, 32–46 (1974).
3. *Gülch, R. W.:* The effect of preload and Ca^{++} ions on the time course of the isometric force and the force-velocity relations: Is V_{max} dependent on the number of cross-bridges? Basic Res. Cardiol. **72**, 102–108 (1977).
4. *Gülch, R. W., R. Baumann, R. Jacob:* Analysis of myocardial action potential in left ventricular hypertrophy of Goldblatt rats. Basic Res. Cardiol. **74**, 69–82 (1979).
5. *Holubarsch, Ch., R. Jacob:* Evaluation of elastic properties of myocardium. Experimental models of fibrosis and contracture in heart muscle strips. Z. Kardiol. **68**, 123–127 (1979).
6. *Holubarsch, Ch.:* Fibrosis type and contracture type of decreased myocardial distensibility in cardiac hypertrophy and hypoxia. Basic Res. Cardiol. **75**, 244–252 (1980).
7. *Jacob, R., Ch. Holubarsch, H. Moser, B. Brenner:* Quantification and interpretation of changes in myocardial elasticity under hypoxia. Experimental models employing whole heart preparations and isolated muscle strips. Advances in Clinical Cardiology, Volume I, G. Witzstrock, Baden-Baden–New York (1980).
8. *Jacob, R., G. Kissling:* Left ventricular dynamics and myocardial function in Goldblatt hypertension of the rat. Biochemical, morphological and electrophysiological correlates. Internat. Sympos. "The heart in hypertension" (München 1979) in press.
9. *Kämmereit, A., R. Jacob:* Alterations in rat myocardial mechanics under Goldblatt hypertension and experimental aortic stenosis. Basic Res. Cardiol. **74**, 389–405 (1979).
10. *Kämmereit, A., I. Medugorac, E. Steil, R. Jacob:* Mechanics of the isolated ventricular myocardium of rats conditioned by physical training. Basic Res. Cardiol. **70**, 495–507 (1975).
11. *Kissling, G., T. Gassenmaier, M. F. Wendt-Gallitelli, R. Jacob:* Pressure-volume relations, elastic modulus, and contractile behaviour of the hypertrophied left ventricle of rats with Goldblatt II hypertension. Pflügers Arch. **369**, 213–221 (1977).

12. *Maughan, D., E. Low, R. Litten, J. Brayden, N. R. Alpert:* Calcium-activated muscle from hypertrophied rabbit hearts. Circulation Res. **44**, 279–287 (1979).
13. *Medugorac, I.:* The myofibrillar ATPase activity and the substructure of myosin in the hypertrophied left ventricle of the rat. Basic Res. Cardiol. (1980) in press.
14. *Meerson, F. Z.:* Insufficiency of hypertrophied heart. Basic Res. Cardiol. **71**, 343–354 (1976).

For reprints:

Prof. Dr. *R. Jacob*, Physiol. Institut II d. Universität Tübingen, Gmelinstraße 5, 7400 Tübingen

Basic Res. Cardiol. **75**, 262–269 (1980)
© 1980 Dr. Dietrich Steinkopff Verlag, Darmstadt
ISSN 0300–8428

Paper, presented at the Erwin Riesch Symposium, Tübingen, April 3–7, 1979

Department of Pediatric Cardiology and Biomedical Engineering,
University of Kiel, FRG

Comparative studies of ventricular ejection phase parameters for the detection of impaired cardiac function*)

Vergleichende Untersuchungen von ventrikulären Auswurfparametern zur Aufdeckung einer kardialen Funktionseinschränkung

J. H. Bürsch, H. H. Hagemann, B. Koch, and *P. H. Heintzen*

With 3 figures

Summary

Experimental studies were carried out in 11 anesthetized pigs in order to compare the sensitivity of left ventricular ejection phase parameters as determined by quantitative angiocardiographic methods, for detection of mild or moderate ventricular dysfunction. The experimental setup implied various degrees of nonadequate muscular hypertrophy in relation to chronic volume overload by aortic insufficiency. Left ventricular stroke volume, flow, ejection fraction and mean circumferential fiber shortening did not demonstrate impairment of ventricular function reserve when studied in the resting state of the circulation, but became indicative to some degree by their abnormal pattern of response to acute afterload stress (angiotensin infusion). Mean normalized systolic ejection rate as well as normalized values of systolic ejection time were found to be the most sensitive indices of ventricular function in this study.

Evaluation of ventricular muscle function constitutes significant problems in clinical as well as in experimental studies. In fact, opinions from the physiology point of view about possibilities and problems of the determination of cardiac performance are controversial (4, 12).

In clinical situations it is generally agreed that the depression of certain parameters like cardiac output, stroke volume and/or ventricular ejection fraction are indicative of advanced cardiac disease and heart failure. Problems, however, arise if mild or moderate myocardial dysfunction shall be detected, because firm hemodynamic criteria for such studies are lacking.

It has been proposed to evaluate ventricular function by increasing resistance to ventricular ejection with angiotensin (11). Although the angiotensin infusion method has been critisized for not yielding reproduc-

---

*) This investigation was supported by the Deutsche Forschungsgemeinschaft

able results (10) its usefulness was demonstrated in several experimental (12) and clinical studies, i.e. for the assessment of left ventricular function in aortic valve incompetence (1). It was clearly demonstrated that comparative determinations of the ejection phase parameters at rest and during stress provide more sensitive measurements for the detection of impaired cardiac function than studies in the basal state of the circulation only.

It is, however, not clear at present which of the various ejection measures like stroke volume, ejection fraction, mean circumferential fiber shortening and others are most sensitive and reliable.

Therefore animal experiments were carried out in order to compare the ejection parameters of the left ventricle as determined by angiocardiographic examinations. The purpose of the study was, firstly, to design an experimental model implying impaired functional reserve of the left ventricle by nonadequate muscular hypertrophy in relation to left ventricular volume overloading (aortic insufficiency), and, secondly, to determine the diverse left ventricular ejection parameters and to evaluate their pattern of response to the elevation of aortic pressure by angiotensin infusion.

It was expected that failure to maintain normal ejection indices would occur in the early phase of ventricular adaption to sustained overload.

Methods

Experiments were performed on 11 pigs weighing 15–20 kg in Urethan-Chloralose anesthesia. Each of the studies included left ventricular and aortic pressure measurements as well as injection of a contrast medium (Urografin 76%) into the left ventricle under resting conditions (basal state) and during increased afterload by infusion of a pressor agent (Angiotensin II, 3 µg/min). At the beginning of the studies all animals were examined immediately before production of aortic valve incompetence (balloon catheter procedure) and served as a control group. Cardiac catheterization was then repeated after 1, 2, and 4 weeks of valvular insufficiency. Biplane video-angiocardiograms were analyzed by a computer-assisted videometry system (6). End-diastolic volumes (EDV) and end-systolic volumes (ESV) were calculated as well as dimensional measures of the ventricular chamber, e.g. the fraction of circumferential shortening (FCF) at the minor equator. The degree of aortic regurgitation was measured by roentgen-videodensitometry in terms of regurgitant fraction (RGF), namely the ratio of regurgitant volume and total stroke volume (2). Systolic ejection time (ET) of the ventricle was measured from the aortic pressure tracings and from this heart rate (HR) was determined.

In addition the following left ventricular parameters were calculated:

Total stroke volume (TSV)	TSV = EDV – ESV
Total flow (TFL)	TFL = TSV * HR
Ejection fraction (EF)	EF = TSV/EDV
Mean normalized systolic ejection rate (MNSER)	MNSER = EF/ET
Mean velocity of circumferential fiber shortening (mean VCF)	mean VCF = FCF/ET

The following numbers (n) of paired measurements (basal state, angiotensin infusion) were obtained in the four individual groups:

	Control	1st week	2nd week	4th week
n	11	6	7	6

Results

The range of aortic RGF values was 10 to 59%. There was, however, no statistically significant change of RGF in each of the individuals, neither with respect to time passing on after production of insufficiency nor to acute elevation of aortic pressure. Heart rate, likewise, did not show statistically significant changes neither with time nor to afterload stress (the means of heart rate and their standard deviations are given in the following table).

HR (l/min)	Control	1st week	2nd week	4th week
Basal st.	115 ± 21	116 ± 28	122 ± 21	125 ± 24
Angioten.	123 ± 23	120 ± 13	117 ± 22	130 ± 19

Ventricular hypertrophy was documented by a significant increase of left ventricular mass (3.78 g/kg body weight) after 4 weeks of valve incompetence as compared to a control group of 13 healthy pigs (2.69 g/kg).

Pressures and volumes in the basal state

As a consequence of regurgitation, the aortic pressure pulse amplitudes were enlarged up to twice of the control group while mean

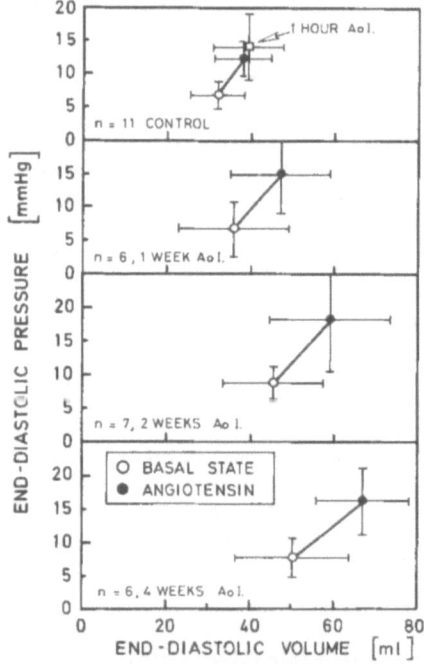

Fig. 1. Relations between left ventricular end-diastolic volumes (EDV) and pressures (EDP) (means with standard deviations) as determined in four consecutive studies (from top to bottom) before and after production of aortic valve incompetence.
The uniform changes of EDV and EDP within each group due to afterload stress are indicated by the straight lines connecting mean data points of the basal state (open circles) with those during angiotensin infusion (closed circles).

aortic pressures remained in the normal range (52–107 mmHg). During the time course of adaption to aortic insufficiency, left ventricular EDV became increasingly higher, but ventricular ejection fraction was maintained (range of the means of EF 54–66%). Quite similar changes were found in end-systolic volumes increasing from 12.5 ml to 23.0 ml in the average. Consequently, total stroke volume rose about 40% above normal and even so did left ventricular total flow.

End-diastolic pressures remained in the normal range (EDP < 10 mm Hg) except for the very acute phase of volume overload during the first hour after production of valvular insufficiency. At this time, both end-diastolic volumes and pressures were significantly increased (fig. 1).

Pressures and volumes during afterload stress

During angiotensin infusion, mean aortic pressure rose on the average somewhat above 50% of basal state. Under these conditions end-diastolic pressures became acutely elevated associated with an increase of EDV and ESV (fig. 1). As a result of this, left ventricular TSV as well as TFL consistently increased during afterload stress.

Ejection phase parameters

The degree of acute increase of TSV and TFL in relation to the elevation of mean aortic pressure by angiotensin was smaller in the 1st and 2nd week of insufficiency than in the control group and in the 4th week of the study. These differences, however, were not statistically significant.

TSV (ml)	Control	1st week	2nd week	4th week
Basal st.	19.2 ± 4.9	23.6 ± 9.4	26.6 ± 8.6	27.3 ± 9.0
Angioten.	24.5 ± 4.9	29.2 ± 7.4	32.4 ± 7.7	36.5 ± 8.4
TFL (l/min)				
Basal st.	2.12 ± 0.35	2.61 ± 0.66	3.09 ± 0.60	3.30 ± 0.77
Angioten.	3.01 ± 0.74	3.39 ± 0.73	3.69 ± 0.65	4.70 ± 0.63

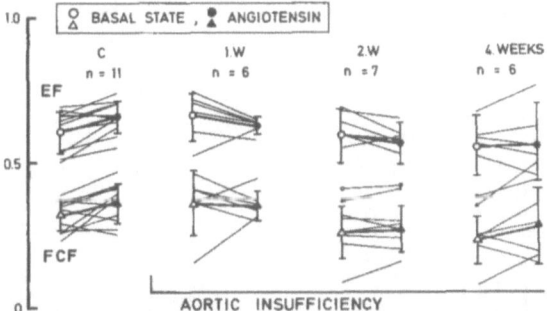

Fig. 2. The response of left ventricular ejection fraction (EF) and the fraction of circumferential shortening (FCF) at the minor equator to afterload stress by angiotensin infusion in the four consecutive studies (left to right). The mean values and standard deviations in each group are indicated. The slight increase of EF and FCF in control studies (C) according to stress is apparently reversed in the first week after acute aortic insufficiency. These differences in response are, however, not statistically significant.

A similar result was obtained when looking at the fractional changes of left ventricular volume as well as internal circumference at the minor equator. As depicted in figure 2, both parameters tend to decrease under angiotensin infusion in the 1st (and 2nd) week while the control group shows increasing values. This pattern again could not be statistically verified. Figure 2 illustrates the individual changes of the parameters within each group. It may be noticed that standard deviations of the circumferential values are higher in relation to their means than those of ejection fraction.

In contrast to these results, the left ventricular ejection time intervals of all individuals clearly changed during stress within the 1- and 2-week study after production of incompetence (fig. 3). These changes were statistically most significant when ET was corrected for heart rate respectively cycle length (CL) by considering the following relationship.

$$ET = 0.09 + 0.33 \, CL$$

This linear equation was obtained from 31 measures out of the control group yielding a correlation coefficient $r = 0.91$.

Combining volume and circumferential data with time measures, it becomes obvious that the resulting MNSER and mean VCF are considerably affected by the stress-induced responses of ET.

MNSER (l/s)	Control	1st week	2nd week	4th week
Basal st.	2.27 ± 0.39	2.63 ± 0.46	2.31 ± 0.43	2.24 ± 0.42
Angioten.	2.39 ± 0.42	2.01 ± 0.25	1.93 ± 0.27	2.32 ± 0.28
meanVCF (l/s)				
Basal st.	1.14 ± 0.20	1.40 ± 0.51	0.96 ± 0.32	0.86 ± 0.32
Angioten.	1.24 ± 0.29	1.14 ± 0.27	0.86 ± 0.28	1.16 ± 0.38

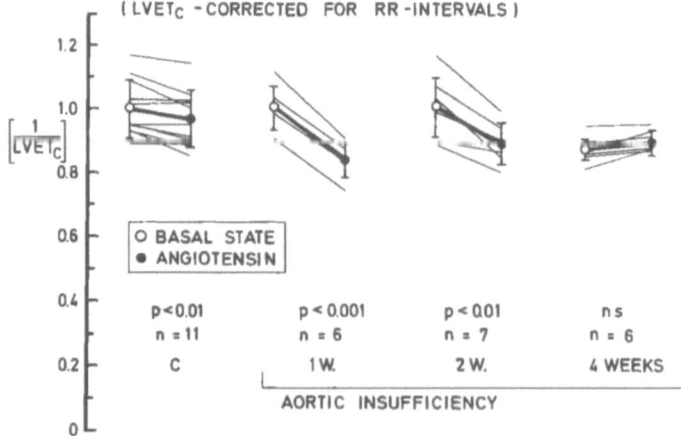

Fig. 3. The response of left ventricular ejection time to afterload stress is demonstrated by the reciprocal values of normalized ejection times $(1/LVET_C)$. $LVET_C$ was determined by the ratio of measured ejection times over calculated times applying the equation
$$ET = 0.09 + 0.33 * RR\text{-Interval}.$$

Statistical analysis revealed a fall of MNSER during increased afterload in the 1st week (p < 0.01) and in the 2nd week (p < 0.05). Corresponding results, however, were not obtained in the mean VCF values. Doubtlessly, the individual changes of mean VCF within each group are not comparable uniformly like those of the MNSER values as indicated by the high standard deviations in relation to the means. Studies of the relationship between volume and dimensional measures of the left ventricular chamber gave evidence that the pattern of contraction was not uniform within this study, thereby influencing the different ejection parameters to a variable degree. Relating fractional changes in volume to those of the circumferences, it appeared that FCF increased over-proportionally with EF. In addition the ventricle became less globular in high EF documented by the positive correlation between EF and the ratio of the length of the ventricular axis to the circumference at the minor equator (r = 0.55, n = 62) as determined for the end-systolic phase. A similar result was obtained relating EF to ventricular elongation.

Conclusions

The experimental model applied in this study may be characterized by the following basic parameters.

1. According to sustained volume overloading after production of aortic insufficiency, a progressive increase in left ventricular end-diastolic and end-systolic volumes was recognized without significant elevation of end-diastolic pressures. These changes in diastolic pressure-volume relationship are presumably combined with changes in ventricular diastolic properties while eccentric muscular hypertrophy develops. Similar conclusions were drawn from animal studies (3) and patients with aortic regurgitation (5).

2. In contrast to this finding, acute increase of end-diastolic volumes and pressures during afterload stress may be interpreted as ventricular response on the basis of the Frank-Starling mechanism.

3. Applying clinical diagnostic criteria, there was no indication of cardiac failure at any time. A more quantitative aspect in this regard is given by the fact that values of ventricular ejection fraction and related parameters were consistently found in the normal range under resting-conditions. Even more, total stroke volume, total flow and ejection fraction did not demonstrate statistically significant differences in response to acute stress in the early phase of volume overloading when compared with data of the control group and those obtained after a four-week period of adaption. Thereby it appears that impairment of ventricular function in this model was detectable only by relatively sensitive ventricular ejection phase indices.

Under consideration of non-adequate muscular hypertrophy during the early stage of ventricular overloading, only two of the parameters were apparently indicative for the detection of temporarily limited ventricular reserve. Mean normalized systolic ejection rate as well as reciprocal values of ejection time (corrected for cardiac cycle length) dropped significantly during afterload stress in the first and second week after production of aortic regurgitation. Circumferential data, however, like mean circumferential fiber shortening appear to be less reliable than the volume data (MNSER), mainly due to effects of variations in ventricular shape (e.g. elongation).

From these findings it may be concluded that the accuracy of simple dimensional and circumferential measures at the ventricular chamber is more limited than volume measurements, even though the best method available for angiocardiographic circumferential measurements had been applied (7). Apparently the specific geometrical consideration of the volume- and/or pressure-overloaded heart has to be more adequately accounted for (8).

In view of this it is worthwhile to notice that systolic ejection time itself has found to be as sensitive as the volume-ejection parameter. It therefore seems promising to account for systolic ejection time measurements in future studies of ventricular function including afterload stress although the determination of systolic time intervals has found to be unreliable for several other applications.

Zusammenfassung

Es wurden experimentelle Untersuchungen an 11 narkotisierten Schweinen mit dem Ziel durchgeführt, die unterschiedliche Empfindlichkeit verschiedener angio-kardiographisch gewonnener Auswurfparameter des linken Ventrikels zur Aufdek-kung einer ventrikulären Funktionseinschränkung zu überprüfen. Die Experimente schlossen Zustände mit akuter und chronischer Volumenbelastung durch Aortenklappeninsuffizienz ein, wobei die Untersuchungen zu verschiedenen Zeiten mit unterschiedlichem Grad der Muskelhypertrophie-Entwicklung durchgeführt wurden. Das linksventrikuläre Schlagvolumen, die Stromstärke, die ventrikuläre Auswurffraktion und die mittlere zirkumferentielle Verkürzungsgeschwindigkeit zeigten unter Ruhebedingungen des Kreislaufs keine Einschränkung der ventrikulären Funktionsreserve an. Sie wurden in gewissem Grade empfindlich durch das abnorme Verhalten der Meßwerte bei Nachlast-Erhöhung durch Angiotensin-Infusion. Die mittlere normalisierte systolische Auswurfrate und die normalisierten Werte der systolischen Austreibungszeit erwiesen sich in dieser Studie als die empfindlichsten Parameter zur Beurteilung der Ventrikelfunktion.

References

1. *Bolen, J. L., E. L. Holloway, J. C. Zener, D. C. Harrison, E. L. Alderman:* Evaluation of left ventricular function in patients with aortic regurgitation using afterload stress. Circulation **53**, 132 (1976).
2. *Bürsch, J. H., P. H. Heintzen, R. Simon:* Videodensitometric studies by a new method of quantitating the amont of contrast medium. Europ. J. Cardiol. **1**, 437 (1974).
3. *McCullagh, W. H., J. W. Covell, J. Ross* Jr.: Left ventricular dilation and diastolic compliance changes during chronic volume overloading. Circulation **45**, 943 (1972).
4. *Elzinga, G., V. Westerhof:* How to quantify pump function of the heart. The value of variables derived from measurements on isolated muscle. Circulat. Res. **44**, 303 (1979).
5. *Gault, J. H., J. W. Covell, E. Braunwald, J. Ross* Jr.: Left ventricular performance following correction of free aortic regurgitation. Circulation **42**, 773 (1970).
6. *Heintzen, P. H., V. Malerczyk, J. Pilarczyk, K. W. Scheel:* On-line processing of the video image for left ventricular volume determination. Comp. Biomed. Res. **4**, 474 (1971).

7. *Heintzen, P. H., K. Moldenhauer, P. E. Lange:* Three-dimensional computerized contraction pattern analysis. Europ. J. Cardiol. **1**, 229 (1974).
8. *Heintzen, P. H., E. Stephan:* Dynamic geometry of the left ventricle in hypertrophy studied by quantitative angiocardiography. Basic Res. Cardiol. **72**, 190 (1977).
9. *Lange, P. E., D. Onnasch, F. L. Farr, P. H. Heintzen:* Angiocardiographic left ventricular volume determination. Accuracy, as determined from human casts, and clinical application. Europ. J. Cardiol. **8**, 449 (1978).
10. *Ronan, J. A., R. B. Steelman, J. P. Schrank, P. T. Cochran:* The angiotensin infusion test as a method of evaluating left ventricular function. Clin. Comm. **89**, 554 (1975).
11. *Ross, J. Jr., E. Braunwald:* The study of left ventricular function in man by increasing resistance to ventricular ejection with angiotensin. Circulation **29**, 739 (1964).
12. *Ross, J., D. Franklin, S. Sasayama:* Preload, afterload and the role of afterload mismatch in the descending limb of cardiac function. Europ. J. Cardiol. **4**, 77 (1976).

Author's address:

Prof. Dr. med. *J. Bürsch,* Abt. Kinderkardiologie und Biomedizinische Technik im Klinikum der CAU, Schwanenweg 20, 2300 Kiel, FRG

Basic Res. Cardiol. **75**, 270–278 (1980)
© 1980 Dr. Dietrich Steinkopff Verlag, Darmstadt
ISSN 0300–8428

Paper, presented at the Erwin Riesch Symposium, Tübingen, April 3–7,1979

Institut für Pathologische Physiologie der Universitätsklinik Essen (GHS)

Maximum contractility of the experimentally hypertrophied heart in situ and survival of the acute coronary occlusion

Maximales Kontraktilitätsverhalten experimentell hypertrophierter Herzen in situ und die Überlebensrate nach akuter Koronarokklusion

K.-O. Bischoff, W. Meesmann, and *K. Stephan*

With 3 figures and 3 tables

Summary

Studies were carried out in dogs with significant moderate left ventricular hypertrophy (LVH) induced by artifical coarctatio aortae to reveal the reserve of performance and the behavior in response to acute ligation of the LCA (left circumflex artery). The hemodynamic data at rest and during catecholamine stimulation were not essentially different, whereas the maximal inotropic state was a little enhanced in LVH dogs ($LVH_1 = 12$; $CG_1 = 6$). The acute maximal pressure rise of the left ventricle – obtained by acute clamping of the aorta ascendens – was nearly the same in both groups ($LVH_2 = 6$; $CG_2 = 6$) when related to 100 g left ventricular wet weight. The LVH hearts react to a rapid volume overload with a slightly higher increase of HR and LVEP indicating a minor adaption to an acute volume overload explained by diminished compliance. In consequence to acute ligation of the LCA ($LVH_3 = 13$; $CG_3 = 11$) LVH hearts showed a higher ($p < 0.05$) survival rate (69%) than controls with comparable collateral status of the coronary collateral vessels because 91% of these developed ventricular fibrillation. To explain this phenomenon we determined the catecholamine-concentration in each part of the heart in a further group ($LVH_4 = 5$; $CG_4 = 6$). Unexpectedly a significant diminution was seen in the non-hypertrophied right ventricle, but the other compartments also showed a decrease of the catecholamine concentration. Subsequent studies have to be done to explore the better electrophysiologic protection of the LVH heart in consequence to acute ligation of the LCA.

In recent years considerable efforts have been made by different investigators to describe and evaluate the chronic pressure-loaded hypertrophy of the heart (2, 6, 8, 9). The results of the different groups are inconclusive. The effect of hypertrophy on the performance and the reserve of contractility of the intact heart in situ is still a matter of dispute. We feel that the extent of hypertrophy and the type of experimental preparation appears to be essential when one deals with the question of whether there is a different functional behavior of chronic pressure-overloaded hearts in response to different acute loads compared to controls. In the present study moderate left ventricular hypertrophy (LVH) was produced in dogs by chronic aortic constriction in order to examine the following questions on the heart in situ:

1. Is the maximum contractility – expressed as (dp/dt)max, t – (dp/dt)max and Vpm in dogs with LVH different from a control group?
2. Is there a significant difference in maximum left ventricular pressure during acute aortic clamping or in reaction to a rapid volume overload in comparison to a control group?
3. Is there a difference in the survival rate following acute occlusion of the left circumflex artery (LCA) between animals with left ventricular hypertrophy and animals without? Both groups met the requirements of the same coronary collateral vessel status.

Methods

40 adult mongrel dogs were prepared for coarctatio aortae during aseptic thoracotomy under anesthesia. A hygroscopic casein cylinder block sleeved by stainless steel was placed around the upper part of the aorta descendens. This prosthesis constricted a mean of about 60% of the lumen of the aorta.

18 of the 40 dogs which survived the coarctation minimum period of 140 days were studied from 144 up to 218 days after operation and compared to a control group of 17 animals with comparable body weight.

The experiments were performed under standardized conditions. Anesthesia was carried out with piritramide and nitrous oxide using artificial respiration.

The heart rate (HR), electrocardiogram, left ventricular (LVP) and aortic pressure (AoP_s, AoP_d), measured by two high-fidelity Millar-catheter-tip-manometers were recorded continuously by a high-speed Honeywell-UV-Recorder.

The "so-called" paramters of contractility – that is (dp/dt)max and peak measured velocity – expressed as the ratio of dp/dt to instantaneous left ventricular pressure – were derived continuously from left ventricular pressure by a differentiator.

In 12 dogs with coarctatio aortae and 6 controls the maximum of contractility – defined by maximal obtained (dp/dt)max – were stimulated by stepwise–increasing doses of combined infusion of isoproterenol and norepinephrine. In earlier investigations we recognized that the heart rate and afterload were nearly constant if the proportion of isoproterenol to norepinephrine was 1:10. The cardiac output was measured by thermodilution. These in situ experiments were done by closed, the following investigations by open chest.

By means of a reversible silk tourniquet, in 6 dogs with left ventricular hypertrophy and 6 control dogs the ascending aorta was occluded acutely and the maximal LVP was measured twice. In these animals the acute volume overload was done by a rapid dextrane (6%) solution injected into the right atrium, with a velocity of 100 ml/min, the total injected volume was 1400 ml.

One to two hours thereafter the left circumflex artery (LCA) was occluded acutely in 13 coarctated dogs and 11 controls. The development of ventricular ectopic beats and the latency – determined as the time from occlusion till the onset of ventricular fibrillation – were monitored in both groups when they occurred.

In 5 animals with coarctatio aortae and 6 control dogs myocardial catecholamines in each part of the heart were assayed spectrofluorometrically by the trihydroxy-indole method according to *van Euler* and *Lishajko* as modified by *Anton* and *Sayre* (1).

24 hours post mortem, a selective coronary angiography was performed to reveal the extent of the collateral vessels of the heart. In a former study the results from

Dr. *Meesmann* (10) clearly revealed the strong positive correlation between early mortality due to ventricular fibrillation and the exclusion of effective collateral vessels of the heart.

All hearts were studied post mortem to determine the presence and degree of left ventricular hypertrophy by weight measuring. The following indices of hypertrophy (8) were calculated: ratio of left ventricular weight to total heart weight subtracted by left ventricular weight and ratio of left ventricular weight to body weight (more methodological details: 3, 10).

Results and discussion

In all dogs with coarctatio aortae, left ventricular heart failure could be excluded by normal left ventricular enddiastolic pressure, the absence of pulmonary edema and ascites. In coarctated dogs the degree of left ventricular hypertrophy – expressed by LVW/BW and LVW/THW-LVW – was significantly greater than that in the controls (s. table 1), therefore a mild left ventricular hypertrophy could be established. Otherwise there was no significant difference in right ventricular weight between both groups.

The average body weight was nearly the same in both groups (LVH = 24.6 ± 4.2 kg; CG = 23.8 ± 4.0 kg).

The mean hemodynamic and contractility data of the 12 LVH dogs and the 6 control dogs at rest and during obtained maximal values of (dp/dt)max stimulated by catecholamines are shown in table 2. As a consequence of the coarctation a significant difference in AoP_s ($p < 0.05$) and AoP_d ($p < 0.01$) at rest occurred. The mildly enhanced stroke volume/10 kg ($p < 0.05$) in the coarctated dogs at rest is explained by the diminished heart rate (–19 b/min) in this group, the cardiac output was nearly the same.

Table 1. Comparison of observed hypertrophy-indices (left ventricular = LV-; right ventricular = RV-; total heart = TH-; and body weight = BW) between aorta-constricted animals (LVH) and control animals (CG).

	LVH_1 n = 12	CG_1 n = 6	LVH_2 n = 6	CG_2 n = 6	LVH n = 18	CG n = 12
coarct. time days	165,7 $^+_-$17	-	217 $^+_-$11	-	180 $^+_-$14	-
LVW g	134,8 ,* $^+_-$19,5	119 $^+_-$20,1	128,3 * $^+_-$9,7	94,3 $^+_-$7,6	133 * $^+_-$16,3	107 $^+_-$13,1
RVW g	43,4 o $^+_-$6,8	42,6 $^+_-$5,2	36,4 * $^+_-$4,3	31,4 $^+_-$4,1	41,4 o $^+_-$5,6	36,4 $^+_-$4,65
LVW THW-LVW	1,99 * $^+_-$0,19	1,72 $^+_-$0,21	1,91 * $^+_-$0,07	1,58 $^+_-$0,14	1,946 * $^+_-$0,15	1,678 $^+_-$0,18
LVW BW	5,32 * $^+_-$0,68	4,6 $^+_-$0,7	5,32 * $^+_-$0,57	4,4 $^+_-$0,38	5,32 * $^+_-$0,7	4,54 $^+_-$0,599

(unpaired t - test ; o = n.s. ;   * = p<0,05) MV $^+_-$ 1 SD

Table 2. Parameter of hemodynamics and contractility at rest and during obtained max. value of (dp/dt)max induced by catecholamine application. Mean values ± SD in dogs with coarctatio aortae compared to a control group. AoPs = systolic, AoPd = diastolic aortic pressure; HR = heart rate; LVEDP = left ventricular enddiastolic pressure; SV/10 kg = stroke volume per 10 kg body weight; parameter of contractility: (dp/dt)max; t-(dp/dt)max, Vpm = velocity peak measured.

	AoP_s mmHg	AoP_d mmHg	HR l/min.	SV/10 kg ml	LVEDP mmHg	$(dp/dt)_{max}$ (mmHg/sec)	$t\text{-}(dp/dt)_{max}$ ms	Vpm cir./sec.
values in rest:								
LVH_1 n=12	149±19	98.8±21	96,5±27	14,2±2,4	4,27±1,86	3362±1180	44,7±5,48	85,3±13,4
	p<0,05	p<0,01	o	p<0,05	o	p<0,05	o	o
CG_1 n=6	132±24	81,7±11	115±18	11,7±1,1	4,5±1,5	2658±873	44,5±11,8	80±12
max. stimulation:								
LVH_1* n=12	157,7±32	92,2±8,04	125,7±15	24,4±1,97	9,5±2,2	10284±2221	26±2,6	135,9±17,5
	o	o	o	p<0,05	o	o	p<0,05	p<0,05
CG_1**	155±13	90±16	122±32	20±2	11±4	10200±3405	30±2	119±14

Mean value ±1 SD ; LVH_1 = left ventric. hypertrophy ; (unpaired t-test) ; control group (CG_1) ; o = no significance
* = (0,1γ Isoproterenol + 1γ Norepinephrine)/kg a. min. ** = (0,25γ Isoproterenol + 2,5γ Norepinephrine)/kg a. min.

The left ventricular enddiastolic pressure was very similar in both groups. In response to exogenous catecholamines only the SV/10 kg was significantly enhanced in the chronic pressure-overloaded group.

Contractility (s. table 2) was assessed by the maximum of the first derivative of the LVP and labeled (dp/dt)max, the time from the beginning till the maximum of (dp/dt)max, and the peak measured velocity (Vpm), a so-called "index of contractility". These parameters were always measured in the isovolumic phase of left ventricular contraction. The parameters of contractility at rest and during maximal catecholamine stimulation are compared. No significant difference was observed in Vpm and t-(dp/dt)max between the two groups at rest, whereas the enhanced (dp/dt)max (p < 0.05) in the LVH group may be explained by a significantly higher afterload. In maximal performed inotropic state, (dp/dt)max was nearly the same in both groups, whereas Vpm and t-(dp/dt)max were significantly changed suggesting enhanced contractility in LVH dogs. We would like to repeat that in this state the heart rate, afterload and the left ventricular enddiastolic pressure were nearly equal. It was evident that the maximum of the nondepressed contractility was attained with a significant, minor concentration of catecholamines (fig. 1). The effective dose of 50% (ED 50) of the maximally reached value of contractility parameters was clearly reduced. It appears that the inotropic actions of isoproterenol and norepinephrine are significantly intensified in the moderate left ventricular hypertrophied heart as compared with normal hearts, a fact which suggests an enhanced β-adrenergic responsiveness of the mildly pressure-overloaded hypertrophied heart. A similar effect was seen by *Kobayashi* et al. (7) who described a clearly intensified inotropic and chronotropic response due to isoproterenol infusion in the nonfailing hypertrophied

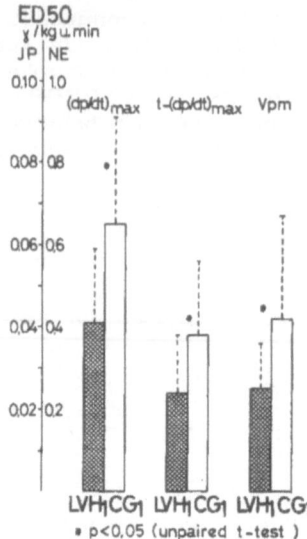

Fig. 1. Effective dose (ED_{50}) at 50% of the maximum value of contractility parameter due to combined doses of isoproterenol (IP) and norepinephrine (NE) (1:10). LVH_1 (n = 12) versus CG_1 (n = 6). Mean ±1SD.

heart. In contrast to this, *Hein* et al. (4) published their findings of restriction of β-adrenergic responsiveness because they found a reduced isoproterenol-induced Ca^{++} uptake of the hypertrophied myocardium. *Ito* et al. (5) otherwise described a normal sarcoplasmic reticular Ca^{++} uptake in the mild, and a reduced Ca^{++} uptake in the severe left ventricular hypertrophy.

Following the subdivision of heart hyperfunction as proposed by *Meerson* (9), acute pressure overload is related to isometrical, whereas acute volume overload corresponds to isovolumic hyperfunction.

After acute occlusion of the ascending aorta, we observed a higher left ventricular peak pressure (fig. 2) in the coarctated animals. However,

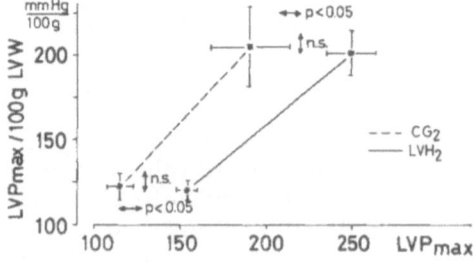

Fig. 2. Mean values (±SEM) of the LVP (left ventricular pressure) – absolutely and per 100 g left ventricular wet weight (LVW) – before and during acute occlusion of the ascending aorta. Dogs with left ventricular hypertrophy (LVH_2, n = 6) compared to control dogs (CG_2, n = 6) (unpaired t test).

when left ventricular peak pressure was calculated per 100 g left ventricular wet weight, the pressure increase was nearly similar in both groups.

On the other hand, during a rapid infusion of 6% dextrane we observed no significant difference in LVEP, and the poorly higher heart rate in the LVH group was also not significant (fig. 3). These results indicate that the chronic pressure-overloaded left ventricle is primarily not adapted to an acute volume overload. A possible explanation may be the diminished compliance of the left ventricular hypertrophied hearts (9).

In a subsequent study we examined the reaction of the hypertrophied heart, especially the early mortality due to ventricular fibrillation in the first arrhythmic phase, that occur in the first 30 minutes following acute ligation of the LCA. This early mortality after acute ligation of the LCA in dogs with coarctatio aortae which is restricted to animals without functional collateral vessels differed markedly from that of the controls. Although many ventricular ectopic beats occurred, 9 of the 13 dogs with LVH survived the early arrhythmic phase following the acute occlusion with an observation time of more than 6 hours. The other 4 died from ventricular fibrillation. In contrast, 10 of the 11 control dogs died of ventricular fibrillation during the first 20 minutes following coronary occlusion. This difference is statistically significant ($p < 0.05$). These findings confirm an earlier comparable study of our laboratory (1a) in which we saw a similar effect in dogs with volume-overloaded hearts induced by running events.

Since ventricular fibrillation as a consequence of acute LCA-ligation decreased significantly in the coarctated dogs, a decrease of the endogenous catecholamines could probably be due in part to this protective mechanism (12). Therefore, the total catecholamines and the norepinephrine concentrations in a fourth group were assayed for each part of the heart. Unexpectedly the catecholamine concentration of the right ventri-

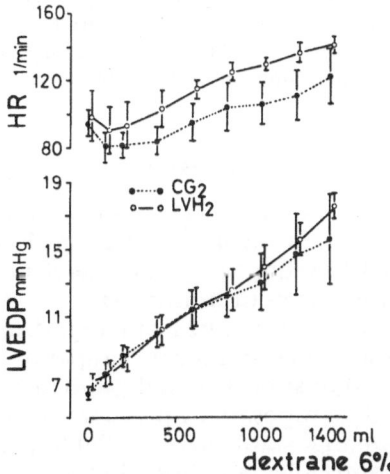

Fig. 3. Mean values (± SEM) of the LVEDP and HR in dogs with coarctatio aortae (LVH$_2$ = 6) compared to controls (CG$_2$ = 6) during rapid infusion of 6% dextrane (100 ml/min). (Unpaired t test; no significance.)

Table 3. Catecholamine-concentration in different parts of the heart. Mean values ± 1 SD in dogs with left ventricular hypertrophy (LVH$_4$, n = 5) compared to a control-group (CG$_4$, n = 6). (ng/g wet weight).

		Total Catecholamines			Norepinephrine		
		LVH$_4$ (n=5)	p	CG$_4$ (n=6)	LVH$_4$ (n=5)	p	CG$_4$ (n=6)
Auricle	l.	1779 ($^+_-$ 255)	ns	1857 ($^+_-$ 242)	1653 ($^+_-$ 241)	ns	1766 ($^+_-$ 241)
	r.	1466 ($^+_-$ 168)	ns	1829 ($^+_-$ 217)	1331 ($^+_-$ 152)	ns	1734 ($^+_-$ 229)
Atrium	l.	1250 ($^±_-$ 136)	ns	1436 ($^+_-$ 132)	1144 ($^+_-$ 127)	ns	1239 ($^+_-$ 102)
	r.	1379 ($^+_-$ 161(	ns	1846 ($^+_-$ 203)	1338 ($^+_-$ 151)	ns	1654 ($^+_-$ 220)
Ventricle	l.	726 ($^+_-$ 22)	ns	748 ($^+_-$ 113)	661 ($^+_-$ 24)	ns	719 ($^+_-$ 112)
	r.	729 ($^+_-$ 67)	s	916 ($^+_-$ 28)	699 ($^+_-$ 71)	s	834 ($^+_-$ 34)

s = p < 0,05 ; ns = no significance (u - test) ; l = left , r = right
Recovery : 63 % (averaged), no correction for this recovery, standard deviations for duplicate analyses : 3,4 %

cle was diminished significantly, however, the catecholamines in all parts were reduced (s. table 3). The mild decrease of the catecholamine concentration in left ventricular hypertrophy suggests that there may be more than one mechanism by which the higher survival rate of the LVH heart could be explained. An additional reason explaining the greater survival rate may be the diminished norepinephrine release from hypertrophied hearts following acute ischemia compared to normal hearts (11). We think that the conditions of ventricular fibrillation are complex and further investigations will be done to explore the reasons as to why the moderately hypertrophied heart has a better electrophysiologic protection against acute ligation of the LCA.

Conclusions

The following conclusions can be drawn from our studies:
1. Moderate pressure-overloaded left ventricular hypertrophy causes no decrease in myocardial function in whole intact hearts. The contractile and pressure reserve force is not diminished.

It is informative to compare results from hypertrophied hearts of intact animals with those from isolated muscle preparations of hypertrophied hearts. In contrast to studies on isolated papillary muscles which indicated a depressed cardiac function in pressure-overloaded hypertrophy, our studies demonstrate that stable myocardial hypertrophy is not associated with depressed ventricular function at rest and acute cardiovascular stress in the intact heart. These results support the thesis that hypertrophy in the absence of cardiac failure is a physiological adaption which enables the heart to meet the demands of chronically increased pressure work.

2. The mild left ventricular hypertrophied heart reacts with an inotropic supersensitivity to exogenous catecholamines.

3. The left ventricular hypertrophied heart is better protected against developing ventricular fibrillation following acute ligation of the LCA. We don't think that the mild depletion of the heart catecholamine concentration is the only mechanism responsible for this protection.

Zusammenfassung

Die Untersuchungen wurden an Hunden mit einer signifikanten, mäßiggradigen, linksventrikulären Hypertrophie unter der Fragestellung der maximalen Leistungsbreite dieser Herzen und des Verhaltens nach akuter Ligatur der linken Koronararterie durchgeführt. Die linksventrikuläre Hypertrophie wurde durch eine Coarctatio aortae erzeugt.

Die hämodynamischen Parameter wurden während der Ausgangsphase und einer stufenweise erhöhten Katecholamin-Infusion gemessen und zu Kontrolltieren (CG = 6) verglichen. Dabei stellte sich heraus, daß die maximale Kontraktilität bei den LVH-Tieren (LVH = 12) gegenüber den Kontrollen gering erhöht war. Bezogen auf 100 g linksventrikuläres Feuchtgewicht ergab sich für beide Gruppen nach akuter Abklemmung der Aorta ascendens ein nahezu identischer maximaler Druckanstieg im linken Ventrikel. Gegenüber einer schnellen Volumeninfusion reagierten die hypertrophierten Herzen mit einem geringgradig höheren Anstieg der Herzfrequenz und des enddiastolischen Druckes, was als Ausdruck einer verminderten Compliance angesehen werden kann.

Nach akuter Ligatur des Ramus circumflexus der linken Kranzarterie (LVH$_3$ = 13, CG$_3$ = 11) zeigte sich eine signifikant (p < 0,05) höhere Überlebensrate bei den Tieren mit linksventrikulärer Hypertrophie und vergleichbarem Kollateralstatus. In einer vierten Gruppe (LVH$_4$ = 5, CG$_4$ = 6) wurde die Katecholaminkonzentration in den verschiedenen Kompartimenten des Herzens als mögliche Erklärungsursache für die unterschiedliche Häufigkeit des Kammerflimmerns nach akuter Koronarligatur bestimmt. Unerwarteterweise sahen wir eine signifikant geringere Katecholaminkonzentration im nicht hypertrophierten rechten Ventrikel der Hypertrophietiere, jedoch waren die Konzentrationen in allen Kompartimenten des hypertrophierten Herzens gering vermindert. Weitere Untersuchungen sind erforderlich, um den besseren elektrophysiologischen Schutz des hypertrophierten Herzens gegenüber einer akuten Koronarligatur zu erklären.

References

1. *Anton, A. H., D. F. Sayre:* A study of the factors affecting the aluminium oxide trihydroxy-indole procedure for the analysis of catecholamines. J. Pharmacol. Exp. Ther. **138**, 360–375 (1962).

1a. *Amann, L., W. Meesmann, G. Schley, F. W. Schulz, K. Stephan, J. Tüttemann, A. Wilde:* Verminderte Mortalität nach akutem experimentellem Koronarverschluß durch körperliches Training. Verh. Dtsch. Ges. Kreislaufforschg. **38**, 276 (Darmstadt 1972).

2. *Badeer, H. S.:* "Contractility" of the nonfailing hypertrophied heart. Amer. Heart J. **73**, 693 (1967).

3. *Bischoff, K.-O., W. Meesmann, K. Stephan:* Untersuchungen zur Kontraktilitäts-, Druck- und Volumenreserve druckhypertrophierter Herzen in situ. Z. Kardiol. **65**, 131–142 (1976).

4. *Hein, B., J. Janke:* Restriction of β-adrenergic responsiveness in hypertrophied ventricular myocardium of rats. Basic Res. Cardiol. **72**, 279–285 (1977).

5. *Ito, Y., C. A. Chidsey:* Intracellular calcium and myocardial contractility. J. Mol. Cell. Cardiol. **4**, 507 (1972).

6. *Kissling, G., M. F. Wendt-Gallitelli:* Dynamics of the hypertrophied left ventricle in the rat. Effects of physical training and chronic pressure overload. Basic Res. Cardiol. **72**, 178–183 (1977).
7. *Kobayashi, T., R. Nakayama, K. Kimura, T. Yoneyama:* Cardiovascular Responses to Intravenous Isoproterenol Infusion in Subjects with and without Left Ventricular Hypertrophy. Jap. Circulat. J. **43**, 575–585 (1970).
8. *Krayenbühl, H. P., E. C. Peirce II, T. Agishi:* Left ventricular Dynamics in the Dog under Chronic Pressure Load from Coarctation of the aorta. Arch. Kreis-l3aufforschg. **56**, 1–25 (1968).
9. *Meerson, F. Z.:* Hyperfunktion, Hypertrophie und Insuffizienz des Herzens. VEB Verlag Volk u. Gesundheit (Berlin 1969).
10. *Meesmann, W., F. W. Schulz, G. Schley, P. Adolphsen:* Überlebensquote nach akutem experimentellen Koronarverschluß in Abhängigkeit von Spontankol-lateralen des Herzens. Z. ges. exp. Med. **153**, 246 (1970).
11. *Shahab, L., A. Wollenberger, E.-G. Krause, S. Genz:* The effect of acute ischaemia on catecholamines and cyclic-AMP levels in normal and hyper-trophied myocardium, in: Effects of Acute Ischaemia on Myocardial Function. Eds.: *Oliver, Julian, Donald* (Livingstone–Edinburgh–London 1972).
12. *Spann, J. F., R. A. Buccino, E. H. Sonnenblick, E. Braunwald:* Contractile state of cardiac muscle obtained from cats with experimentally produced ventricular hypertrophy and heart failure. Circulat. Res. **21**, 341 (1967).

Authors' address:

Dr. *K. O. Bischoff,* Kardiologische Abt. der Med. Klinik u. Poliklinik d. Universität (GHS), Hufelandstr. 55, 4300 Essen

Basic Res. Cardiol. **75**, 279–280 (1980)
© 1980 Dr. Dietrich Steinkopff Verlag, Darmstadt
ISSN 0300-8428

Paper, presented at the Erwin Riesch Symposium, Tübingen, April 3–7, 1979

Medizinische Universitätsklinik, Tübingen, Germany

Influence of acute alcohol intoxication on the left ventricular pressure-volume relations of the rat heart

Einfluß der akuten Alkoholintoxikation auf die linksventrikulären Druck-Volumen-Beziehungen am Rattenherzen

A. Hepp, H. Schier, and *K. Kochsiek*

With 1 table

Summary

In 17 Wistar rats isovolumetric pressure-volume diagrams, the rate of pressure rise, and the resting tension curve were recorded prior to and during acute alcohol intoxication. Ethyl alcohol was infused intravenously; parameters were recorded at blood alcohol levels between 0.6% and 0.2%. The following results were obtained.
1. In agreement with other authors, even slight amounts of alcohol induce significant cardiodepression.
2. At high blood alcohol levels the isovolumetric pressure-volume relation is shifted to higher enddiastolic volumes and pressures.
3. The alcohol-induced cardiodepression is dose-dependent. There is a linear correlation between the maximum rate of pressure rise and the blood alcohol level.

Cardiac depression is a known feature of acute and chronic alcohol intoxication (1). This has been confirmed by some authors. There are only few investigations, however, about the influence on the pressure-volume relations of the left ventricle and about the assumed dose-dependent cardiac depressant effect. This study was designed to test to what extent acute alcohol intoxication causes a dose-related cardiac depression.

Methods

17 young healthy male Wistar rats with an average body weight of 320 g were anesthetized with Urethane i.p.; tracheotomy and thoracotomy were performed, ventilation was maintained by a respirator, and a cannula was inserted into the left ventricle for pressure recordings. Left ventricular pressure (LVP), left ventricular enddiastolic pressure (EDP), rate of pressure rise (dp/dt) and an Ecg were recorded in situ under isovolumetric cardiac performance before and after alcohol infusion at different blood alcohol levels, and the resting tension curve was constructed (EDV = enddiastolic volume).

After intravenous infusion of ethyl alcohol the initial blood alcohol level of 0.6% fell to 0.2% within one hour.

Statistical analysis was done with the paired t-test.

Results

In acute alcohol intoxication the isovolumetric systolic pressure-volume curve is shifted to a higher enddiastolic volume as compared with controls, i.e., at any enddiastolic pressure the intoxicated rats develop a lower systolic pressure. The optimum of the pressure-volume relation (= point of maximal systolic pressure), however, is shifted to higher enddiastolic pressure and volume only for high blood alcohol levels.

At a blood alcohol level of 0.55% dp/dt_{max} is diminished by 45%, LVP by 28%, EDP is increased by 44%, EDV by 11% at the optimum. The change of LVP and dp/dt_{max} induced by alcohol intoxication is significant even at a blood alcohol level of 0.2%.

The maximum rate of pressure rise proves to be the most sensitive parameter for cardiac depression caused by acute alcohol intoxication; dp/dt_{max} corresponds to blood alcohol level in a linear correlation.

The resting tension curve is not altered by acute alcohol intoxication.

Table 1.

Values at the optimum of pressure volume diagram

n = 17 $\bar{x} \pm s\bar{x}$		LVP mmHg	EDP mmHg	EDV µl	dp/dt_{max} mmHg/sec
Controls		282 ± 4	5.6 ± 0.6	302 ± 7	11 580 ± 383
Alcohol	0.2 %	273 ± 4	4.5 ± 0.2	281 ± 6	10 574 ± 471
	0.45%	244 ± 7	5.7 ± 0.5	310 ± 9	8 191 ± 617
	0.55%	202 ± 13	8.1 ± 0.9	334 ± 10	6 382 ± 385

According to these findings it is concluded that
1. in agreement with other authors even small amounts of alcohol produce significant cardiac depression.
2. at higher blood alcohol levels the isovolumetric pressure-volume relation is shifted to higher enddiastolic pressure and volume.
3. cardiac depression in acute alcohol intoxication is dose-dependent, as expressed in the linear correlation of blood alcohol level and dp/dt_{max}.

Zusammenfassung

Bei 17 Wistarratten wurden vor und während akuter Alkoholintoxikation isovolumetrische Druck-Volumen-Diagramme, Druckanstiegsgeschwindigkeit und die Ruhedehnungskurve registriert. Der Äthylalkohol wurde intravenös infundiert; die Messungen erfolgten bei Blutalkoholspiegeln zwischen 0,6% und 0,2%.

Dabei ergaben sich folgende Ergebnisse:
1. In Übereinstimmung mit anderen Autoren führen bereits geringe Mengen zu einer signifikanten Kardiodepression.
2. Bei hohem Blutalkoholspiegel ist die isovolumetrische Druck-Volumen-Beziehung zu höheren enddiastolischen Volumina und Drücken verschoben.
3. Die alkoholinduzierte Kardiodepression ist dosisabhängig. Maximale Druckanstiegsgeschwindigkeit und Blutalkoholspiegel zeigen eine lineare Korrelation.

References

1. *Kuhn, H.* und *F. Loogen:* Die Wirkung von Alkohol auf das Herz einschließlich der Alkoholkardiomyopathie. Internist **19,** 97–106 (1978).

For reprints:

Dr. A. Hepp, Medizinische Universitätsklinik, 7400 Tübingen

Basic Res. Cardiol. **75**, 281–288 (1980)
© 1980 Dr. Dietrich Steinkopff Verlag, Darmstadt
ISSN 0300-8428

Paper, presented at the Erwin Riesch Symposium, Tübingen, April 3–7, 1979

*Department of Physiology and Biophysics, University of Nebraska College of
Medicine, Omaha, Nebraska*

The contribution of neural pathways to blood volume homeostasis in the subhuman primate*)

Der Beitrag nervaler Einflüsse zur Homöostase des Blutes bei Primaten

J. P. Gilmore and *I. H. Zucker**)*

With 5 figures

Summary

Studies are presented which indicate that the neural components of an atrio-
renal reflex appear to be present in the primate and thus presumably in man.
However, this reflex does not appear to contribute importantly to blood volume
homeostasis in the primate. It is our hypothesis that it is the high-pressure
baroreceptors, i.e., those in the carotid sinus and those in the aortic arch which play
the major role in the neural control of blood volume in the primate and thus in man.
This apparent evolutionary change in the importance of high pressure vs. low
pressure receptors in the neural modulation of blood volume may be related to the
assumption of an upright or semi-upright posture.

In 1956 *Henry* and associates demonstrated that distention of the left
atrium of the dog was associated with a significant diuresis which could
not be accounted for on the basis of the associated hemodynamic changes.
The results of their study led them to conclude that stretch receptors in the
left atrium and terminal pulmonary veins are involved in a mechanism
which links changes in the actively circulating blood volume with
homeostatic responses of the kidney. Subsequent studies by other investigators demonstrated that the afferent pathway of the atrio-renal reflex
was via the vagus and that the efferent component appeared to involve
both hormonal and neural mechanisms. The former conclusion was based
on the observation that either cooling, or section of, the vagi inhibited the
diuretic response to distention of the left atrium (12). A number of investigators have shown that distention of the atrium is associated with a
decrease in the circulating levels of ADH (2, 3) and possibly the circulating
levels of renin (16) and thus presumably aldosterone. And finally, distention of the atrium is associated with an inhibition of renal nerve activity
(13) and a substantial tachycardia (14), particularly in the conscious dog or
in the anesthetized dog whose basal heart rate is within normal limits.
Figure 1 is a schematic of how these responses to atrial distention may

*) The material presented was supported by NIH Grant No. HL13427
**) Dr. *Zucker* is an Established Investigator of the American Heart Association

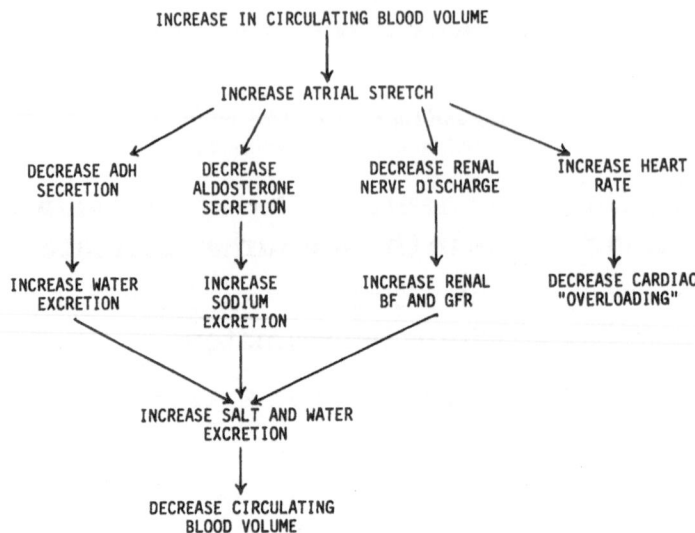

Fig. 1. Schematic of homeostatic response to an increase in circulating blood volume.

play an important role in blood volume homeostasis. An increase in circulating blood volume will lead to an increase in the extent of atrial stretch thereby stimulating the so-called atrial volume receptors. This, in turn, will lead to a decrease in the secretion of ADH and aldosterone. As a result there will be an increase in both salt and water excretion thereby decreasing circulating blood volume returning it to its normal level. The decrease in renal nerve discharge will presumably increase renal blood flow and glomerular filtration rate thereby adding to the increased salt and water excretion and thus decrease in circulating blood volume. The increase in heart rate resulting in a decrease in the time available for cardiac filling will prevent diastolic overloading of the heart.

Except for the effect on aldosterone secretion, the mechanisms shown in figure 1 have been reasonably well documented in the dog. However, the extent to which this atrio-renal reflex may play an important homeostatic role in the primate and thus in man has not been well documented. Several years ago, while carrying out studies designed to characterize various factors which may alter the electrical discharge from atrial receptors, we undertook experiments to determine whether or not one could demonstrate the presence of this reflex in the subhuman primate and, if so, to determine its physiologic significance. The first series of experiments were undertaken to determine if it was possible to demonstrate by recording from vagal afferents receptor activity in the atrium which was specifically responsive to increases in atrial volume and thus atrial distention. Figure 2 is a tracing of an original recording from a typical left atrial stretch receptor obtained from an open-chest monkey (17). The activity from the receptor is seen only during the period of atrial filling, i.e., during the period of the v-wave of the atrial pressure pulse.

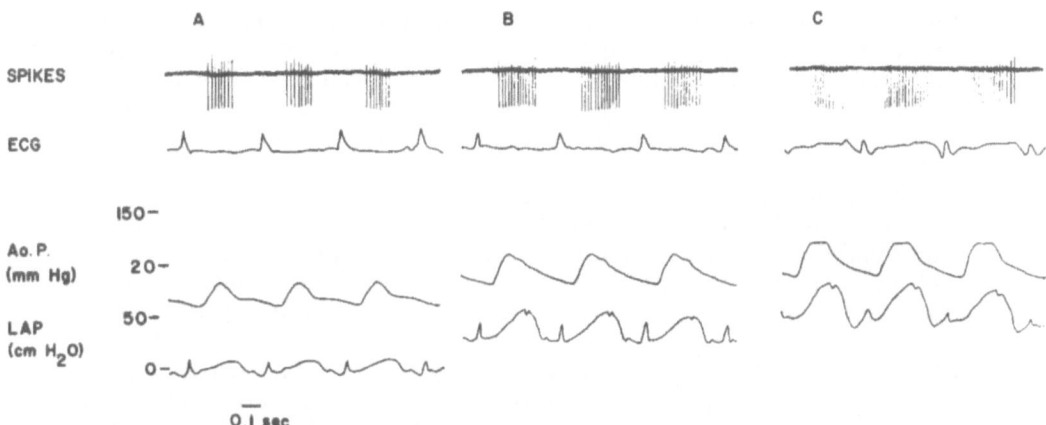

Fig. 2. Recording from a monkey showing discharge from a left atrial receptor (spikes) electrocardiogram (Ecg) aortic pressure (AoP) and left atrial pressure (LAP). Between A and B and B and C intravenous isotonic saline was given in order to increase LAP. Reprinted with permission (17).

Also note that at the time the atrio-ventricular valve opens, i.e., when the v-wave descends, electrical activity stops completely. Between panels A and B and B and C an intravenous infusion of isotonic saline was administered in order to increase left atrial pressure. With each increase in atrial pressure there was an increase in receptor discharge. Although these experiments demonstrated the presence of volume or stretch responsive receptors in the left atrium of the monkey, they did not provide quantitative information concerning their sensitivity. Therefore we undertook a

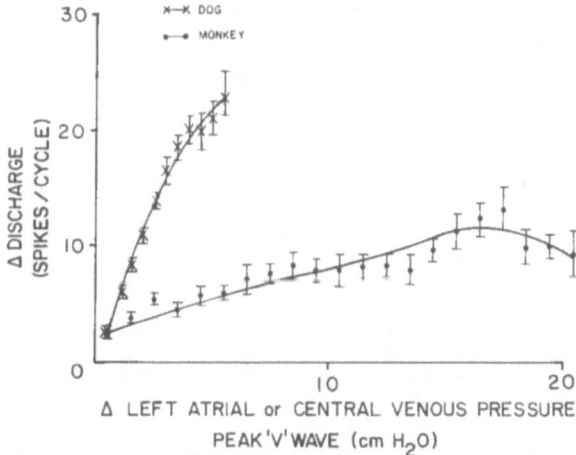

Fig. 3. The relationship between the change in discharge from left atrial receptors and the change in left atrial or central venous pressure for the dog (X–X; n = 24) and monkey (●–●; n = 24). Atrial pressure was increased by the IV administration of isotonic saline. Vertical bars are ± S.E.M. Reprinted with permission (17).

series of experiments to compare the sensitivity of these receptors in the monkey with those in the dog. Figure 3 shows the results of these experiments (17). Note how exquisitely sensitive the atrial receptors are in the dog. Small changes in left atrial pressure elicits very large changes in left atrial receptor activity. In contrast, in the monkey the receptors are considerably less sensitive.

Since it has been clearly shown by a number of investigators that increasing atrial stretch or distention is associated with a diuresis, we undertook experiments to determine if a similar response either quantitatively or qualitatively could be demonstrated in the subhuman primate (7). Before doing this, however, we assured ourselves that in our laboratory, atrial distention in the dog would indeed induce a diuresis (18). Figure 4 compares the renal responses of the monkey and those of the dog to atrial distention accomplished by inflating a balloon in the left atrium. This maneuver partially obstructs the mitral valve, producing a functional stenosis thereby increasing left atrial pressure and thus increasing the extent of left atrial stretch. Although significant elevations in left atrial pressure consistently induced a diuresis in the dog which could be

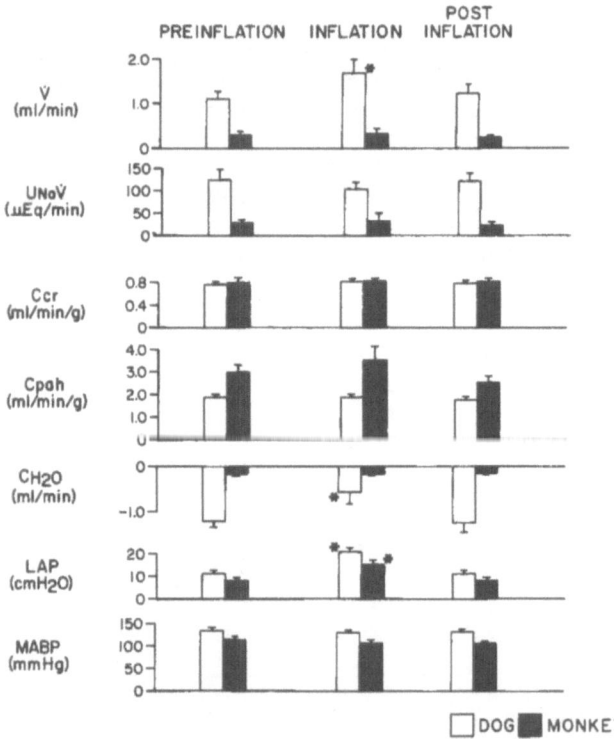

Fig. 4. Comparison of the renal responses to left atrial balloon inflation between the dog and monkey. $\dot{V}$ = urine flow, $U_{NA}\dot{V}$ = sodium excretion, C_{cr} = creatinine clearance, C_{pah} = para-aminohippuric acid clearance, C_{H_2O} = free water clearance, LAP = left atrial pressure, MABP = mean arterial blood pressure. Asterisk indicates a significant change from the preinflation value. Bars are ± S.E.M.

accounted for primarily on the basis of alterations in free water clearance, such an intervention had no significant influence on renal function of the primate, a finding consistent with the low sensitivity of the primate atrial receptors as indicated by the previous figure.

Distending a balloon in the atria of an animal is a very artificial way in which to increase atrial pressure. It has been shown that head-out water immersion of the human in the vertical position induces a very substantial natriuresis and diuresis (6). This maneuver is associated with a translocation of blood from the periphery to the thorax and substantial increases in heart volume and central venous pressure (4, 1). Since it has been hypothesized that the natriuretic and diuretic responses to head-out immersion in man are secondary to the stimulation of atrial receptors (1), we undertook experiments to determine the contribution of cardiopulmo-

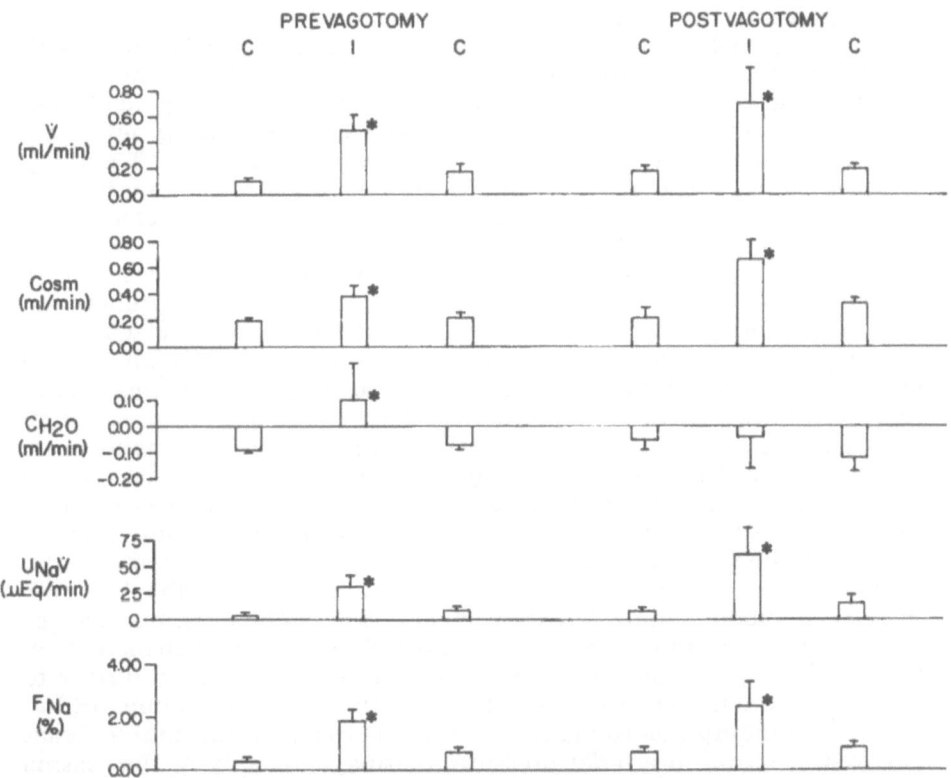

Fig. 5. Influence of bilateral cervical vagotomy on the renal responses to head-out immersion in the monkey. C = control with monkey sitting in a chair in the immersion tank without water; I = period during which tank was filled to the suprasternal notch. The first control values were obtained during the 10-minute period preceding immersion, the immersion values were obtained during the last 10 minutes of a 40-minute immersion period and the control after immersion 20 minutes after emptying the tank. Bars are ± S.E.M. Asterisk indicates a significant change from the control, $\dot{V}$ = urine flow, C_{osm} = osmolal clearance, C_{H_2O} = free water clearance, $U_{NA}\dot{V}$ = sodium excretion; F_{NA} = fractional sodium excretion.

nary receptors to the renal responses to head-out immersion in the nonhuman primate (8). As shown in figure 5, we observed that as in conscious man, head-out immersion of the anesthetized primate is associated with a substantial natriuresis and diuresis, the natriuresis being accounted for primarily by an increased fractional excretion of sodium. However, as is also shown in figure 5, bilateral cervical vagotomy had no substantial influence on the renal responses to immersion indicating that cardiopulmonary receptors whose axons traverse the vagal nerves are not necessary for the homeostatic adjustments to central hypervolemia in the primate and also presumably in man.

Head-out immersion of man is not associated with a tachycardia (1) despite the substantial increases in central venous pressure suggesting that the Bainbridge reflex, which is so easily demonstrable in the dog, has little functional importance in man. Further substantiation of this position is suggested by the results of a study by *Sanghvi* and associates who compared the hemodynamic responses of a group of normal patients with patients with coronary artery disease to acute intravascular volume expansion using low molecular weight dextran (15). In the normal patients, left ventricular end-diastolic pressure increased by 10.4 mm Hg, while the increase in the patients with coronary artery disease was 8.9 mm Hg. Despite these substantial elevations in left ventricular end-diastolic pressure and presumably left atrial pressure no significant changes in heart rate occurred in either group.

If atrial receptors play an important role in modulating the plasma level of ADH in response to changes in intravascular volume in the primate and man, one would predict that increases in intravascular volume which are associated with substantial increases in central venous pressure would also be associated with a decrease in the circulating levels of antidiuretic hormone. Experiments were therefore carried out in a group of six monkeys anesthetized with pentobarbital sodium (9). Measurements were made of arterial pressure, left ventricular end diastolic pressure as an index of left atrial pressure, plasma osmolality and plasma ADH concentrations. Intravascular volume was increased in two steps using isotonic-isooncotic dextran with each step consisting of a 7.5% increase in the estimated blood volume of the animal. In response to the first-step increase in blood volume, left ventricular end-diastolic pressure increase from a value of 4.3 to 18.5 cm of water and with the second-step increase in blood volume left ventricular end-diastolic pressure increased further to 20.7 cm of water. However, despite these substantial elevations of left ventricular end-diastolic and presumably left atrial pressure no significant changes occurred in arterial pressure, plasma osmolality or the plasma concentration of ADH in response to either infusion. These results are consistent with those of *Goetz* et al. who demonstrated that a non-hypotensive hemorrhage of 500 ml in man produces no changes in the circulating levels of antidiuretic hormone or renin (10). In these experiments, it is important to note that no changes in arterial pressure occurred as was the case in our experiments in which plasma volume was expanded.

We have recently completed experiments to determine the influence of atrial pressure on renal nerve activity. Monkeys were anesthetized with pentobarbital sodium and a balloon catheter inserted through the left atrial appendage after the animal had been prepared by thoracotomy. Efferent renal nerve activity was measured using standard electrophysiologic techniques. Elevations of atrial pressure induced by inflation of the atrial balloon produced variable changes in renal nerve activity in the neurally intact monkey. However, when the animals were baroreceptor-denervated, there was a consistent inhibition of renal nerve activity in response to the elevation of left atrial pressure.

Conclusions

Taken together, the data presented above indicate:
1) that the neural components of an atrio-renal reflex appear to be present in the primate and thus presumably in man:
2) Although present, this reflex does not appear to contribute importantly to blood volume homeostasis in the primate.
3) It is our hypothesis that it is the high pressure baroreceptors, i.e., those in the carotid sinus and those in the aortic arch, that play the major role in the neural control of blood volume in the primate and thus in man. This apparent evolutionary change in the importance of high pressure *vs.* low pressure receptors in the neural modulation of blood volume may be related to the assumption of an upright or semi-upright posture.
4) The differences between the dog and the primate raise questions as to the usefulness of the dog as a model for man in studying the neural control of blood volume.

Zusammenfassung

Die Ergebnisse der vorgelegten Studie weisen darauf hin, daß beim Primaten und wahrscheinlich auch beim Menschen eine nervale Komponente eines atrio-renalen Reflexes vorhanden ist. Jedoch scheint dieser Reflex beim Primaten nicht wesentlich zur Homöostase des Blutvolumens beizutragen. Beim Primaten (und somit auch beim Menschen) spielen nach unserer Hypothese die Druckrezeptoren im Karotissinus und im Aortenbogen die Hauptrolle bei der nervalen Kontrolle des Blutvolumens. Diese entwicklungsgeschichtliche Änderung in der Bedeutung der Druckrezeptoren im arteriellen System, verglichen mit den Rezeptoren des Niederdrucksystems, bezüglich einer nervalen Regelung des Blutvolumens könnte mit der aufrechten oder halbaufrechten Körperhaltung in Zusammenhang gebracht werden.

References

1. *Arborelius, M., U. I. Balldin, B. Lilja, C. E. G. Lundgren:* Hemodynamic changes in man during immersion with the head above water. Aerospace Med. **43**, 592–598 (1972).
2. *Baisset, A., P. Montastruc:* Polyurie par distension auriculaire chez le chien: rôle de l'hormone antidiuretique. J. Physiol. (Paris) **49**, 33–36 (1957).
3. *De Torrente, A., F. L. Robertson, K. M. McDonald, R. W. Schrier:* Mechanism of diuretic response to increased left atrial pressure in the anesthetized dog. Kidney int. **8**, 355–361 (1975).
4. *Echt, M., L. Lange, O. H. Gauer:* Changes of peripheral venous tone and central transmural venous pressure during immersion in a thermo-neutral bath. Pflügers Arch. **352**, 211–217 (1974).

5. *Echtenkamp, S. F., J. P. Gilmore:* Left atrial balloon-induced changes in efferent renal nerve activity in the nonhuman primate. Fed. Proc. **38**, 1201 (1979).
6. *Epstein, M.:* Cardjovascular and renal effects of head-out water immersion in
   man: Application of the model in assessment of volume homeostasis. Circulat.
   Res. **39**, 619–628 (1976).
7. *Gilmore, J. P., I. H. Zucker:* Failure of left atrial distension to alter renal
   function in the non-human primate. Circulat. Res. **42**, 267–270 (1978).
8. *Gilmore, J. P., I. H. Zucker:* Contribution of vagal pathways to the renal
   responses to head-out immersion in the non-human primate. Circulat. Res. **42**,
   263–267 (1978).
9. *Gilmore, J. P., I. H. Zucker, M. J. Ellington, M. A. Richards, L. Share:* Failure of
   acute intravascular volume expansion to alter plasma ADH in the non-human
   primate M. fascicularis. (Submitted for publication 1979.)
10. *Goetz, K. L., G. C. Bond, W. E. Smith:* Effect of moderate hemorrhage in
    humans on plasma ADH and renin. Proc. Soc. Exp. Biol. Med. **145**, 277–280
    (1974).
11. *Henry, J. P., O. H. Gauer, J. L. Reeves:* Evidence of the atrial location of
    receptors influencing urine flow. Circulat. Res. **4**, 85–90 (1956).
12. *Henry, J. P., J. W. Pearce:* The possible role of cardiac atrial stretch receptors in
    the induction of changes in urine flow. J. Physiol. **131**, 572–585 (1956).
13. *Karim, F., C. Kidd, C. M. Malpus, P. E. Penna:* The effects of stimulation of the
    left atrial receptors on sympathetic efferent nerve activity. J. Physiol. **227**,
    243–260 (1972).
14. *Ledsome, J. R., R. J. Linden, W. J. O'Connor:* The mechanisms by which
    distension of the left atrium produces diuresis in anaesthetized dogs. J. Physiol.
    159, 87–100 (1961).
15. *Sanghvi, V. R., F. Khaja, A. L. Mark, J. O. Parker:* Effects of blood volume
    expansion on left ventricular hemodynamics in man. Circulation **46**, 780–787
    (1972).
16. *Zehr, J. E., J. A. Hasbargen, K. D. Kurz:* Reflex suppression of renin secretion
    during distension of cardiopulmonary receptors in dogs. Circulat. Res. **38**,
    232–239 (1976).
17. *Zucker, I. H., J. P. Gilmore:* Responsiveness of type B atrial receptors in the
    monkey. Brain Res. **95**, 159–169 (1975).
18. *Zucker, I. H., L. Share, J. P. Gilmore:* Renal effects of left atrial distension in
    dogs with chronic congestive heart failure. Amer. J. Physiol. **236**, H554–H560
    (1979).

Authors' address:

Dr. *J. P. Gilmore* and Dr. *I. H. Zucker,* Department of Physiology and Biophysics,
University of Nebraska College of Medicine, Omaha, Nebraska 68105, U.S.A.

Basic Res. Cardiol. **75,** 289–293 (1980)
© 1980 Dr. Dietrich Steinkopff Verlag, Darmstadt
ISSN 0300–8428

Paper, presented at the Erwin Riesch Symposium, Tübingen, April 3–7, 1979

Marien-Hospital Düsseldorf and Med. Univ.-Klinik Tübingen

Electrolyte and water balance in cardiac insufficiency. Recent clinical and experimental data

Elektrolyt- und Wasserhaushalt bei Herzinsuffizienz.
Neue klinische und experimentelle Ergebnisse

K. Hayduk, G. Riegger, and *A. Hepp*

With 3 figures

Summary

The reasons for the disturbances of electrolyte and water balance in cardiac failure are not yet clarified. The decrease of cardiac output in cardiac insufficiency causes humoral regulatory mechanisms such as increased activity of the renin-angiotensin-aldosterone system and increased secretion of antidiuretic hormone. These mechanisms in turn lead to an enhancement of renal sodium and water reabsorption. The humoral disturbances can be interpreted as ineffective regulatory mechanisms for hemodynamic changes in cardiac insufficiency; in fact, the humoral disturbances increase cardiac failure. In addition, an increased sodium content of the arteries may contribute to the hemodynamic changes in cardiac insufficiency.

The mechanisms involved in the disturbances of electrolyte and water balance in cardiac insufficiency are still poorly defined. In congestive heart failure, decreased cardiac output may cause humoral disturbances, such as increased activity of the renin-angiotensin-aldosterone system and enhanced release of antidiuretic hormone. These mechanisms result in an increased renal sodium and water retention.

The humoral factors may indicate compensatory mechanisms for hemodynamic changes in congestive heart failure. There are a lot of definitions of congestive heart failure (CHF), but there is no agreement as to which definition meets all kinds of heart failure. There is agreement that in CHF the heart is not able to keep up with the requirements of the periphery. The starting point of CHF is in fact the hemodynamic failure of the heart or at least the disability of the heart to compensate for increased hemodynamic requirements of the periphery (for example, anemia or arterial hypertension). The decreased cardiac output induces changes in the renin-angiotensin-aldosterone system (RAAS) and in the secretion of antidiuretic hormone (ADH).

These mechanisms may be primarily compensatory, but lead in fact by a vicious circle to a worsening of CHF. There are a lot of experimental

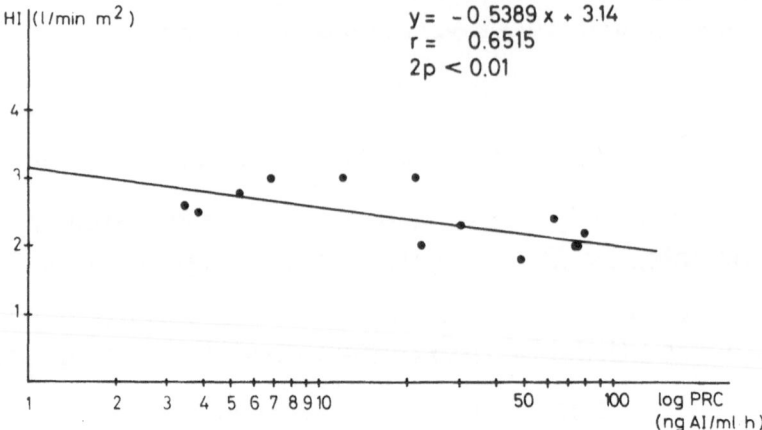

Fig. 1. Correlation between cardiac index and plasma renin concentration.

models of CHF. However, it should be kept in mind that different models of CHF (11) and studies in different species may result in quite controversial results and conclusions.

I. Renin-angiotensin-aldosterone system and sympathetic nervous systems

When cardiac output decreases, the activity of the sympathetic nervous system increases as shown directly by high plasma norepinephrine and

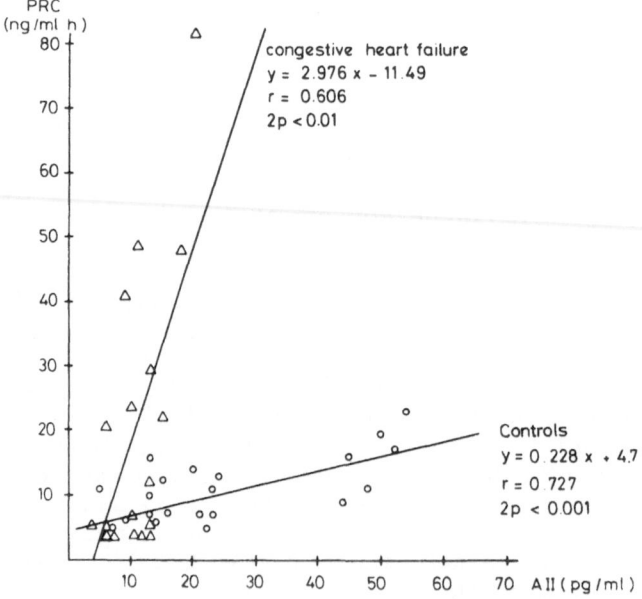

Fig. 2. Correlations between plasma renin concentration and angiotensin II in normal controls and patients with congestive heart failure.

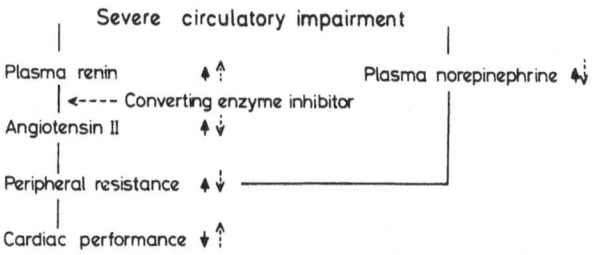

Fig. 3. Present concept of CEI in congestive heart failure.

possibly indirectly and multifactorially by an increase of heart rate and total peripheral resistance (11).

At the same time a redistribution of blood flow to the different organs occurs. The renal perfusion drops, the renal blood flow is redistributed from a prevalence of the outer cortex to the juxtamedullary zone. Renin secretion should increase when renal perfusion drops. However, in this point there is some controversy (2, 6, 10).

In 6 dogs with CHF and ascites caused by total tricuspidectomy we found a slightly higher plasma renin concentration (PRC) than in control dogs (n = 10; 1.38 ± 0.41 vs. 0.74 ± 0.25 ng angiotensin/ml·h incubation, mean ± SE). Surprisingly, renal renin concentration (RRC) was lower in dogs with CHF than in controls (19.0 + 1.0 vs. 49.7 ± 8.0 µg angiotensin/g renal cortex·h incubation; p < 0.05). RRC corresponded with the juxta-glomerular index (6.6 ± 0.8 vs. 11.5 ± 1.0; p < 0.01). The discrepancy between elevated PRC and suppressed RRC cannot be explained at present. Possibly, renin degradation is delayed because of hepatic congestion in CHF.

In men with severe CHF we studied the correlations between PRC and plasma angiotensin II (AII) and cardiac index (*Riegger, G.* et al., in preparation). There was a negative correlation between cardiac index and PRC (fig. 1) and AII, the correlation being closer to PRC than to AII (y = −0.4918x + 3.11; r = 0.5721; p < 0.02). Patients with CHF had low AII in correlation to their PRC compared with normal controls (fig. 2). Preliminary studies of our group indicate that the increased circulation time in CHF may cause higher degradation of AII in peripheral blood resulting in relatively low AII levels. Two effects of AII may be involved in development and maintenance of CHF: stimulation of aldosterone secretion and direct vasoconstrictory effect. A good correlation between PRC and aldosterone was shown several years ago (6, 9). Possibly, besides elevated aldosterone secretion a diminished aldosterone degradation by the congested liver may add to the enhancement of aldosterone in CHF. However, elevated aldosterone could not be demonstrated in CHF under steady-state conditions, aldosterone being augmented in developing CHF only.

A new and highly fascinating view on the role of RAAS is provided by the studies with converting enzyme inhibitors (CEI). High activity of AII at the arteriolar level (this has to be differentiated from plasma level of AII or pressor response to AII infusion) could account, together with increased activity of the sympathetic nervous system, for the vasoconstriction well known in CHF. After application of CEI total peripheral resistance (3, 5) and plasma norepinephrine (3) dropped. Plasma renin increased in both studies, whereas the predictory value of baseline PRC was somewhat controversial. Figure 3 summarizes the present data on CEI in congestive heart failure. The concordant changes of AII and norepinephrine support the old hypothesis that the action of AII is mediated by liberation of NE from sympathetic nerve endings (4).

There are some striking similarities in the role of RAAS in CHF and in arterial hypertension. In CHF, angiotensin-induced vasoconstriction may prevent hypotension and by overcompensation may be deleterious; in hypertension, primary angiotensin-induced vasoconstriction may produce hypertension. In both disorders CEI can restitute normal conditions.

II. Antidiuretic hormone (ADH)

The other axis which may induce disturbances of water metabolism in CHF is ADH. However, there are few studies on ADH in CHF, possibly because the measurement of ADH is still far from being established. In dogs with CHF and ascites after total tricuspidectomy there was a significant higher plasma ADH level compared to control values before tricuspidectomy and to values in dogs with tricuspidectomy but without severe CHF (1).

III. Electrolyte and water content in arterial tissue

Electrolyte and water balance may be disturbed in CHF at the vascular level as well. In dogs with CHF we studied sodium, potassium and water content in several vascular beds (mesenteric, saphenous, femoral, carotid, and renal arteries and thoracic aorta). Besides in the carotid artery, sodium content was higher in all arteries of dogs with CHF than in control dogs, potassium and water content showing no essential differences (8). The increased vascular sodium content which was demonstrated by other investigators as well (12) may contribute to vascular stiffness in CHF. Experimental studies on electrolytes, especially on potassium and magnesium in heart tissue, may add to the understanding of cardiac function in chronic electrolyte disturbance in man (7).

Zusammenfassung

Die Ursachen der Störungen des Elektrolyt- und Wasserhaushaltes bei Herzinsuffizienz sind noch weitgehend ungeklärt. Das verminderte Herz-Zeit-Volumen bei Herzinsuffizienz löst humorale Regulationsmechanismen wie eine gesteigerte Aktivität des Renin-Angiotensin-Aldosteron-Systems und eine vermehrte Freisetzung von antidiuretischem Hormon aus. Diese Mechanismen führen zu einer gesteigerten renalen Natrium- und Wasserretention. Die humoralen Faktoren können als ineffektive Kompensationsmechanismen für die gestörte Hämodynamik bei Herzinsuffizienz interpretiert werden; sie führen jedoch letztlich zu einer Verstärkung der Herzinsuffizienz. Daneben dürfte ein erhöhter Natriumgehalt der Arterien zu den hämodynamischen Veränderungen bei Herzinsuffizienz beitragen.

References

1. *Belleau, L., H. Mion, S. Simard, P. Granger, E. Bertranou, W. Nowaczynski, R. Boucher, J. Genest:* Studies on the mechanism of experimental congestive heart failure in dogs. Can. J. Physiol. Pharmacol. **48**, 450–456 (1970).
2. *Brown, J. J., D. L. Davies, V. W. Johnson, A. F. Lever, J. I. S. Robertson:* Renin relationships in congestive cardiac failure, treated and untreated. Amer. Heart J. **80**, 329–342 (1970).
3. *Curtiss, C., J. N. Cohn, T. Vrobel, J. A. Franciosa:* Role of the renin-angiotensin system in the systemic vasoconstriction of chronic congestive heart failure. Circulation **58**, 763–770.
4. *Distler, A., H. Liebau, H. P. Wolff:* Action of angiotensin on sympathetic nerve endings in isolated blood vessels. Nature **207**, 764–765 (1965).
5. *Gavras, H., D. P. Faxon, J. Berkoben, H. R. Brunner, T. J. Ryan:* Angiotensin converting enzyme inhibition in patients with congestive heart failure. Circulation **58**, 770–776 (1978).
6. *Genest, J., P. Granger, J. de Champlain, R. Boucher:* Endocrine factors in congestive heart failure. Amer. J. Cardiol. **22**, 35–42 (1968).
7. *Haddy, F. J.:* Potassium deficiency and heart function. J. Chron. Dis. **26**, 467–469 (1973).
8. *Hayduk, K., H. M. Brecht, A. Vladutiu, S. Simard, J. M. Rojo-Ortega, L. Belleau, R. Boucher, J. Genest:* Renin activity and norepinephrine, cation, and water contents of cardiovascular tissue of dogs with congestive heart failure and ascites. Can. J. Physiol. Pharmacol. **48**, 463–468 (1970).
9. *Judson, W. E., O. M. Helmer:* Relationship of cardiorenal function to renin-aldosterone system in patients with valvular heart disease. Circulation **44**, 245–253 (1971).
10. *Krause, D. K., E. Rosskamp, K. A. Meurer, W. Kaufmann:* Zur Reagibilität des Renin-Angiotensin-Systems bei kardialer Hydropsie: Hinweise auf eine vom Gesamtnatriumbestand abhängige Regulation der Reninfreisetzung. Klin. Wschr. **50**, 311–326 (1972).
11. *Yaron, M., C. M. Bennett:* Renal sodium handling in acute right-sided heart failure in dogs. Mineral Electrolyte Metab. **1**, 303–314 (1978).
12. *Zelis, R., C. S. Delea, H. N. Coleman, D. T. Mason:* Arterial sodium content in experimental congestive heart failure. Circulation **41**, 213–216 (1970).

For reprints:

Prof. Dr. *Karl Hayduk*, Marien-Hospital, Rochusstraße 2, 4000 Düsseldorf 30, FRG

ACKNOWLEDGEMENT

The authors would like to express their gratitude to the Erwin Riesch Stiftung whose generous support has made this symposium possible.

We would also like to thank the following contributors for additional assistance:

Byk Gulden, Konstanz
Cassella AG, Frankfurt/Main
Chemiewerk Homburg, Frankfurt/Main
Ciba-Geigy, Wehr/Baden
Giulini Pharma, Hannover
Gödecke, Berlin
Hellige, Freiburg
IDEE-Kaffee, Hamburg
Kanoldt, Höchstädt
Paul-Martini-Stiftung, Frankfurt/Main
Pfizer, Karlsruhe
Pharma Schwarz, Monheim
Thomae, Biberach
Tönnies, Freiburg

SUBJECT INDEX

(Numbers refer to the first page of respective articles)